# Coercive Treatment in Psychiatry

# Coercive Treatment in Psychiatry

Clinical, Legal and Ethical Aspects

**Editors: Thomas W. Kallert, Juan E. Mezzich and John Monahan**

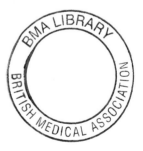

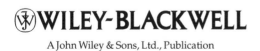

A John Wiley & Sons, Ltd., Publication

*Library of Congress Cataloging-in-Publication Data*

Coercive treatment in psychiatry : clinical, legal and ethical aspects / editors, Thomas Kallert, Juan Mezzich and John Monahan.
  p. cm.
 Includes index.
 ISBN 978-0-470-66072-0 (cloth)
 1. Involuntary treatment–Moral and ethical aspects. I. Kallert, Thomas W. II. Mezzich, Juan E. III. Monahan, John.
 R727.35.C64 2012
 174.2'9689–dc22

                                                                          2010054029

A catalogue record for this book is available from the British Library.

This book is published in the following electronic formats: ePDF 978-0-470-97854-2; Wiley Online Library 978-0-470-97857-3; ePub 978-0-470-97865-8

Set in 10.5/13pt Times by Thomson Digital, Noida, India
Printed and bound in Singapore by Markono Print Media Pte Ltd

First Impression   2011

# Contents

# List of Contributors

**Paul S. Appelbaum**
Elizabeth K. Dollard Professor
  of Psychiatry, Medicine and Law
Columbia University, Department
  of Psychiatry
Director
New York State Psychiatric Institute,
  Division of Law, Ethics, and
  Psychiatry
1051 Riverside Drive, Unit 122
New York, NY, 10032
USA

**Julio Arboleda-Flórez**
Professor Emeritus
Queen's University, Department
  of Psychiatry and Department
  of Community Health and
  Epidemiology
Kingston, ON, K7L 3N6
Canada

**Dorothea S. Buck-Zerchin**
Honorary Chair
German Federal Association of (ex-)
  Users and Survivors of Psychiatry
Brummerskamp 4
Hamburg, 22457
Germany
www.dorothea-buck.de

**Tom Burns**
Professor of Social Psychiatry
University of Oxford, Warneford
  Hospital
Oxford, OX3 7JX
UK

**Dorothy M. Castille**
Health Scientist Administrator
National Institutes of Health,
  National Institute on
  Minority Health and Health
  Disparities
6707 Democracy Boulevard,
  Suite 800
Bethesda, MD, 20892
USA
(work completed while
  at Columbia University
  and New York State Psychiatric
  Institute, New York)

**John Dawson**
Professor of Law
University of Otago, Faculty of Law
PO Box 56
Dunedin 9016
New Zealand


**Wolfgang Gaebel**
Professor of Psychiatry, Director of the
    Department of Psychiatry and
    Psychotherapy
Heinrich-Heine University, Department
    of Psychiatry and Psychotherapy,
    Medical Faculty
Bergische Landstrasse 2
Düsseldorf, 40629
Germany


**Thomas W. Kallert**
Head of the Department of Psychiatry,
    Psychosomatic Medicine and
    Psychotherapy
Park Hospital Leipzig
Morawitzstrasse 2
Leipzig, 04289
Germany


Medical Director
Soteria Hospital Leipzig
Morawitzstrasse 4
Leipzig, 04289
Germany


Professor of Psychiatry
Dresden University of Technology,
    Faculty of Medicine
Fetscherstrasse 74
Dresden, 01307
Germany

**Lars Kjellin**
Associate Professor, Research Manager,
    Psychiatric Research Centre
Örebro University, School of Health and
    Medical Sciences
PO Box 1613
Örebro, SE-701 16
Sweden


**Robert Klitzman**
Professor of Clinical Psychiatry
    (in Sociomedical Sciences)
Columbia University, Department
    of Psychiatry and Mailman School
    of Public Health
Director, Masters
    of Bioethics Program
New York State Psychiatric
    Institute, HIV Center,
    Ethics, Policy and Human
    Rights Core
1051 Riverside Drive, Unit 15
New York, NY, 10032
USA


**Peter Lepping**
Visiting Professor, Associate
    Medical Director and Consultant
    Psychiatrist
Betsi Cadwaladr University Health
    Board and Glyndŵr University,
    Wrexham Academic Unit
Ffordd Croesnewydd
Wrexham LL13 7YP, Wales
UK


**Charles W. Lidz**
Research Professor
    of Psychiatry
University of Massachusetts
    Medical School

55 Lake Avenue North
Worcester, MA, 01655
USA

**Bruce G. Link**
Professor, Epidemiology and Sociology
Columbia University, New York State
  Psychiatric Institute
722 West 168th Street, 16th Floor
New York, NY, 10032
USA

**Juan E. Mezzich**
President 2005–2008, World Psychiatric
  Association
President, International Network
  for Person-centered Medicine
Professor of Psychiatry
New York University, Mount Sinai
  School of Medicine
5th Avenue and 100th Street, Box 1093
New York, NY, 10029-6574
USA

**John Monahan**
John S. Shannon Distinguished
  Professor of Law, and Professor of
  Psychology and of Psychiatry and
  Neurobehavioral Sciences
University of Virginia
580 Massie Road
Charlottesville, VA, 22903
USA

**Kristina H. Muenzenmaier**
Associate Clinical Professor of
  Psychiatry and Behavioral Medicine
Albert Einstein College of Medicine
1500 Waters Place
Bronx, NY, 10461
USA

**David W. Oaks**
Executive Director of MindFreedom
  International (MFI), Board of
  Directors of the United States
  International Council on Disabilities
  (USICD) and the Oregon Consumer/
  Survivor Coalition (OCSC)
MindFreedom International
454 Willamette St, Suite 216,
  PO Box 11284
Eugene, OR, 97440-3484
USA

**Ahmed Okasha**
Professor and Director of WHO
  Collaborating Center for Training
  and Research
Ain Shams University,
  Institute of Psychiatry, Faculty
  of Medicine
3 Shawarby Street, Kasr El Nil
Cairo, 11211
Egypt

**Tarek Okasha**
Professor of Psychiatry
Ain Shams University, Institute
  of Psychiatry, Faculty of Medicine
3 Shawarby Street, Kasr El Nil
Cairo, 11211
Egypt

**Dirk Richter**
Nursing Research Professor
Bern University of Applied Sciences,
  School of Health Sciences
Murtenstrasse 10
Berne, CH-3008
Switzerland

**Jasna Russo**
Consultant Researcher
Mental Disability Advocacy Centre
Hercegprímás utca 11
Budapest, H-1051
Hungary

**Tilman Steinert**
Head of Dept. General Psychiatry and
    Psychotherapy, Research Director
Ulm University, Centre for Psychiatry
    Suedwuerttemberg
Ravensburg-Weissenau 88214
Germany

**Rael Strous**
Director Chronic Inpatient Unit, Beer
    Yaakov Mental Health Center
Associate Professor of Psychiatry,
    Sackler Faculty of Medicine
Tel Aviv University
70350 Beer Yaakov, PO Box 1
Tel Aviv
Israel

**George Szmukler**
Professor of Psychiatry and Society
King's College London, Institute
    of Psychiatry
De Crespigny Park
London SE5 8AF
UK

**Jan Wallcraft**
Honorary Fellow
University of Birmingham, Centre for
    Excellence in Interdisciplinary
    Mental Health
Muirhead Tower
Birmingham, B15 2TT
UK
Visiting Fellow
University of Hertfordshire, Centre
    for Mental Health Recovery
College Lane
Hatfield, Herts AL10 9AB
UK

**Harald Zäske**
Psychologist
Heinrich-Heine University, Department
    of Psychiatry and Psychotherapy,
    Medical Faculty
Bergische Landstrasse 2
Düsseldorf, 40629
Germany

# Introduction

## Thomas W. Kallert,[1,2,3] Juan E. Mezzich[4] and John Monahan[5]

[1]*Park Hospital Leipzig, Department of Psychiatry, Psychosomatic Medicine and Psychotherapy, Leipzig, Germany*
[2]*Soteria Hospital Leipzig, Leipzig, Germany*
[3]*Dresden University of Technology, Faculty of Medicine, Dresden, Germany*
[4]*New York University, Mount Sinai School of Medicine, New York, NY, USA*
[5]*University of Virginia School of Law, Charlottesville, VA, USA*

The relevance of coercive treatment for psychiatry has been underestimated for a long period in the history of this discipline. It is only within the last two decades that it has been viewed as an increasingly important area for clinical and research initiatives. There may be a number of reasons behind this change of interest.

First, it has become clear that clinical procedures summarized under the term 'coercive treatment' are still more frequent than desired. Recent international studies showed that from 3% (Portugal) to 30% (Sweden) of all psychiatric inpatient episodes consist of involuntary hospital admission of general psychiatric patients [1]; these rates vary by a factor of 10 internationally, leading to speculations about the impact of specific features of national mental health service configuration and mental health legislation. A time series from the 1990s in 15 member states of the European Union indicated an overall tendency towards more-or-less stable rates of 10 to 20% in most countries [1]. As shown in another European multi-site study, approximately one-third of legally involuntarily admitted patients are currently subjected to individual coercive measures such as mechanical restraint, seclusion or forced medication within the first four weeks after admission; again, variation across clinical sites is enormous and rates can be as high as 60% [2]. A broad and robust base of empirical knowledge on such elements of service provision does not exist, however [3].

Second, interest in exploring the issue of coercive treatment has expanded beyond the psychiatric hospitals and now concentrates on diverse institutionalized settings for patient groups with high vulnerability regarding the use of coercive measures, such as forensic mental health hospitals, old-age homes, long-term care homes for chronically severely mentally ill or mentally disabled persons, and also general medical hospitals [4]. In the era of deinstitutionalization and community-orientation of service provision, new legal and clinical concepts involving elements of coercion such as outpatient commitment and leverage [5,6] were developed; evaluating their effects is an increasingly important and challenging field of services research.

Third, the complex and internationally diverse linkage of all forms of coercive measures to mental health legislation has become a field which must be assessed in much more detail, in particular when new forms of coercive treatment are to be introduced and existing legal frameworks must be adapted to such needs (see Chapter 7) [7].

Fourth, coercive measures are more and more seen as a sensitive human rights issue, and recent internationally binding documents like the UN Convention on the Rights of Persons with Disabilities [8] have been published which emphasize this position. The effects of protecting human rights in providing mental health care on population-based mental health outcomes are an area of interest for future research.

Fifth, ethical issues [9] associated with clinical practice and research on coercive measures have become of utmost importance. They range from exploring undue influences on research, and questions of properly assessing the ability to give informed consent (see Chapter 17) to attitudes of professionals towards coercive measures [10] and uncertainties about how psychiatric advance directives should be respected in emergency situations [11] which might require the use of coercive measures. The need to address such fields comes from different sources. These include historical examples like the criminal perversion of mental health care during the Nazi era (see Chapter 10), and the recent international movement to develop evidence-based guidelines on how to use coercive measures, for example in the context of the short-term management of disturbed/violent behaviour in psychiatric inpatient settings and emergency departments [12].

Sixth, the development and critical analysis of strategies to reduce the use of coercive measures in different settings (e.g. [13]) are areas of high relevance for public mental health care and research.

Seventh, coercive measures are not only critical for shaping public opinion regarding psychiatry, but are the main area in which this medical discipline faces increasing criticism, particularly from the human rights perspective [14] voiced by users of mental health services and prominent international political bodies such as the Council of Europe.

Eighth, and most important from the point of view of the editors of this volume, coercive measures constitute and symbolize a core element of the relationship of individual mental health professionals with their patients and of the dialogue of professional bodies, such as the World Psychiatric Association (WPA), with the different national and international users' organizations. Subjective experiences of coercive measures and outcomes of coercive measures in terms of adherence to treatment and satisfaction with treatment are important issues for this kind of relationship, and important clinical fields in themselves. That the needed, but long-neglected dialogue on this issue at the level of organizations was a realistic option was demonstrated by the successful WPA Thematic Conference *Coercive Treatment in Psychiatry: A Comprehensive Review*, 6–8 June 2007 in Dresden, Germany, which may have been the first international scientific event dedicated to this sensitive issue [15]. Whereas, traditionally, critical users' groups mount protests outside conference venues, this time most of them decided to come inside and engage in discussions with the conference organizers and other professionals. This rendered the conference a landmark for the WPA in pursuing dialogue between the treaters and the treated.

Organizing a volume that comprehensively explores important clinical, legal and ethical aspects of the highly sensitive and hotly debated issue of coercive treatment in psychiatry presented many challenges. Therefore, the editors conceptualized a book containing original chapters written by international authors from different cultural backgrounds. All are highly experienced and very well respected in the fields or research issues addressed in their contributions. Thus, the volume reflects the current state of the art in the individual themes and is subdivided into five sections:

• *Conceptual and clinical aspects of coercive treatment*
• *Legal aspects of coercive treatment*
• *Ethical aspects of coercive treatment*
• *Users' views on coercive treatment*
• *Coercion and undue influence in decisions to participate in psychiatric research.*

Additionally, the volume could be seen as a starting point for future international discussions and initiatives in this field aiming to minimize coercion. Its importance could go beyond its content, as a symbol of the commitment of psychiatrists globally to deal with a serious and sensitive issue responsibly and creatively.

   The section on *conceptual and clinical aspects of coercive treatment* contains five chapters.

Juan E. Mezzich, the President of the WPA 2005–2008, during which period the WPA Dresden Thematic Conference took place, addresses *the issue of coercion and cooperation and psychiatry for the person*, and demonstrates convincingly that the framework of Psychiatry for the Person, a major WPA initiative, can be helpful for such analyses. This initiative's fundamental goals involve the promotion of a Psychiatry of the Person (of the totality of the person and his/her health, ill and positive aspects included), a Psychiatry by the Person (with clinicians extending themselves as full human beings and professionals with high ethical aspirations), a Psychiatry for the Person (assisting the fulfilment of each person's life project) and a Psychiatry with the Person (in respectful collaboration with the person presenting for care). The conceptual and ethical bases of this initiative are enlightening, and its specific implications to improve diagnosis, clinical care and public health represent nothing less than a paradigmatic shift in our field.

Wolfgang Gaebel and Harald Zäske address the question of whether there is a *link between coercive treatment and stigma of mental illness.* They argue that there is a complex connection. The fact that compulsory treatment is administered within the treatment of mentally ill persons, but not of patients with somatic illness, shapes the public's impression that mentally ill persons are different from others, and potentially unpredictable and dangerous. In Germany, coercive treatment is subject to strict legal regulations. Nevertheless, occasions and justifications for coercive treatment in clinical practice may vary due to individual tolerance limits and competence in de-escalation techniques which in turn are influenced by beliefs, attitudes and professional experiences of the ward staff. Finally, this contribution considers whether the frequency of compulsory admissions and coercive treatment measures can be reduced by educational and stigma-orientated interventions.

John Monahan deals in much detail with the issue of *mandated psychiatric treatment in the community* and demonstrates the forms, prevalence, outcomes and controversies associated with this approach. He argues that much of the international debate on 'outpatient commitment' or 'community treatment orders' assumes that court-ordered treatment in the community is simply an extension of long-existing policies authorizing involuntary commitment as a hospital inpatient. In fact, outpatient commitment is only one of many forms of 'leverage' being used to mandate adherence to psychiatric treatment in community settings. In the social welfare system, benefits disbursed by money managers, and the provision of subsidized housing are both used to assure treatment adherence. Similarly, for people who commit a criminal offence, adherence to psychiatric treatment may be made a condition of probation. Favourable disposition of a case by a mental health court may also be tied to treatment participation. Psychiatric advance directives can be thought of as a form of 'antidote' to treatment mandated by others. This chapter does four things. First, it illustrates a new and broader perspective on requiring adherence to outpatient mental health services, called 'mandated community treatment'. Second, it provides estimates of the frequency with which various forms of leverage are applied to psychiatric outpatients in the United States, as well as of the use of psychiatric advance directives. Third, it summarizes preliminary empirical findings on the outcomes attributable to the different forms of leverage. Finally, it addresses two controversial issues that often arise in discussions of mandated community treatment: the extent to which the use of leverage amounts to 'coercion', and the role of culture in understanding people's views of the legitimacy of mandated community treatment.

Tilman Steinert and Peter Lepping emphasize that the definition of a *best practice standard for coercive treatment in psychiatry* could ensure that unavoidable interventions are performed with the least possible harm to both patients and staff. They outline three different approaches that have been used to define a best practice standard: a viewpoint of personal virtue and wisdom; evidence; and consensus. Each has advantages and drawbacks. Personal virtue and wisdom has been the motor of most humanitarian reforms in psychiatry but is not a valid and reliable method. Empirical evidence is insufficient to provide answers for many ethical challenges. Consensus is highly dependent on the personal views of opinion leaders. A carefully balanced combination of evidence and consensus of multidisciplinary experts can currently be considered as the best approach to define best practice standards. However, each such standard can be valid only for the conditions of the time and will have to take into account cultural and historical aspects.

Dirk Richter explores the issue of *how to de-escalate a clinical risk situation to avoid the use of coercion.* This chapter outlines organizational and personal approaches for nonphysical interventions. After a review of current empirical research on de-escalation efforts, it gives a brief overview of the situational dynamics as the main cause of aggression and violence in psychiatric care. A general strategy is recommended which is based upon the following issues: safety and security assessment; establishing a rapport and a working relationship; identifying and dealing with substantive problems; dealing with feelings and emotions; and generation and exploration of options and alternatives. Several specific techniques (e.g. verbal and nonverbal interventions) are introduced and discussed.

The section on *legal aspects of coercive treatment* contains three chapters.

Julio Arboleda-Flórez analyses whether *the fields of psychiatry and the law agree in their views on coercive treatment.* He emphasizes that coercion is an element of some treatments in psychiatry, and it is contemplated in legislation, which often dictates parameters for involuntary admissions and use of restrictive treatments. A trend in recent years has been to widen the parameters required for commitment, thereby extending coercive elements of psychiatric treatments to less-immediate situations and into the community, as in assertive community treatment strategies and, most pointedly, in community treatment orders. Elements of coercion could appear in different ways that range from voluntary acceptance to seeming adherence to outright refusal and force. The author outlines how these elements comport with legal mandates and how they are justified in psychiatry and in law in a balance between needs for protection and individuality and autonomy. Further, the ethics of coercion are reviewed from a point of view of human and civil rights, both negative and positive rights of mental patients.

George Szmukler and John Dawson propose *the 'fusion' of incapacity and mental health legislation to reduce discrimination in mental health law.* They argue that mental health legislation, as conventionally conceived, discriminates against people with a mental illness. The 'rules' governing involuntary treatment of patients with a 'mental' disorder are quite distinct from those governing involuntary treatment of patients with a 'physical' disorder. The latter respect the autonomy of the person who has decision-making capacity, while the former do not. In this chapter, they propose a legal framework for comprehensive legislation based on decision-making capacity that would cover all persons with impaired capacity, from whatever cause. They examine the contexts and distinct functions and characteristics of the common forms of (1) incapacity legislation and (2) mental health (or civil commitment) legislation. Principles are then proposed for their 'fusion' into a single scheme. They show that a statute combining the particular, and complementary, strengths of both incapacity and civil commitment schemes can be readily constructed, based on the incapacity criteria found in the Mental Capacity Act 2005 for England and Wales. Such legislation would be an important step in reducing unjustified legal discrimination against mentally disordered persons and in providing a sound basis for 'coercive' treatments in psychiatry. Consistent ethical principles would be applied across all medical law.

Thomas Kallert explores the issue of whether *the fields of mental health care and patients' rights are currently compatible.* In detail, this chapter addresses the following questions from a European perspective: first, are the human rights of mental health patients sufficiently guaranteed and respected? The European Convention on Human Rights, the UN Convention on the Rights of Persons with Disabilities, and the practice of the European Court of Human Rights serve as examples to analyse if and how these rights are considered. Second, do new approaches in the field of mental health care endanger patients' rights? Outpatient commitment and laws on mental health care reporting are taken as examples. Third, can promising initiatives for improving patients' rights be identified? Revisions of national mental health laws, the elaboration of best practice guidelines for the use of coercive measures, and the formulation of psychiatric advance directives are analysed regarding their potential to improve patients' rights. Fourth, is autonomy still the supreme principle guiding recent socio-legal developments with regard to mental health care? The right of the individual patient to choose a so-called personal (financial) health care budget for chronic mental illness (as defined in the German socio-legal system) and the concept of leverage from the social welfare system are two examples examined. Fifth, are there legal areas that need clearer definitions in order to respect patients' rights? The patient's freedom to choose a psychiatric hospital for inpatient care, and involuntary placement and treatment in long-stay care homes are two examples from Germany of such areas of concern. In general, the analysis of the five questions presented in this chapter demonstrates that compatibility of mental health care and patients' rights seems to be more of a general aim for health politics and the field of psychiatry, albeit an extremely important intention, than a reality at present.

The section on *ethical aspects of coercive treatment* contains three chapters.

Ahmed Okasha and Tarek Okasha address the issue of *cross-cultural perspectives on coercive treatment in psychiatry* and demonstrate that individual autonomy is valued in European and American cultures but is not empowering for the traditional, family-centred societies in Arab, sub-Saharan African, Indian and Japanese cultures. This difference may affect the use of involuntary hospital admission and informed consent, amongst other practices, in traditional versus Western societies. In traditional societies, the decision for involuntary or voluntary admission for children and adolescents is totally the responsibility of the family. Neither the judicial system nor the civil law has a role. In some traditional societies in Africa, South East Asia and the Middle East, the perception of mental illness varies between rural and urban areas. In rural areas it is still considered to be due to possession by evil spirits, magic, the evil eye or the wrath of ancestors. To use coercive treatment and restraint to exorcise the evil eye spirit is socially acceptable and if not applied the society will consider the family as negligent. The patients' acceptance of their family decision on involuntary placement in non-Western cultures may surprise Western practitioners. Patients are often grateful to their family for pursuing the path to get rid of the evil influence. Although there are no scientific studies of patient's perception in those cultures available, it is the impression of the authors that it does not leave any scar or anger or rejection, as the patients perceive themselves as being led back to the path of virtue. Thus, this chapter discusses the transcultural ethical aspects of implementing coercive management of psychiatric disorders, with special emphasis on the conflict between the human rights values of Western culture and the social and religious conformity of some traditional societies.

Rael Strous explores the theme of *historical injustice in psychiatry*, presents examples from Nazi Germany and others, and derives ethical lessons for the modern professional from his analysis. He argues that along with the tremendous responsibility of the psychiatry profession comes tremendous power. Unfortunately, although this occurs relatively rarely, this power inherent in clinical and research psychiatry may be abused. History does provide us with some important examples of crossing the boundaries of ethical health care in individuals with mental illness. Much of this unethical behaviour emanates from boundary violations. It is thus critical to learn basic concepts of ethical practice during training. However, learning the concepts alone is not enough. Ethics training without a focus on clinical and research psychiatric practice with examples from history would be fundamentally lacking. As a model to explain concepts of medical ethics, a brief explanation of four cardinal ethical principals is presented as well as examples from the past where these concepts have been ignored or violated. Providing vivid historical examples of unethical practice increases the chance that lessons may be learned and that concepts will be applied in a more appropriate manner.

Tom Burns addresses the issue of *paternalism in mental health*. He shows that mental health legislation has received enormous attention internationally in the era of deinstitutionalization, particularly as societies become more risk averse. The response has been framed within a libertarian tradition and the language is almost exclusively about autonomy and partnership. Apart from risk, patient autonomy has gone from being one of the principles in the discourse surrounding mental health legislation to being the principle one. Paternalism and beneficence are discarded as discredited. Practice, however, is still recognisably paternalistic in most developed countries. This disjunction between the public language and common practice leads to sometimes tortured and unconvincing definitions (to permit current practice) and unhelpful confusion in the public mind about what psychiatry is. Contrary to the widespread belief within mental health that everyone else has abandoned paternalism, there are cogent and respectable critiques of autonomy as a dominant ethical principle. These critiques encourage a less damning view of paternalism, seeking to place it alongside other ethical goals in society. These challenges come from within economics, the law, political philosophy and, perhaps most surprisingly, from some feminist authors. These critiques are briefly outlined with the modest ambition of encouraging debate in this area. While patient autonomy is important, it does not preclude the legitimate consideration of restriction of liberty in a patient's best interests. A debate which reflects more accurately what we do (rather than think we ought to do) may be more helpful in informing policy and legislation.

The section on *users' views on coercive treatment* contains four chapters.

David W. Oaks offers thorough reflections on *the moral imperative for dialogue with organizations of survivors of coerced psychiatric human rights violations*. He describes how coerced mental health procedures sever the human relationship between mental health professionals and mental health clients, creating an insurmountable power imbalance and immense human suffering. While some individual mental health professionals question this inequality, there are barriers to institutional change. David W. Oaks argues that one possibility to begin to address this power imbalance is open, mediated dialogue between representatives of organizations of mental health professionals and representatives of organizations of psychiatric survivors, that is, individuals who identify as having experienced coerced human rights violations while undergoing psychiatric care. Civil dialogue could explore three categories of coercive psychiatry: (1) physically forced psychiatric care, for example involuntary electroconvulsive therapy against the clearly expressed wishes of the subject; (2) allegations that some mental health professionals provide fraudulent information, such as inaccurate descriptions of the effects of psychiatric medications; (3) the necessity for more choices for mental health care, especially peer-run alternatives, beyond the conventional medical model approach.

Jasna Russo and Jan Wallcraft address in much detail the *service user/survivor perspective on research on coercion,* and particularly explore some of the structural obstacles to including service user/survivor perspectives in psychiatric research on coercion. Without aiming to provide a systematic or complete review, they take a closer look at several psychiatric studies on coercion, and discuss their overall approaches and the methodologies applied. The standpoints of the authors of this chapter are informed by their own research practice, by their activism in the international movement of psychiatric survivors, and by their personal experiences of forced or coercive treatment. This contribution aims to extend the debate on the ethics of coercion beyond the notions of 'treatment effectiveness' and 'perceived coercion' by raising questions about how coercive methods impact individual lives. The second part of the chapter outlines some of the principles and values that the authors consider essential for comprehensive and responsible research on coercion.

The editors are extremely grateful for Dorothea S. Buck-Zerchin's contribution which is entitled '*Seventy Years of Coercion in Psychiatric Institutions, Experienced and Witnessed*'. Dorothea Buck was born in Germany in 1917 and can therefore be called a contemporary witness. She had five stays in psychiatric hospitals between 1936 and 1959 and was subjected to various forms of coercion, such as forced sterilization, cold wet sheet packs and forced injections, and was never granted a single conversation to inform her about the origin or meaning of her psychotic episodes. Facing the historical development of psychiatry and its effects on today's mental health system, she challenges biological psychiatry, which rejects communication with patients, and demands a paradigm shift toward a psychosocial system based on the wealth of patients' experiences that provides alternatives to psychiatry, such as the therapeutic principles of 'Soteria' and Yrjö Alanen's 'need-adapted treatment'.

Dorothy Castille, Kristina H. Muenzenmaier and Bruce Link contribute an original research paper entitled *Coercion: point, perception, process,* with a clear focus on users' views. They investigated the implications of outpatient commitment for perceptions of coercion in a sample of people committed and voluntarily presented to outpatient psychiatric treatment through New York State's Kendra's Law. Using a perceived coercion scale that shows evidence of reliability and validity, they found no significant difference in perception of coercion between those with and without court-ordered treatment. To understand this finding, the authors conducted open-ended interviews of 11 persons without court orders and 9 persons with court orders. Qualitative interviews revealed three perspectives that helped to understand why there were no differences in perceived coercion between these groups: the ubiquity of coercion, conformity over confrontation, and valued services. Study participants stressed the importance of a collaborative, mutually respectful relationship with the case manager, flexibility in application of the treatment plan, and goal-directed recovery orientation as amongst the factors that made even people who were objectively coerced feel less so.

The volume's final section on *coercion and undue influence in decisions to participate in psychiatric research* contains two chapters.

Lars Kjellin's chapter presents *ethical issues of participating in psychiatric research on coercion*, and discusses these in the context of international declarations on ethics of medical research and current issues in psychiatric research ethics. Experiences from a large European multi-centre study and a Nordic study of coercion in psychiatry are presented. Researchers have to be careful and sensitive when approaching involuntarily admitted patients, in particular, to ask for informed consent to participate in research. The author argues that possible benefits for future psychiatric patients, subjected to coercive measures in psychiatric care, from methodologically and ethically sound studies will most likely be greater than the possible risks of harm to participating patients.

In their chapter on *coercion and undue influence in decisions to participate in psychiatric research*, Paul Appelbaum, Charles W. Lidz and Robert Klitzman outline a theory of voluntary consent to research and of factors that may constrain it, based on the doctrine of informed consent. From this perspective, only influences that are external, intentional, illegitimate and causal may negate voluntariness. Of particular concern in the research setting are offers, pressures and threats, which may unduly influence or coerce potential subjects. Assessment of coercion and undue influence in research settings is challenging because of the need to take contextual factors into account. Research on the nature and prevalence of constraints on voluntariness is limited, with many gaps in current knowledge. In particular, it is unclear whether patients with psychiatric and substance use disorders are particularly susceptible to influences that constrain voluntariness. The discipline of psychiatry stands at the beginning of systematic study of voluntariness, coercion and undue influence in research, which promises to provide answers to many important questions in research ethics.

By comprehensively exploring important clinical, legal and ethical aspects of coercive treatment in the way outlined above, the editors very much hope

- to increase the visibility of the issue within the discipline of psychiatry, but also for all individual persons, bodies and organizations involved or interested in dealing with the themes addressed in the volume;

- to decrease resistance from various circles of diverse professions to deal competently with all the sensitive and controversial issues referred to as coercive treatment;
- to encourage further open discussions, at different levels, including the one of representatives of organizations of mental health professionals and representatives of organizations of psychiatric users/survivors;
- to stimulate further, urgently needed empirical research in the individual themes addressed;
- to increase activities towards defining better standards and procedures on how to deal with the challenges of this issue; and
- to give a crystal clear signal that it is absolutely essential, for all clinical and research work in the field of coercive treatment in psychiatry, to act according to the highest ethical standards in the best interest of our patients.

## References

1. Salize, H.J. and Dressing, H. (2004) Epidemiology of involuntary placement of mentally ill people across the European Union. *British Journal of Psychiatry*, **184**, 163–168.
2. Raboch, J., Kališová, L., Nawka, A. *et al.* (2010) Use of coercive measures during involuntary hospitalization: findings from ten European countries. *Psychiatric Services*, **10**, 1012–1017.
3. Kallert, T.W., Glöckner, M. and Schützwohl, M. (2008) Involuntary vs. voluntary hospital admission – a systematic review on outcome diversity. *European Archives of Psychiatry and Clinical Neuroscience*, **258**, 195–209.
4. Kallert, T.W. (2008) Coercion in psychiatry. *Current Opinion in Psychiatry*, **21**, 485–489.
5. Swartz, M. and Swanson, J. (2008) Outpatient commitment: when it improves patient outcomes. *Current Psychiatry*, **7**, 25–35.
6. Bonnie, R.J. and Monahan, J. (2005) From coercion to contract: reframing the debate on mandated community treatment for people with mental disorders. *Law and Human Behavior*, **29**, 485–503.
7. Kallert, T.W. and Torres-González, F. (eds) (2006) *Legislation on Coercive Mental Health Care in Europe. Legal Documents and Comparative Assessment of Twelve European Countries*, Peter Lang, Frankfurt am Main.
8. UN Convention on the Rights of Persons with Disabilities (13 December 2006).
9. Helmchen, H. and Sartorius, N. (eds) (2010) *Ethics in Psychiatry. European Contributions*, Springer Verlag, Berlin.
10. Steinert, T. (2007) Ethical attitudes towards involuntary admission and involuntary treatment of patients with schizophrenia. *Psychiatrische Praxis*, **34** (Supplement 2), S186–S190.
11. Swanson, J.W., van McCrary, S., Swartz, M.S. *et al.* (2007) Overriding psychiatric advance directives: factors associated with psychiatrists' decisions to preempt patients' advance refusal of hospitalization and medication. *Law and Human Behavior*, **31**, 77–90.
12. National Institute for Health and Clinical Excellence (2005) *Violence: The Short-Term Management of Disturbed/Violent Behaviour in Psychiatric In-patient Settings and Emergency Departments*, NICE Clinical Guideline 25, Royal College of Nursing, London.

Available at http://guidance.nice.org.uk/CG25/NICEGuidance/pdf/English (accessed 22 November 2010).

13. Smith, G.M., Davis, R.H., Bixler, E.O. *et al.* (2005) Pennsylvania state hospital system's seclusion and restraint reduction program. *Psychiatric Services*, **56**, 1115–1122.
14. Dudley, M. Silove, D. and Gale, F. (eds) Mental Health and Human Rights, Oxford University Press, Oxford, in press.
15. Kallert, T.W. Monahan, J. and Mezzich, J. (eds) (2007) World Psychiatric Association (WPA) Thematic Conference: Coercive Treatment in Psychiatry: A Comprehensive Review. Meeting abstracts, Dresden, Germany. 6–8 June 2007, *BMC Psychiatry*, **7** (Supplement 1).

# Section 1

## Conceptual and clinical aspects of coercive treatment

# 1 Person-centred psychiatry perspectives on coercion and cooperation

## Juan E. Mezzich

*New York University, Mount Sinai School of Medicine, New York, NY, United States*

## 1.1 Introduction

The topic of coercive treatment in psychiatry is both complex and sensitive. It is complex as it involves, *inter alia*, clinical, public health, ethical and legal issues. And it is sensitive as it deals with delicate aspects of human experience and interpersonal relations. In order to offer a frame of reference to address such complexity and sensitivity, this chapter first summarizes an ongoing initiative on person-centred psychiatry and medicine. It then discusses the place for *dialogue*, partnership and trust in implementing person-centred care and dealing with the tension between social control and personal autonomy, between coercion and cooperation in health care.

*Coercive Treatment in Psychiatry: Clinical, Legal and Ethical Aspects*, First Edition.
Edited by Thomas W. Kallert, Juan E. Mezzich and John Monahan.
© 2011 John Wiley & Sons, Ltd. Published 2011 by John Wiley & Sons, Ltd.

## 1.2    Psychiatry for the whole person

The basic thrust of person-centred clinical care is to place the person in context at the centre of health care. It involves shifting the focus of the field from disease to patient to person [1,2].

### 1.2.1    Origins and early developments

The roots of person-centred care can be traced back to ancient civilizations both Eastern (e.g. Chinese and Ayurvedic) and Western (principally Hellenistic) which employed a broad concept of health and organized treatments in a personalized manner. Such a broad concept of health (full wellbeing and not only the absence of disease) has been incorporated into the World Health Organization (WHO) definition of health.

In response to disease-based distortions in modern medicine [3], pioneering developments on person-centred perspectives emerged in the twentieth century, illustrated by Tournier's *Medicine de la Personne* in Switzerland [4], Rogers' person-centred approach focused on open communication and empowerment in the US [5], McWhinney's family medicine movement in the UK and Canada [6], Brera's person-centred medicine programme in Italy [7], and Alanen's need-adaptive assessment and treatment approach in Finland [8]. There has been, as well, increasing recognition of the key role of a collaborative clinician–patient relationship. Tasman pointed out in his American Psychiatric Association presidential address [9] that this relationship must start from the first encounter and represents the fundamental matrix for the whole of care. It must ensure empathetic listening, comprehensive diagnosis beyond symptom checklists, appreciation for symbolic meaning, and effective therapeutic partnerships instead of narrow and reductionistic approaches.

In a related development, *recovery-orientated* concepts emerged from a coalescence of efforts from both mental health service users and professional groups. On one hand, individuals who suffered and recovered from mental illnesses formed a recovery movement and a national and international community of activists (e.g. [10,11]) who expressed their criticism against negatively experienced psychiatric treatment, and demanded to be considered active protagonists and partners rather than passive recipients of care. On the other hand, well-known experts in the field of psychosocial rehabilitation (e.g. [12]) have welcomed the statements of service users and the need to attend to their subjective experiences, in contrast to traditional rehabilitation which appeared focused on improving functioning and adaptation and not on the fulfilment of the individual human being. At least since the beginning of the 1990s, many professionals in rehabilitation and other mental health fields, and various service user groups have started substantial collaboration through joint publications and conferences [13].

Also public health policy developments have been moving in a person- and people-centred direction. In a landmark study [14], the Institute of Medicine in the United States concluded that the American health system was seriously flawed and required a new framework with particular aims and rules, a key one being person-centeredness. Along the same lines, a US Presidential Commission on Mental Health diagnosed a state of disarray in national mental health care and proposed a thorough transformation to be driven by the patient and the community in a recovery orientation manner [15]. Likewise, the World Health Organization European Office [16] held a ministerial event which concluded that integration of mental health services should be organized by the involvement of patients and caregivers; that is, collectively tackling stigma, discrimination and inequality, and empowering and supporting people with mental health problems and their families to be actively engaged in this process; furthermore, recognizing the experience and knowledge of service users and caregivers as an important basis for planning and developing services.

Most recently, the WHO World Health Assembly formulated innovative resolutions for primary health care [17], two pillars of which are people-centred care and health systems responsiveness to human and social aspirations.

### 1.2.2    Emergence of person-centred psychiatry and medicine

As elucidated by historians Garrabe and Hoff from the proceedings of the First World Congress of Psychiatry of September 1950 [18], the World Psychiatric Association (WPA) revealed since its inception a keen interest on articulating science and humanism as the seeds of a person-centred psychiatry. But it was only in 2005 that the WPA General Assembly established an Institutional Program on Psychiatry for the Person: from Clinical Care to Public Health (IPPP). This initiative affirmed the *whole person in context* as the centre and goal of clinical care and health promotion, at both individual and community levels. It pointedly argued for the articulation of the scientific method and humanism to optimize attention to the ill and the positive aspects of a person's health, the integration of all relevant health and social services, and the advancement of pertinent public health policies.

The person-centred approach promotes clinical care *of* the person (the totality of the person's health, including its ill and positive aspects), *for* the person (to assist in the fulfilment of the person's life project), *by* the person (with clinicians extending themselves as full human beings, scientifically grounded and with high ethical aspirations), and *with* the person (in respectful and empowering collaboration with persons who present for care). The person is conceptualized with its full pluralistic richness and within its life context in line with Ortega y Gasset's dictum *I am I and my circumstance*. This approach represents a paradigmatic shift from the disease to the person as the main target and centre of medicine and health care [19,20].

Amongst the key elements of person-centred care are the following: (1) A broad biological, psychological, socio-cultural and spiritual framework. (2) Attention to both ill health and positive health. (3) Person-centred research on the process and outcome of clinician–patient–family communication, diagnosis, clinical care and health promotion. (4) Promotion of and respect for the autonomy, responsibility and dignity of every person involved.

Person-centeredness, in addition to its ethical relevance, may be shown to enhance the effectiveness and outcome of the various aspects of clinical care, from interviewing the person who consults and pertinent family members, to comprehensive diagnosis, and to the various aspects of treatment and health promotion. Illustratively, person-centred diagnosis [21,22] is primarily aimed at optimizing treatment planning, and involves pointed attention to health status, to experience of health and illness and to contributory agents including risk and protective factors, and it employs descriptive categories, dimensions and narratives, and activates the interaction of clinicians, the patient and family members. A perspective has been articulated recently to integrate conventional disease-centred or nosological diagnosis within a broad, person-centred diagnosis [23].

Person-centred medicine training programmes are emerging in several countries, such as those at Ambrosiana University Medical School in Milan, Italy, Birmingham University in the UK (A. Miles, Medical School Dean, personal information, 1 December 2009), and at Cayetano Heredia Peruvian University in Lima (J. Saavedra, Professor of Psychiatry, personal information, 18 December 2009). Curricula are being developed at the listed medical schools and through the International Network for Person-centered Medicine (INPCM) [24]. Additionally to be noted are Conferences on Psychiatry for the Person in London (co-organized by the WPA Institutional Program on Psychiatry for the Person (IPPP) and the UK Department of Health), October 2007, Paris (co-organized by the WPA IPPP and the Association of WPA French Member Societies) February 2008, and Prague (WPA XIV Congress of Psychiatry), September 2008, and the Geneva Conferences on Person-Centered Medicine in May 2008 and 2009 [25].

The person-centred medicine academic programmes and events listed above pointedly involve also research activities. These include both conceptual explorations [1,26] as well as the presentation of empirical research on topics such as clinical communication [27,28] and Person-Centred Integrative Diagnosis [21,22].

## 1.3    The WPA Dresden conference – reviewing coercion and cooperation

A key element of the above outlined initiative is to promote a psychiatry and medicine *with* the person; that is, the affirmation of the personhood of the patient and the commitment to work in respectful and collaborative partnership with the person who consults. This includes, first, work with individuals highlighting the ethical underpinnings of this effort. It also encompasses work with patient groups including those critical of psychiatry.

It is on these grounds that the WPA Thematic Conference held in Dresden on 6–8 June 2007 represented a crucial opening for dialogue. The conference had an intriguing and sensitive overall topic, *Coercive Treatment in Psychiatry: A Comprehensive Review*. Professor John Monahan, Scientific Committee chair, anticipated on his invitation letter that

> while the fissures in this area run so deep and are so long-standing that achieving consensus is unlikely, our aspiration is that this historic meeting will sharpen moral issues, clarify political viewpoints, identify evidence-based practices, and share cutting-edge data on one of the most contested topics of our time.

In fact, as reported by Professor Thomas Kallert, Organizing Committee chair, the Conference succeeded in attracting participants from 36 different countries, with virtually all world experts on this field attending and speaking at it, all leading to an absolutely top-quality scientific programme.

But there was, additionally, a surprising event that marked the Dresden Conference indelibly for all its organizational and individual participants. Many of the user groups critical of psychiatry (but not all), which traditionally would be expected to protest outside, decided to come in and engage in a discussion of serious concerns. This opening had a crucial value for global psychiatry as this substantially broadened the range of its patients/users interlocutors which also encompass groups (including self-help groups) with which psychiatric organizations have been interacting for a long time.

In a historic encounter on 6 June, requested formally and with the endorsement of the WHO by Mind Freedom International, the European Network of (ex-)Users and Survivors of Psychiatry and world networks of current and past users of psychiatric services (ENUSP, World Network of Users and Survivors of Psychiatry WNUSP), the president and other top leaders of the WPA met with four representatives of the user organizations. The encounter, originally scheduled to last one hour, spontaneously extended to three. A range of issues were discussed, and possibilities for continuing the dialogue in congresses and other settings were explored. As reported by David Oaks [29], Director of Mind Freedom International, 'This conversation was different than usual. Yes, once more, the proof will be in the results. But all involved felt they were heard and respected in this discussion'.

During the following day, the WPA Executive Committee temporarily suspended its official business meeting in order to attend the keynote lecture by Ms Dorothea Buck on '70 Years of Coercion in German Psychiatric Institutions, Experienced and

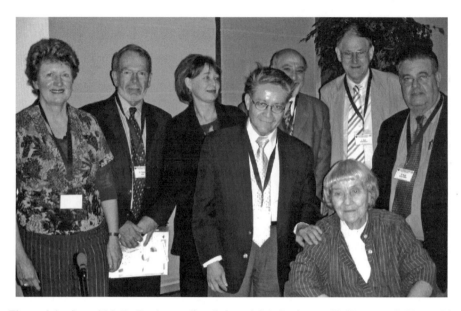

**Figure 1.1**   Seated Ms D. Buck; standing (left to right): Professors H. Herrman, S. Tyano, M. Amering, J. E. Mezzich, M. Jorge, J. Cox and P. Ruiz at the WPA Thematic Conference, Dresden, 7 June 2007.

Witnessed'. On the basis of her personal history, she challenged a psychiatry that neglects communication with patients, and demanded a paradigm shift based on the wealth of patients' experiences. After her lecture, the WPA president offered a thank-you speech for Ms Buck's articulate and moving lecture, and greeted her in the company of all present members of the WPA Executive Committee and the session chair (see Figure 1.1).

At an immediately ensuing press conference, representatives of the WPA, Council of Europe, and user organizations sitting at the main table held a lively exchange of questions, answers and comments with press representatives and the general audience (Figure 1.2). The issues experienced globally by service users, the patterns and diversity of their organizations, and prospective opportunities for continuing the Dresden dialogue and for user participation in activities of global and national psychiatry activities were broadly discussed.

## 1.4   Evolving developments for enhancing cooperation

The current volume on *Coercive Treatment in Psychiatry* represents a principal follow-up of the 2007 Dresden Conference. Many of its speakers, including multidisciplinary scholars and users, are present again through its pages. The topics covered comprise a comprehensive clinical, public health, ethics and legal review of

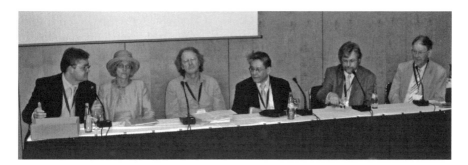

**Figure 1.2**   (Left to right): Professor T. Kallert (conference organizer), Dr V. Pimenoff (Council of Europe representative), Mr P. Lehmann (author and German User Network representative), Professor J. E. Mezzich (president of the WPA and of the conference), Mr D. Oaks (Mind Freedom International Director) and Professor J. Cox (WPA Secretary General), seated at the press conference of the WPA Thematic Conference in Dresden, 7 June 2007.

the volume's complex and sensitive theme. As a group they encompass both intellectual and experiential, scientific and humanistic perspectives. They can be conceived, therefore, as representing a *person-centred* approach.

Some steps have been undertaken in the years that followed Dresden in terms of invitations to user and family representatives to speak at person-centred conferences in Paris (February 2008), Prague (September 2008) and Geneva (May of 2008, 2009 and 2010). Joint studies involving users, families and professionals are evolving as well [13,30]. The room for further collaborative work, however, is ample indeed.

Additionally, one can list some recent innovative developments that may contribute directly or indirectly to addressing usefully and helpfully the tension between coercion and cooperation. They refer in various degrees to clinical care and public health.

One such development is the ongoing preparation of a Person-Centred Integrative Diagnosis model undertaken by the INPCM [24]. This comprehensive diagnosis model covers both ill health, through a nosological diagnosis component based on the WHO International Classification of Diseases, and positive health (self-awareness, resilience, sense of control and transcendence, resources, well-being), attends to the person's experience and values as well as to risk and protective health factors, employs categories, dimensions and narratives as descriptive instruments, and engages the patient, family and clinicians in partnerships for shared diagnostic understanding and shared commitment to care [22]. Extending the practical prospects for person-centred diagnosis, a number of national and regional developments incorporating such approaches are being developed in Europe [31] and Latin America [32].

Based on the resolutions of the WHO [17] World Health Assembly promoting people-centred primary health care, the WHO and the INPCM are planning the

Fourth Geneva Conference on Person-Centered Medicine for 2–4 May 2011, which will include presentation of an evolving study on the systematic conceptualization and measurement of person- and people-centred care. This may open new horizons for addressing control–cooperation issues in a diversity of countries.

Applicable to all aspects of health care are research and development efforts towards enhancing clinical communication. They facilitate direct acquaintance, fluid exchange of information, and presentation of helpful intentions and attitudes [27,33]. As such, they can powerfully foster empathy and trust, crucial elements of person-centred care and relevant to understanding and addressing usefully the tension between coercion and cooperation.

## 1.5   Concluding remarks

We have briefly reviewed broad historical and contemporary perspectives on person-centred care, and global psychiatry and medicine's evolving scientific and humanistic response to them. A renewed commitment to the clinician–patient relationship appears crucial, as well as building an effective dialogue with service users and families, respecting the diversity of their perspectives. Let's take advantage of the Dresden opening and developments that followed to find creative paths to jointly address specific coercion–cooperation issues and cultivate a shared commitment to promote health in individuals and communities across the world.

## References

1. Mezzich, J.E., Snaedal, J., van Weel, C. and Heath, I. (eds) (2010) Introduction to conceptual explorations on person-centered medicine. *International Journal of Integrated Care*, **10** (Supplement), e022.
2. Christodoulou, G.N., Fulford, K.M.W. and Mezzich, J.E. (2007) Conceptual bases of psychiatry for the person. *International Psychiatry*, **5**(1), 1–3.
3. Heath, I. (2005) Promotion of disease and corrosion of medicine. *Canadian Family Physician*, **51**, 1320–1322.
4. Tournier, P. (1940) *Medicine de la Personne*. Delachaux et Niestle, Neuchâtel.
5. Rogers, C.R. (1961) *On becoming a Person: A Therapist's View of Psychotherapy*, Houghton Mifflin, Boston.
6. McWhinney, I.R. (1989) *A Textbook of Family Medicine*, Oxford University Press, Oxford.
7. Brera, G.R. (1992) Epistemological aspects of medical science. *Medicine and Mind*, **7**, 5–12.
8. Alanen, Y.O. (1997) *Schizophrenia: Its Origins and Need-adaptive Treatment*, Karnak, London.
9. Tasman, A. (2000) Presidential Address: The doctor-patient relationship. *American Journal of Psychiatry*, **157**, 1763–1768.
10. Chamberlin, J. (1979) *On Our Own: Patient-controlled Alternatives to the Mental Health System*, McGraw-Hill, New York.

11. Deegan, P. (1992) The independent living movement and people with psychiatric disabilities: taking back control over our own lives. *Psychosocial Rehabilitation Journal*, **15**, 3–19.
12. Anthony, W. (1993) Recovery from mental illness. The guiding vision of the mental health service system in the 1990s. *Psychosocial Rehabilitation Journal*, **16**, 11–23.
13. Amering, M. and Schmolke, M. (2009) *Recovery in Mental Health: Reshaping Scientific and Clinical Responsibilities*, John Wiley & Sons, Ltd, Chichester.
14. Institute of Medicine (2001) *Crossing the Quality Chasm: A New Health System for the 21st Century*, National Academies Press, Washington, DC.
15. New Freedom Commission on Mental Health (2003) Achieving the Promise: Transforming Mental Health Care in America. Final Report. DHHS Pub. No. SMA-03-3832, US Department of Health and Human Services, Rockville, MD.
16. World Health Organization European Office (2005) Mental Health Action Plan for Europe: Facing the Challenges, Building Solutions. WHO European Ministerial Conference on Mental Health. Helsinki, Finland, 12–15 January 2005. EUR/04/5047810/7, WHO Regional Office for Europe, Copenhagen
17. World Health Organization (2009) Resolution WHA62.12. Primary health care, including health system strengthening, in Sixty-Second World Health Assembly, Geneva, 18–22 May 2009: Resolutions and Decisions. WHA62/2009/REC/1, World Health Organization, Geneva, pp. 16–19.
18. Garrabe, J. and Hoff, P. (2010) Historical views on psychiatry for the person. *Psychopathology*, in press.
19. Mezzich, J.E. (2007) Psychiatry for the Person: articulating medicine's science and humanism. *World Psychiatry*, **6**, 1–3.
20. Mezzich, J.E., Snaedal, J., Van weel, C. and Heath, I. (2010) Toward person-centered medicine: from disease to patient to person. *Mount Sinai Journal of Medicine*, **77**, 304–306.
21. Mezzich, J.E. and Salloum, I.M. (2009) Towards a person-centered integrative diagnosis, in *Psychiatric Diagnosis: Challenges and Prospects* (eds I.M. Salloum and J.E. Mezzich), John Wiley & Sons, Ltd, Chichester, p. 297.
22. Mezzich, J.E., Salloum, I.M., Cloninger, C.R. *et al.* (2010) Person-centred integrative diagnosis: conceptual bases and structural model. *Canadian Journal of Psychiatry*, **55**(11), 701–708.
23. Mezzich, J.E. (2010) New developments on classification and diagnostic systems. *Canadian Journal of Psychiatry*, **55**(11), 689–691
24. Mezzich, J.E., Snaedal, J., van Weel, C. and Heath, I. (2009) The International Network for Person-centered Medicine: background and first steps. *World Medical Journal*, **55**, 104–107.
25. Mezzich, J.E. (2009) The Second Geneva Conference on Person-centered Medicine. *World Medical Journal*, **55**, 100–101.
26. Cox, J., Campbell, A. and Fulford, K.M.W. (2006) *Medicine of the Person*, Kingsley Publishers, London.
27. Finset, A. (2010) Emotions, narratives and empathy in clinical communication. *International Journal of Integrated Care*, **10** (Supplement), e020.
28. Zwaanswijk, M., Tates, K., van Dulmen, S. *et al.* (2007) Young patients', parents' and survivors' communication preferences in paediatric oncology: Results of online focus groups. *BMC Pediatrics*, **7**, 35.
29. Oaks, D. (2007) World Psychiatric Association meets with psychiatric survivor movement groups. www.mindfreedom.org/campaign/global/wpa-meets-with-movement (accessed 15 November 2010).

30. Wallcraft, J., Schrank, B. and Amering, M. (2009) *Handbook of Service User Involvement in Mental Health Research*, JohnWiley & Sons, Ltd, Chichester.
31. Botbol, M. (2010) French developments on person-centered diagnosis. Presented at the Third Geneva Conference on Person-centered Medicine. International Network for Person-centered Medicine, Geneva, May 2, 2010.
32. Otero, A., Saavedra, J.E., Mezzich, J.E. and Salloum, I.M. (2010) La Guia Latinoamericana de Diagnostico Psiquiatrico (GLADP) y su Revision. *Revista de la Asociación Psiquiátrica de América Latina*, in press.
33. Shiryaev, O.U., Gayvoronskaya, E.B. and Shapovalov, D.L. (2008) *Separate Aspects of Psychology and Pedagogy*. Voronezh N. N. Burdenko State Medical Academy, Voronezh, Russia.

# 2 Coercive treatment and stigma – is there a link?

**Wolfgang Gaebel and Harald Zäske**

*Heinrich-Heine University, Department of Psychiatry and Psychotherapy, Medical Faculty, Düsseldorf, Germany*

## 2.1 Introduction

Involuntary admissions as well as coercive measures such as seclusion, (physical) restraint and forced medication are immanent elements of psychiatric care; nevertheless they are fundamental encroachments of human rights. In the following, the term 'coercive measures' will be used as an umbrella term for involuntary admissions and placements, and coercive treatments such as seclusion, restraint or forced medication.

In this chapter, the relationship between coercive measures and the stigma of mental illness will be discussed. The stigma of mental illness incriminates those suffering from mental illness, aggravating the course of the illness, hampering social functions and offending against equal opportunities [1–4].

As coercive measures are 'understudied issues' themselves [5], it is not surprising that their relationship to the stigma of mental illness is not yet well studied, as demonstrated by a retrieval of the PUBMED database (www.ncbi.nlm.nih.gov/pubmed): the search 'stigma AND mental illness' results in 1798 hits, whereas the search 'stigma AND (coercion OR coercive OR involuntary)' reveals only 58 hits

*Coercive Treatment in Psychiatry: Clinical, Legal and Ethical Aspects*, First Edition.
Edited by Thomas W. Kallert, Juan E. Mezzich and John Monahan.
© 2011 John Wiley & Sons, Ltd. Published 2011 by John Wiley & Sons, Ltd.

(retrieval from the 22nd February 2010). Thus literature on this topic is scarce, but nevertheless, some valuable findings will be presented here.

In the first section, coercive measures concerning epidemiological and legal issues will be discussed. Most available empirical data concern involuntary admissions, presumably because they are far easier to assess than data about coercive treatments. For example, in Germany involuntary admissions are threefold regulated: the 'protective' placement according to the German Civil Code, Section 1906; placements because of a threat of public safety or to oneself according to Federal State laws, such as the *Gesetz über Hilfen und Schutzmaßnahmen bei psychischen Krankheiten (Psych-KG)* from North Rhine-Westphalia [law on aids and protection measures in the case of mental illness: Mental Health Act], and placements in the context of penal imprisoning (*StGB* [criminal code]). Coercive treatments usually comprise seclusion, medication and physical restraint. In Germany, the legal prerequisites are defined in the *FamFG (Gesetz über das Verfahren in Familiensachen und in den Angelegenheiten der freiwilligen Gerichtsbarkeit* [law on the procedure of family matters and of matters of voluntary jurisdiction]). Thus physical restraint is allowed only in the case of averting a danger, and if other effective measures are not available. A judicial approval is obligatory (*post hoc*, if necessary), as well as the duty of documentation.

In Section 2.2, we will focus on the question of which attributes are characteristic for involuntarily admitted patients, and discuss the comparability of data from different countries. Furthermore, legal regulations and long-term trends will be considered.

In Section 2.3, stigma will be discussed as a contributing factor in coercive measures. Stigmatizing attitudes towards people with mental illness such as negative stereotypes and high social distance are related to a positive attitude towards coercive measures. The question is, whether these attitudes also affect the evaluations of psychiatrists as well as the decisions of judges concerning coercive placements and treatments, respectively.

Further topics to be discussed in Sections 2.4 and 2.5 are illness-related behaviour that might facilitate coercive measures and consequences of coercive measures. These are to be differentiated into subjective consequences (e.g. perceived coercion, traumata) and objective consequences (e.g. loss of custody of own children, job loss).

Finally, in Sections 2.6 and 2.7, strategies to fight against stigma and discrimination due to mental illness are presented and discussed regarding their impact on the prevention and practice of coercive measures. Hence a global human rights perspective on these issues is important to ensure long-term achievements in the fight against the stigma and to minimize negative consequences of coercive measures against people with mental illness.

## 2.2    Coercive treatment – epidemiology and international comparisons

Before starting the discussion about the relation between stigma and coercive measures, it seems helpful to elaborate what is covered by the term 'coercive measures'. The complexity of this issue might be a reason for the low number of empirical studies in this domain. In general, causes for involuntary admissions and coercive treatment comprise several issues which can be subsumed under two conditions (see Table 2.1): someone endangers himself, or someone endangers other people. For example, suicidal intentions potentially endanger oneself, as well as under-nourishment, manic episodes or disorientation. Obviously, the mental state itself is not a reason for coercive admissions but only the resulting potential danger he or she is exposed to. The same applies for endangerment of other people, as in the case of homicide-suicide incidents, or (being delusional or not) threats of violence.

Characteristics of patients who are involuntarily admitted into a hospital have been described in a case study by Längle *et al.* [6]. According to their German sample ($N = 47$), involuntary admissions predominantly concern persons with a diagnosis of schizophrenia and happen usually outside of the regular working hours. Further characteristics such as sex, age, living situation or nationality do not correlate with involuntary admissions. However, validity of these results is limited due to the small sample and, of much more importance, the fact that the situation of Germany is not representative for other countries, neither in the European Union. Numbers of involuntary placements in European Union member states differ significantly; furthermore differences in developmental trends can be observed between some of these states [7]. Thus an absolute increase of involuntary placements between 1990 and 2000 has been recorded in some of the analysed countries (Austria, Finland, Sweden, as well as Germany and France), but in other countries the numbers remained rather constant (Denmark, Ireland, Luxemburg and England).

Additionally, if set in relation to the countries' population numbers, the rate of involuntary placements differs substantially between these countries (Figure 2.1);

**Table 2.1**   Causes for involuntary admissions and coercive treatment

| *Endangerment of oneself* | *Endangerment of others* |
| --- | --- |
| Suicidal intentions | Threat of violence |
| Disorientation | |
| Undernourishment | |
| Manic episode | |
| Homicide-suicide | |

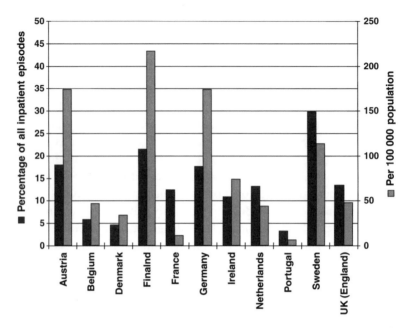

**Figure 2.1**   Rates of involuntary placements in European Union countries. Numbers refer to the years 1998, 1999 or 2000. Adapted from [7].

with the lowest figures in Portugal (6 per 100 000) and France (11), and the highest figures in Finland (215), Austria and Germany (both 175). A rather similar distribution appears for the percentage of involuntary placements in relation to all inpatient episodes in these countries (Figure 2.1). The authors discuss three explanations for these findings [7]: first, no operational descriptions for the basic judicial definitions are available. Second, in different countries, different concepts and definitions of involuntary placement (with different historical backgrounds of national legal systems and mental health care systems) exist. And third, the rate of patients whose status changed during hospitalization from voluntary to involuntary placement was not included in most countries.

Regarding the situation in Germany, some further interesting findings arise concerning the epidemiology of involuntary admissions: in a catchment area in Berlin, the ratio between the number of involuntary admissions and the rate of total admissions has been found to be constant over a period of 15 years (approximately 13% between 1988 and 2003; [8]). For Germany, Salize and Dressing provide rather constant ratios between 1993 (13.5%) and 1999 (15.9%) [7]. In other European countries, the ratio is also relatively constant over time, although on different levels (between 4.5 in Denmark and 20 in Finland). Nevertheless, for Germany, a constant rise of absolute numbers of admissions in total, and of involuntary admissions, has been recorded in the 1990s (probably due to a higher patient turnover because of shorter length of hospital stays; see [8]). Hence the ratio seems to be unaffected by the development of regulations to reduce involuntary admissions and treatments since the 1970s in Germany: the (ongoing) transition process toward a decentralized, community-orientated mental health care system [9]; further development of laws regulating involuntary placement and treatment on federal and state level (e.g. German Civil Code and Mental Health Acts); implementation of hospital inspection commissions as governmental control systems; and the development of guidelines and recommendations in the German Association for Psychiatry and Psychotherapy (DGPPN).

On the European level, legal regulations also seem not to affect numbers of involuntary placements (per 100 000 inhabitants) or involuntary placement rates (percentage of all inpatient cases; [10]). Both numbers and rates differ substantially between 12 analysed European countries, but the differences are not closely related to the legal practices in these countries such as, for example, whether dangerousness is used explicitly as a criterion for involuntary placement or not (as is the case in Italy, Spain or Sweden), or whether countries have detailed legal regulations for involuntary placements, as in Austria, Denmark, Germany, the Netherlands and Sweden. The Austrian example will elucidate this finding: in 1991, the Civil Commitment law (*Unterbringungsgesetz*) was implemented in Austria, which includes restrictive rules for involuntary admissions, namely that two psychiatrists must assess the patient and that provision of legal assistance is mandatory [11]. Despite these strict regulations, a high and increasing rate of involuntary admissions is found in Austria [10]. Moreover, in countries with very low rates of involuntary placements, legal regulations may differ substantially, for example in Portugal (only about 3% of all admissions are involuntary) with a restrictive judicial system vs. Denmark (with a rate of 4–5%), where the regulations are more treatment orientated and no judicial approval is needed [10]. As Schanda states [11], intended changes and improvements through laws (or their reforms, respectively) and real effects of their practical implementation may show high discrepancies, at least in the field of mental health care.

In sum, no stringent correlation between the kind of detailed legal regulations and rates of involuntary admissions can be observed across Europe. Nevertheless, such regulations are necessary to provide a reliable mental health care system, ensuring predictability of legal decisions in a constitutional state. Now the question arises, what other factors might influence the practice of involuntary psychiatric hospital admissions and coercive treatments in psychiatry? In terms of decision-making, a multitude of medical, social, cultural and psychological factors bear on the decision of whether to apply coercive measures. From an international point of view, the related decision-making process varies between countries: mostly, the psychiatrist is expert witness, counselling the judge who decides about the admission, but in some countries (e.g. in Denmark) the psychiatrist himself decides about involuntary admissions.

However, independent of the question of legal responsibility, diverse objectives and attitudes might play a role for those who are involved in the decision: intentions such as the prevention of self-harm and care for the patients might play a role as well as paternalistic attitudes (which are somewhat double-edged: on the one hand, they express an attentive attitude towards patients; on the other hand they might result in the unintended suppression of the patients' self-empowering resources). A second cluster of influencing factors relates to the perceived dangerousness of the concerned patient to himself (the evaluation of the seriousness of suicidal intentions is one of the most important diagnostic tasks) as well as to others (influencing factors such as public safety concerns and current political sentiments are important, especially in the second case). A third point concerns the symptom severity of a mental disorder. Even though, legally, the severity of symptoms is not the decisive cause for a decision for involuntary admittance, physicians might be influenced in their decision-making, because the patients' communicative behaviour is influenced by their symptoms, at least in some cases. Beyond these clinical, societal and attitudinal factors, we assume that the prevailing stigma against individuals with mental disorders affects the practice of coercive measures. This issue will be examined in the following section.

## 2.3   Stigma as a contributing factor in coercive measures

A persistent stigmatizing myth about psychiatry is that in psychiatric hospitals people are commonly treated against their will (if treated at all). The negative picture of psychiatric institutions is underpinned by scientific debates on the arbitrariness of psychiatric diagnoses, for example in the framework of the 'Rosenhan experiment' (for a current contribution to this topic, see [12]) and a common theme in mass media representations, as for example in the melodramatic movie *One Flew Over The Cuckoo's Nest* (1975), representing psychiatric hospitals as authoritarian and oppressive systems. Moreover, the stigma of mental illness is far more complex, and concerns also illness-specific prejudices, lay theories of the genesis of mental disorders, and attitudes towards psychiatric treatment settings and institutions. Such attitudes and cognitions can be found in the general public and in specific groups, for example in persons who work in psychiatric institutions (mental health professionals). We will show that some of these attitudes towards coercive measures correlate with attitudes directly associated with the stigma of mental illness.

As demonstrated in a British representative survey, stigmatizing attitudes in the population are differentiated concerning different mental illnesses ([13]; see Figure 2.2). Hence, negative attitudes such as perceived dangerousness and

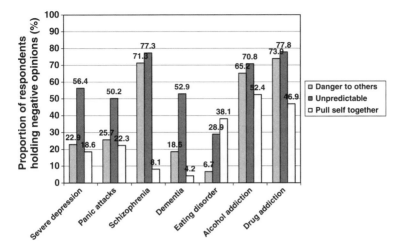

**Figure 2.2**   Public opinions on different mental illnesses. UK: representative household survey (1998; $N = 1737$; illnesses were presented with labels). Adapted from [13].

unpredictability relate predominantly to persons suffering from schizophrenia and substance or drug abuse disorders. Hence up to 75% of interviewees endorse negative statements about persons with schizophrenia. An overall lower frequency (approximately 40–50%) of negative attitudes in the population is found in mental disorders such as depression, anxiety disorders and eating disorders.

The stereotype that people with severe mental illness are dangerous is a crucial issue for stigma research, not only because of its high prevalence (more than 70% of the British population think that persons with schizophrenia or with alcohol or drug addictions are dangerous), but in particular because of its associated implications. As Lauber and colleagues have shown [14], stigmatizing attitudes towards people with mental illness in terms of negative stereotypes (with assumed dangerousness being a key stereotype) and the acceptance of coercive measures (namely compulsory admissions) correlate significantly which each other. Thus one central message of antistigma programmes is to set the alleged dangerousness of people with a severe mental illness, especially schizophrenia, into a more realistic context, that persons with schizophrenia are not more dangerous than the average population (if they are professionally treated), and that the increased risk (for persons not adequately treated, and for those having an additional diagnosis of substance abuse) of being violent or having a related criminal record is comparable with that of young male adolescents, compared to the average. Additionally, persons with a severe mental illness are more often victims of violent assaults than offenders (see [15]).

Before continuing to report further empirical data, a methodological issue needs to be clarified. A general obstacle in psychiatric stigma research is to measure it.

Direct observation of stigmatizing behaviour is methodologically complicated; hence proxy measures are used to assess the tendency to stigmatize in the sense of a behavioural intention. A commonly used stigma proxy is the adapted concept of social distance that was originally developed to assess attitudes towards ethnic minorities [16]. Several predictors or correlates of social distance towards people with mental illness, especially to those suffering from schizophrenia, are reported in the research literature. Apparently, the most prevalent one is the above-reported stereotype of dangerousness, which is closely associated with further negative stereotypes such as eeriness and unpredictability [17]. Further correlates of social distance are the kind of symptoms and the course of illness, perceived strangeness and impaired social skills (e.g. [18]), ascribed responsibility and lack of personal contact (e.g. [19]), and lack of knowledge about a mental illness (e.g. [20]). Two correlates of social distance will be discussed in more detail: lay theories on the genesis of mental disorders, and attitudes towards psychiatric treatment settings.

Theories about the genesis of mental disorders are a key issue, because they are guessed to affect further stigma-relevant attitudes, that is, about treatment options for mental illnesses, the course of the illness, and ascribed responsibility. Furthermore, lay concepts of the genesis of mental illness are correlated with the desire for social distance towards mentally ill people. In a German representative survey by the authors, genetic models for schizophrenia were related to the extent of desire for social distance towards people with schizophrenia [21]. On average, the lowest values of social distance were found in persons who ascribed biological and psychosocial causes to schizophrenia, in contrast to persons who named only psychosocial causes or only biological causes, who showed higher values of social distance.

Attitudes towards treatment settings and treatment methods are closely correlated with social distance towards people with mental illness. In a German representative survey by the authors [17], nearly a third of the interviewed thought that it would be harmful (in contrast to useful and neither/nor) for persons with schizophrenia to be treated on a closed ward. Other services like open psychiatric wards (3.3%), psychiatric day hospitals (2.0%) and group homes (2.1%) were much less frequently regarded as harmful. Persons who think closed wards are harmful have, on average, lower values of social distance and think less frequently that people with schizophrenia are dangerous (with both effects being independent of each other, as confirmed in a multiple correlation analysis). It seems that a benevolent attitude towards persons with schizophrenia is related to a negative attitude towards closed psychiatric wards. It might be by chance, but in another survey conducted in Germany, a third of the population (30%) are of the opinion that patients in a psychiatric hospital receive no treatment but are only calmed down [22]. However, it is not reported whether these respondents also have a more benevolent attitude towards psychiatric patients. The concurrent negative view on psychiatric hospitals is also illustrated by 24% of the interviewees, who think that patients in a psychiatric hospital receive no treatment but that their state worsens during their stay.

The empirical findings discussed so far focus on attitudes of the general population. Nevertheless, as recent empirical data about discrimination experiences indicate [23], some people with mental illness feel stigmatized particularly by mental health professionals. Since mental health professionals are socialized in the same environment as the general population, they share society's norms and values with other people. Thus they make experiences within their work, which additionally shape their attitudes towards people with mental illness. On the other hand, mental health professionals are opinion makers and leaders potentially affecting the public opinion and should therefore scrutinize their own attitudes [24]. Nevertheless, there is empirical evidence that attitudes of mental health professionals (of psychiatrists and psychologists) towards coercive measures correspond with those of lay people. In a vignette study by Steinert et al. [25], a case report of a 19-year-old man was presented, who had a first episode of paranoid delusions, ideas of being poisoned, marked social withdrawal and represented a moderate danger to himself, while several attempts to provide treatment by outpatient services and by means of persuasions had failed. The subjects (the sample was drawn from different mental health professions and lay people) rated whether they agreed with coercive measures (neuroleptic treatment and admission). They reported that 63% of the psychiatrists (59% of the psychologists) agreed with coercive medical treatment; 76% (77%) agreed with coercive admission. The agreement rates in the group of lay people (67% for coercive medical treatment, 73% for coercive admission) were rather similar. The only professional group with markedly lower agreement rates was social workers (48% and 55%, respectively).

Concerning stereotypes towards people with mental illness, the picture is somewhat different. In a survey comparing attitudes between mental health professionals and the general public [26], psychiatrists showed, on average, a higher extent of negative stereotypes compared with other mental health professions and the general population. Negative stereotypes included such items as dangerousness, unpredictability or stupidity. It is possible that these negative stereotypes are a consequence of the selective sample of patients and illness states that psychiatrists have to deal with (i.e. more severe and acute cases).

## 2.4  Behavioural markers and their impact on coercive measures

Some people with a severe mental illness show deviating communication behaviour due to their illness (see [27]), that might irritate others because lay people do not know and hence are not able to understand the causes for this odd behaviour. From the stigma perspective, we need to question, whether such illness-related behaviour endorses stigmatizing attitudes or coercive measures against those who show it. An experimental study from Penn and colleagues suggests this assumption: patients with schizophrenia were videotaped during conversation probe role-play tests [18]. Lay people rated their wish of social distance towards them, and clinicians rated several psychiatric symptoms, social skills and attractiveness. One single main variable predicting social distance was identified, namely 'strangeness'. Strangeness itself was correlated with several variables related to communicative behaviour, such as affective expressiveness, speech clarity, eye contact or involvement of the conversation. In a further study [28], videotapes of people with different mental disorders and of persons without a psychiatric diagnosis were analysed concerning affective flattening assessed with the corresponding SANS (Scale for the Assessment of Negative Symptoms) subscale [29] and social distance. In a series of multiple regression analyses of the different diagnostic groups (healthy control, depression, remitted schizophrenia, acute schizophrenia), significant correlations were found only in the schizophrenia groups. Hence persons with schizophrenia sometimes seem to show a communicative behaviour style which is related to the wish for social distance towards them. Obviously, this distance-evoking communication style is the result of symptoms of or disabilities caused by the illness schizophrenia. Though therapeutic techniques are being developed to regain communication skills [30], it is possible that impaired communication skills can provoke or aggravate critical situations and thus contribute to coercive measures.

## 2.5 Consequences of coercive measures

In a case study [6], Längle *et al.* interviewed the patients being involuntarily committed one year afterwards or later. The results are noteworthy, although, due to the small sample size and the local sample, they are not supposed to be representative. Less than 50% of the patients in Längle's study thought that the commitment had a positive effect on their illness course. Approximately 80% thought, in retrospection, that with the right strategies the commitment could have been avoided, and 70% perceived the commitment as strongly coercive, whereas only 20% saw their commitment with relief. The most stressful consequences the patients perceived were to remain on a closed ward (43%), side effects of medication (34%) and feelings of helplessness (23%). These 'subjective' consequences of coercive measures are of such high importance because they shape the image of inpatient psychiatry in the public eye. Furthermore, 15% of the patients also reported 'objective' consequences of the coercive measures, that is, loss of independence, loss of custody of children, and fewer social contacts. Adverse consequences in their jobs were reported by 11%.

The patients' perspective sometimes differs from that of professionals. Bindman *et al.* examined the perception of coercion in a consecutive English sample of inpatients at the time of admission [31]. Using the Admission Experience Interview (AEI), they examined associated factors of a high subjectively perceived coercion. These were a diagnosis of schizophrenia or any other psychosis, objective coercion (detention under the English Mental Health Act or involvement of the police during admission), a lower insight score, and high scores of the AEI subscales 'experiences of negative pressures' being exerted during admission and 'experiences of process exclusion' (feelings of not being heard and considered in arriving at the decision to admit to hospital). A further finding was the lack of knowledge about their own legal status and rights, even though these rights are clearly established within the Mental Health Act.

Beyond that, the question arises of whether patients' future treatment adherence and treatment might be influenced by negative subjective experiences of coercion during former hospital stays. In the survey of Bindman *et al.* [31], no significant predictors for treatment engagement in a 10-month follow-up were identified, as well as in another 1-year-follow-up study from the United States [32]. Since such long-term studies face the problem of controlling external effects, an approach assessing the patients' behaviour retrospectively might be more promising. Swartz *et al.* found, in a survey with patients with schizophrenia, that previous involuntary hospitalizations, as well as perceived coercion in outpatient treatment (i.e. whether someone has experienced forced threats and other pressures to seek treatment), are significantly associated with a delay in seeking medical help for mental health or alcohol/drug problems [33].

## 2.6   Evolving strategies – international guidelines for coercive measures and advocacy of non-discrimination

Psychiatry is a rapidly developing science; hence the first strategy to reduce the stigma of mental illness is to improve psychiatric treatment methods and to reduce the occurrence of coercive measures. Internationally harmonized guidelines to regulate coercive measures might be an important part of this. The European Council (EC) [34] adopted five criteria that must all be fulfilled to justify involuntary placement (Box 2.1). Further articles of the European Council recommendation define criteria for involuntary treatment and principles of how involuntary treatment should be implemented. All European Union (EU) member states are committed to these criteria. For this purpose, the states are to monitor the 'compliance with standards . . . [by] conducting visits and inspections of mental health facilities' (EC recommendations, Article 37) and provide 'systematic and reliable anonymized statistical information' (EC recommendations, Article 38) available to the public.

**Box 2.1** International Guidelines for Involuntary Placements and Treatments [34].

*Article 17 – Criteria for involuntary placement*

1. A person may be subject to involuntary placement only if all the following conditions are met:

    i. the person has a mental disorder;
    ii. the person's condition represents a significant risk of serious harm to his or her health or to other persons;
    iii. the placement includes a therapeutic purpose;
    iv. no less restrictive means of providing appropriate care are available;
    v. the opinion of the person concerned has been taken into consideration

[. . .]

*Article 18 – Criteria for involuntary treatment*

A person may be subject to involuntary treatment only if all the following conditions are met:

    i. the person has a mental disorder;
    ii. the person's condition represents a significant risk of serious harm to his or her health or to other persons;
    iii. no less intrusive means of providing appropriate care are available;
    iv. the opinion of the person concerned has been taken into consideration

*Article 19 – Principles concerning involuntary treatment*

1. Involuntary treatment should:

    i. address specific clinical signs and symptoms;
    ii. be proportionate to the person's state of health;
    iii. form part of a written treatment plan;
    iv. be documented;
    v. where appropriate, aim to enable the use of treatment acceptable to the person as soon as possible.

2. In addition to the requirements of Article 12.1 above[1] the treatment plan should:
    i. whenever possible be prepared in consultation with the person concerned and the person's personal advocate or representative, if any;
    ii. be reviewed at appropriate intervals and, if necessary, revised, whenever possible in consultation with the person concerned and his or her personal advocate or representative, if any.

3. Member states should ensure that involuntary treatment only takes place in an appropriate environment.

The second strategy is to fight the stigma of mental illness in its manifestations, affecting not only those suffering from a mental illness, their relatives and friends, but also the people working in psychiatric and mental health care services, as well as psychiatric treatment methods. As stated in the UN Convention on the Rights of Persons with Disabilities [35], non-discrimination due to disability is a fundamental human right (Box 2.2).

---

**Box 2.2** The UN Convention on the Rights of Persons with Disabilities [35].

*Preamble*

The States Parties to the present Convention,

a. Recalling the principles proclaimed in the Charter of the United Nations which recognize the inherent dignity and worth and the equal and inalienable rights of all members of the human family as the foundation of freedom, justice and peace in the world,
b. Recognizing that the United Nations, in the Universal Declaration of Human Rights and in the International Covenants on Human Rights, has proclaimed and agreed that everyone is entitled to all the rights and freedoms set forth therein, without distinction of any kind,
c. Reaffirming the universality, indivisibility, interdependence and interrelatedness of all human rights and fundamental freedoms and the need for persons with disabilities to be guaranteed their full enjoyment without discrimination,

[. . .]

Have agreed as follows:

*Article 1 – Purpose*

The purpose of the present Convention is to promote, protect and ensure the full and equal enjoyment of all human rights and fundamental freedoms by all persons with disabilities, and to promote respect for their inherent dignity.

[. . .]

*Article 3 – General principles*

The principles of the present Convention shall be:

a. Respect for inherent dignity, individual autonomy including the freedom to make one's own choices, and independence of persons;
b. Non-discrimination;
c. Full and effective participation and inclusion in society;
d. Respect for difference and acceptance of persons with disabilities as part of human diversity and humanity;
e. Equality of opportunity;
f. Accessibility;
g. Equality between men and women;
h. Respect for the evolving capacities of children with disabilities and respect for the right of children with disabilities to preserve their identities.

**Article 5 – Equality and non-discrimination**

1. States Parties recognize that all persons are equal before and under the law and are entitled without any discrimination to the equal protection and equal benefit of the law.
2. States Parties shall prohibit all discrimination on the basis of disability and guarantee to persons with disabilities equal and effective legal protection against discrimination on all grounds.
3. In order to promote equality and eliminate discrimination, States Parties shall take all appropriate steps to ensure that reasonable accommodation is provided.
4. Specific measures which are necessary to accelerate or achieve *de facto* equality of persons with disabilities shall not be considered discrimination under the terms of the present Convention.

## 2.7   Human rights and antistigma programmes

Member states that ratified the convention are obliged to 'ensure and promote the full realization of all human rights and fundamental freedoms for all persons with disabilities without discrimination of any kind on the basis of disability' (UN Convention, Article 4.1). The scope of disability includes 'those who have long-term physical, mental, intellectual or sensory impairments which in interaction with various barriers may hinder their full and effective participation in society on an equal basis with others' (UN Convention, Article 1).

The concept of human rights adopted by the UN lays special emphasis on social participation and inclusion of people with disabilities, which is reflected in several articles of the convention, especially in Article 8 (awareness-raising about the issues of people with disabilities), Article 9 (ensuring access to the physical environment, to transportation, to information and communications, including information and communications technologies and systems), and further on:

- Article 19 – Living independently and being included in the community
- Article 21 – Freedom of expression and opinion, and access to information
- Article 24 – Education
- Article 27 – Work and employment
- Article 29 – Participation in political and public life
- Article 30 – Participation in cultural life, recreation, leisure and sport.

International antistigma programmes such as, for example, the Global Programme Against Stigma And Discrimination Because Of Schizophrenia – 'Open The Doors' [1,36] – pursue a strategy adapted to the local situation of persons with mental illness, addressed at specific target groups such as school children, teachers, journalists, police officers, and so on, and which employs specific methods to counteract the stigma (e.g. to involve persons with mental illness in planning and organizing of interventions; to provide information about causes, symptoms and treatment methods of mental illnesses; and to seek for empathy and tolerance for people who are different from the majority). A central issue is to involve people with personal experiences of mental illness in the antistigma work; as Meise *et al.* showed [37], antistigma interventions involving mental health care users provide better results in terms of attitudinal change than interventions without.

The German Open the Doors Programme was set up in 2000. Seven centres located in six different cities implemented local and partially nationwide antistigma interventions in the above-described sense. Efficacy of these antistigma interventions has been examined with quasi-experimental panel design representative population surveys undertaken by the authors in the context of the German Network on Schizophrenia Research, funded by the German Federal Ministry of Research and Education [17]. In this study, social distance towards people with schizophrenia was assessed in inhabitants of different German cities, some of them where antistigma interventions were located, and some of them where this was not the case. The surveys were repeated after three years of interventions in the same cities with the same interviewees. Social distance towards people with schizophrenia decreased significantly from 2001 to 2004. In further multiple regression analyses, the decrease was significantly related to those cities where antistigma interventions were located, and to persons who were aware of such antistigma interventions. Though the effect size of the social distance decrease as well as of the regression analyses was small (in a sample of $N = 4624$), and the design was only quasi-experimental, this study was the first providing evidence for the efficacy of antistigma interventions on a population level in Germany.

These encouraging results facilitated the foundation of the German Alliance for Mental Health. Members of Open the Doors Germany were initiators, as well as the German Association for Psychiatry and Psychotherapy (DGPPN; [38]). Under the patronage of the German Federal Minister of Health, and together with the federal associations of users (Bundesverband Psychiatrie-Erfahrener; BPE) and relatives (Bundesverband der Angehörigen psychisch Kranker; BApK), the Alliance started work in 2005. The German Alliance is a long-term engagement of the participating groups, confederating local and nationwide antistigma projects and initiatives conjointly with societal institutions (e.g. political, church, work, health care, sports). It addresses different mental illnesses with the target of improving the situation of mental health care users through the joint fight against the stigma of mental illness. Current information about the Alliance and its activities can be obtained via the Internet (www.seelischegesundheit.net).

## 2.8   Summary and future prospects

The relationship between stigma of mental illness and coercive measures in psychiatry has been elucidated in this chapter. Evidently, the issues are interlinked, but if, in terms of the details, this relationship is characterized by complexity and is not yet well studied, nevertheless there is evidence that the stigma might contribute to frequency and practice of coercive measures, and that frequency and practice of coercive measures affect the image of psychiatry and the corresponding stigma of mental illness.

From an epidemiological perspective, absolute frequencies of coercive admissions are rising in parallel to rising total numbers of psychiatric admissions in many EU countries. Hence the quota of involuntary vs. voluntary admissions remains constant. However, absolute and relative frequencies of involuntary admissions vary significantly across EU member states. As regards epidemiology and clinical practice of coercive treatments, there is further need for differentiation, also to enable international comparisons. The variability between countries in the EU is so high that it seems that other factors than legal definitions of involuntary admissions or dangerousness as explicitly stated criterion for involuntary admissions are of the same or even of more importance: for example the historical background of national mental health care systems.

However, the frequency of coercive measures is not yet a stand-alone criterion for the quality of psychiatric health care; hence practical procedures need to be controlled to establish equal human rights' standards in psychiatric institutions all over Europe. Best practice, such as adoption of a transparent communication style in the context of coercive measures, duty of documentation, or systematic debriefings of patients (and staff!) after incidents where coercive measures had to be applied, may contribute to a better image of psychiatry and thus a reduction of stigma. It is a kind of self-amplifying process: patients experiencing coercive measures in a less traumatic way may afterwards develop a more differentiated perspective on coercive measures. If coercive measures themselves get rid of the image of arbitrariness and punishment, they might also reduce the stigmatizing potential that the patients additionally suffer from.

The stigma of mental illness (in terms of high social distance and negative stereotypes) is related to a positive attitude towards coercive measures, as has been shown in many population-based surveys. But also some mental health professionals show negative attitudes towards people with mental illness; hence antistigma interventions targeted directly at mental health professionals are of utmost importance, though not yet well established.

Furthermore, illness-related behaviour such as impaired communication skills may amplify negative attitudes. In contrast to these risks, personal contact with persons with mental illness is generally a stigma-reducing factor. In personal contact, mental illness becomes a more normal state of life and persons with a mental illness become people like ourselves. Consequently, antistigma programmes involve mental health care users in their activities and contribute successfully to a better knowledge of mental illness and thus a stigma reduction. Several programmes exist on an international level ('Open the Doors' from the World Psychiatrists Association), national level (e.g. 'Time to Change' in England; German Alliance for Mental Health) and regional level (e.g. Open the Doors local centres in Germany).

From the European perspective, the harmonization and implementation of professional and legal guidelines for coercive measures as well as the creation of a reliable and valid database are of utmost interest. However, coercive measures will be unavoidable in the near future. They should be applied under the most transparent and skilled, least harmful and most humane conditions possible, and under circumstances where other preventive measures are not available.

These assertions should be taken for granted, but they are obviously not. A possible explanation would be that sometimes mental health professionals have to find their own professional role in the context of coercive measures. Hence the need for justification of such measures might stand in contrast to their own ethical standards (see [39]), thus counteracting an open and confident handling of coercive measures. Such a conclusion would need empirical validation. Nevertheless it is crucial to address both topics, stigma and coercion, in regular further education for mental health professionals, because people with mental illness have the right to treatment respecting human rights, and mental health professionals have the means to make this possible in most cases. In those cases where this is not possible, everything has to be done to minimize human rights violations and to minimize possible negative consequences for the patients treated coercively.

## Notes

1 Article 12.1: Persons with mental disorder should receive treatment and care provided by adequately qualified staff and based on an appropriate individually prescribed treatment plan. Whenever possible the treatment plan should be prepared in consultation with the person concerned and his or her opinion should be taken into account. The plan should be regularly reviewed and, if necessary, revised.

## References

1. World Psychiatric Association (1998) *Fighting Stigma and Discrimination because of Schizophrenia*, World Psychiatric Association, New York.

2. Gaebel, W., Möller, H.J. and Rössler, W. (eds) (2005) *Stigma – Diskriminierung – Bewälti-gung. Der Umgang mit sozialer Ausgrenzung psychich Kranker* [Stigma – discrimination – coping. The coping with social exclusion of people with mental illnesses], W. Kohlhammer, Stuttgart.

3. Sartorius, N. and Schulze, H. (2005) *Reducing the Stigma Of Mental Illness. A Report from a Global Programme of the World Psychiatric Association*, Cambridge University Press, New York.

4. Thornicroft, G. (2006) *Shunned. Discrimination Against People With Mental Illness*, Oxford University Press, Oxford.

5. Kallert, T.W., Glöckner, M., Onchev, G. *et al.* (2005) The EUNOMIA project on coercion in psychiatry: study design and preliminary data. *World Psychiatry*, **4**, 168–172.

6. Längle, G., Renner, G., Günthner, A. *et al.* (2003) Psychiatric commitment: patients' perspectives. *Medicine and Law*, **22**, 39–53.

7. Salize, H.J. and Dressing, H. (2004) Epidemiology of involuntary placement of mentally ill people across the European Union. *British Journal of Psychiatry*, **184**, 163–168.

8. von Haebler, D., Beuscher, H., Fähndrich, E. *et al.* (2007) Compulsory psychiatric admissions in two districts of Berlin – how open are the psychiatric services? *Deutsches Ärzteblatt*, **104**, A 1232–A 1236.

9. Deutscher Bundestag (1975) *Bericht über die Lage der Psychiatrie in der Bundesrepublik Deutschland: Zur psychiatrischen und psychotherapeutischen/psychosomatischen Versorgung der Bevölkerung*. Drucksache 7/4200, Deutscher Bundestag, Bonn.

10. Dreßing, H. and Salize, H.J. (2004) Nehmen Zwangsunterbringungen psychisch Kranker in den Ländern der Europäischen Union zu? [Is there an increase in the number of compulsory admissions of mentally ill patients in European Union Member States?]. *Gesundheitswesen*, **66**, 240–245.

11. Schanda, H. (2005) Die aktuelle Psychiatriegesetzgebung in Österreich: Zivil- und Strafrecht aus psychiatrischer Sicht. *Recht & Psychiatrie*, **23**, 159–165.

12. Spitzer, R.L., Lilienfeld, S.O. and Miller, M.B. (2005) Rosenhan revisited: the scientific credibility of Lauren Slater's pseudopatient diagnosis study. *The Journal of Nervous and Mental Disease*, **193**, 734–739.

13. Crisp, A.H., Gelder, M.G., Rix, S. *et al.* (2000) Stigmatisation of people with mental illnesses. *British Journal of Psychiatry*, **177**, 4–7.

14. Lauber, C., Nordt, C., Falcato, L. and Rössler, W. (2002) Public attitude to compulsory admission of mentally ill people. *Acta Psychiatrica Scandinavica*, **105**, 385–389.

15. Walsh, E., Moran, P., Scott, C. *et al.* (2003) Prevalence of violent victimisation in severe mental illness. *British Journal of Psychiatry*, **183**, 233–238.

16. Bogardus, E.M. (1925) Measuring social distance. *Journal of Applied Sociology*, **9**, 299–308.

17. Gaebel, W., Zäske, H., Baumann, A.E. *et al.* (2008) Evaluation of the German WPA "program against stigma and discrimination because of schizophrenia–Open the Doors": results from representative telephone surveys before and after three years of antistigma interventions. *Schizophrenia Research*, **98**, 184–193.

18. Penn, D.L., Kohlmaier, J.R. and Corrigan, P.W. (2000) Interpersonal factors contributing to the stigma of schizophrenia: social skills, perceived attractiveness, and symptoms. *Schizophrenia Research*, **45**, 37–45.

19. Kurihara, T., Kato, M., Sakamoto, S. *et al.* (2000) Public attitudes towards the mentally ill: a cross-cultural study between Bali and Tokyo. *Psychiatry and Clinical Neurosciences*, **54**, 547–552.

20. Gaebel, W., Baumann, A., Witte, A.M. and Zaeske, H. (2002) Public attitudes towards people with mental illness in six German cities: results of a public survey under special consideration of schizophrenia. *European Archives of Psychiatry and Clinical Neuroscience*, **252**, 278–287.
21. Gaebel, W. (2006) "Antistigma" in Forschung und Praxis – Wo stehen wir heute? Lecture, DGPPN Annual Conference, Berlin, November 22–25, Germany.
22. Angermeyer, M.C. (ed) (1994) Das Bild der Psychiatrie in der Öffentlichkeit, in *Versorgungsstrukturen in der Psychiatrie*. Tropon Symposium, Volume IX (ed F. Reimer), Springer, Berlin.
23. Thornicroft, G., Brohan, E., Rose, D. *et al.* for the INDIGO Study Group (2009) Global pattern of experienced and anticipated discrimination against people with schizophrenia: a cross-sectional survey. *Lancet*, **373**, 408–415.
24. Lauber, C., Nordt, C. and Rössler, W. (2006) Attitudes and mental illness: consumers and the general public are on one side of the medal, mental health professionals on the other. *Acta Psychiatrica Scandinavica*, **114**, 145–146.
25. Steinert, T., Lepping, P., Baranyai, R. and Hoffmann, M. (2005) Compulsory admission and treatment in schizophrenia: a study of ethical attitudes in four European countries. *Social Psychiatry and Psychiatric Epidemiology*, **40**, 635–641.
26. Nordt, C., Rössler, W. and Lauber, C. (2006) Attitudes of mental health professionals toward people with schizophrenia and major depression. *Schizophrenia Bulletin*, **32**, 709–714.
27. Grant, P.M. and Beck, A.T. (2009) Evaluation sensitivity as a moderator of communication disorder in schizophrenia. *Psychological Medicine*, **39**, 1211–1219.
28. Baumann, A., Craigie, E., Zäske, H. and Gaebel, W. (2005) Interpersonal factors contributing to the desire for social distance. Lecture, XIII World Congress of Psychiatry, Cairo, September 10–15, Egypt.
29. Andreasen, N.C. (1989) The Scale for the Assessment of Negative Symptoms (SANS): conceptual and theoretical foundations. *British Journal of Psychiatry. Supplement*, (7), 49–58.
30. Frommann, N., Streit, M. and Wölwer, W. (2003) Remediation of facial affect recognition impairments in patients with schizophrenia: a new training program. *Psychiatry Research*, **117**, 281–284.
31. Bindman, J., Reid, Y., Szmukler, G. *et al.* (2005) Perceived coercion at admission to psychiatric hospital and engagement with follow-up – a cohort study. *Social Psychiatry and Psychiatric Epidemiology*, **40**, 160–166.
32. Rain, S.D., Williams, V.F., Robbins, P.C. *et al.* (2003) Perceived coercion at hospital admission and adherence to mental health treatment after discharge. *Psychiatric Services*, **54**, 103–105.
33. Swartz, M.S., Swanson, J.W. and Hannon, M.J. (2003) Does fear of coercion keep people away from mental health treatment? Evidence from a survey of persons with schizophrenia and mental health professionals. *Behavioral Sciences & The Law*, **21**, 459–472.
34. Council of Europe (2004) Recommendation Rec(2004)10 of the Committee of Ministers to member states concerning the protection of the human rights and dignity of persons with mental disorder (Adopted by the Committee of Ministers on 22 September 2004 at the 896th meeting of the Ministers' Deputies). Council of Europe, Strasbourg.
35. United Nations (2006) Convention on the Rights of Persons with Disabilities, United Nations, New York.
36. World Psychiatric Association (2003) *Fighting Stigma and Discrimination because of Schizophrenia. Training Manual Version II*, World Psychiatric Association, New York.

37. Meise, U., Sulzenbacher, H., Kemmler, G. *et al.* (2000) "... nicht gefährtlich, aber doch furchterregend". Ein Programm gegen Stigmatisierung von Schizophrenie in Schulen. *Psychiatrische Praxis*, **27**, 340–346.
38. Gaebel, W., Zäske, H. and Baumann, A. (2004) Stigmatisierung und Diskriminierung psychisch Erkrankter als Herausforderung für die Gesundheitsversorgung in Deutschland. *Deutsches Ärzteblatt*, **101**, A 3253–A 3255.
39. Vuckovich, P.K. and Artinian, B.M. (2005) Justifying coercion. *Nursing Ethics*, **12**, 370–380.

# 3 Mandated psychiatric treatment in the community – forms, prevalence, outcomes and controversies

## John Monahan

*University of Virginia School of Law, Charlottesville, VA, USA*

Treating people with mental disorder who do not want to be treated for mental disorder has always and everywhere been the most contentious issue in mental health law. For centuries, unwanted treatment took place solely in mental hospitals. What has changed in recent decades is the locus of unwanted treatment. What was once hidden from sight in closed institutions has increasingly shifted into plain view in the open community.

Outpatient commitment – a civil court order requiring a person to adhere to psychiatric treatment in the community, at the risk of being hospitalized if the order is defied – has grown rapidly in the past two decades, being adopted in Australia in 1986, in Israel in 1991, in New Zealand in 1992, in Ontario, Canada, in 2000, in Scotland in 2005, and in England and Wales, Taiwan and Sweden in 2008 [1]. But perhaps nowhere has outpatient commitment grown as fast, and with as much controversy, as in the United States. Since New York State introduced the first modern outpatient commitment statute in 1999, many other American jurisdictions

*Coercive Treatment in Psychiatry: Clinical, Legal and Ethical Aspects*, First Edition.
Edited by Thomas W. Kallert, Juan E. Mezzich and John Monahan.
© 2011 John Wiley & Sons, Ltd. Published 2011 by John Wiley & Sons, Ltd.

have followed suite with new or strengthened laws, including California in 2003; Florida, Michigan and West Virginia in 2005; Illinois, Idaho and Virginia in 2008; and New Jersey and Maine in 2010 [2].

Much of the strident policy debate on outpatient commitment treats it as if it were simply an extension of inpatient commitment, viewing it within the same conceptual and legal framework historically used to analyse commitment to a mental hospital. Increasingly, however, it is becoming apparent that concepts developed within an institutional setting do not translate well to the much more open-textured context of the community. It was for good reason that Goffman [3] famously described mental hospitals as 'total institutions': a single source supplied an individual's lodging, administered welfare benefits, maintained order and provided treatment. In the community, in contrast, one source supplies an individual's lodging (a housing agency), another administers benefits (a welfare agency), a third maintains order (the criminal justice system), and a fourth provides treatment (the mental health system). Outpatient commitment, rather than being seen as a diluted form of mental hospitalization, may be better considered as one of a growing array of legal tools from the social welfare and judicial systems being used as 'leverage' to ensure adherence to psychiatric treatment in the community [4].

This chapter does four things. First, it illustrates a new and broader perspective on requiring adherence to outpatient mental health services, called 'mandated community treatment'. Second, it provides estimates of the frequency with which various forms of leverage are applied to psychiatric outpatients in the United States, as well as of the use of psychiatric advance directives. Third, preliminary empirical findings on the outcomes attributable to the different forms of leverage are summarized. Finally, the chapter addresses two controversial issues that often arise in discussions of mandated community treatment: the extent to which the use of leverage amounts to 'coercion', and the role of culture in understanding people's views of the legitimacy of mandated community treatment.

## 3.1  The forms of mandated community treatment

It is primarily through the social welfare and legal systems that leverage can be applied to people with mental illness to increase the likelihood that they will adhere to treatment in the community. People with serious mental disorder may qualify under American law to receive assistance from the social welfare system. Two forms of assistance for which some people with mental illness qualify are financial benefits and subsidized housing. In addition, people with serious mental disorder are sometimes required to comply with treatment by judges or by other officials acting under judicial authority (e.g. probation or parole officers). Even without a formal judicial order, people with mental illness may agree to adhere to treatment in the community in the hope of avoiding an unfavourable resolution of their case, such as being sentenced to jail, or being committed to a mental hospital.

### 3.1.1   Money as leverage

Recipients of government disability benefits in the United States typically receive checks made in their own names. The law, however, provides for the appointment of a 'representative payee' to receive the checks if it is determined to be in the beneficiary's best interests to do so. For example, a representative payee might be appointed for a beneficiary who is in a coma, or who is a young child. An estimated one million Americans with a mental disability also receive federal government benefits through a representative payee [5]. Some of these people with mental disability who have a representative payee appointed for them believe that there is a quid-pro-quo relationship between their adherence to outpatient treatment and their receipt of what they consider to be 'their' money [6]. For example, the patient brochure on representative payee services used by one state agency states: 'You are receiving benefits based on the mental health and physical problems that you have. The Social Security Administration requires that you be involved in mental health services and work with your program so that you will feel better' [7].

### 3.1.2   Housing as leverage

A recent survey of the United States reported that 'there is not one state or community in the nation where a person with a disability receiving [federal disability] payments can afford to rent a modest... one-bedroom or efficiency housing unit' [8]. To avoid widespread homelessness, federal and state governments provide a number of housing options in the community for people with mental illness. No one questions that property owners can impose generally applicable requirements – such as not disturbing neighbours – on their tenants. However, proprietors sometimes proactively impose the additional requirement on a tenant with mental disorder that he or she be actively engaged in treatment [9]. Agencies that manage housing programmes for people with mental disorders may consider the programmes primarily as 'residential treatment' and only incidentally as lodging. For example, the standard lease used by one housing provider reads, 'Refusing to continue with mental health treatment means that I do not believe I need mental health services... I understand that since I am no longer a consumer of mental health services, it is expected that I will find alternative housing. I understand that if I do not, I may face eviction' [4].

### 3.1.3    Jail as leverage

Making the acceptance of mental health treatment in the community a condition of sentencing a defendant to probation rather than to jail has long been an accepted judicial practice [10]. For example, Chapter 18, Section 3563 of the United States Code states that a federal court may impose as a condition of probation that an offender 'undergo available medical, psychiatric, or psychological treatment'. In addition to this general provision of treatment as a condition of probation, an entirely new type of criminal court – called, appropriately, a 'mental health court' – has been developed that makes even more explicit the link between avoiding criminal punishment and accepting treatment in the community. Adapted from the drug court model, a mental health court offers the defendant intensely supervised outpatient treatment as an alternative to jail [11].

### 3.1.4    Hospitalization as leverage

Outpatient commitment, as described above, refers to a court order directing a person with a serious mental disorder to adhere to a prescribed plan of treatment in the community, under pain of being hospitalized for failure to do so, if the person meets the statutory criteria. There are three types of outpatient commitment in use in the United States today. In the first type, *conditional discharge*, a psychiatric inpatient continues to meet commitment criteria, but is offered hospital discharge on the condition that he or she continue with treatment in the community. In the second type, *alternative to hospitalization*, a person in the community meets inpatient commitment criteria, but is offered outpatient commitment in lieu of admission to a psychiatric hospital. In the final and most controversial type, *preventive commitment*, a person does *not* meet inpatient commitment criteria, but is believed to be deteriorating to the point that – unless treatment in the community is obtained – he or she soon will qualify for involuntary hospitalization [7].

Only two randomized clinical trials of outpatient commitment exist [12,13], and these two American studies reached opposite conclusions. A third randomized clinical trial, in the United Kingdom, is currently under way [14]. One review of 72 studies undertaken in six countries concluded that 'it is not possible to state whether [outpatient commitment] orders are beneficial or harmful to patients' ([15]; but see [16]). This lack of agreement in the data has not kept advocacy groups from making unequivocal empirical judgments (see Table 3.1 comparing the views of the leading American patient advocacy group, the Bazelon Center, and the leading American family advocacy group, the Treatment Advocacy Center).

**Table 3.1** American advocacy groups' opposing views of existing data on outpatient commitment (OPC).

| Issue | Bazelon Center [17,18] | Treatment Advocacy Center [19,20] |
| --- | --- | --- |
| Overall research findings | 'The studies, relatively few in number, clearly show that [OPC] confers no benefit beyond access to effective community services – access that is too often nonexistent on a voluntary basis.' | 'Studies and data from states using AOT[a] prove that it is effective in reducing ... homelessness, arrests and incarcerations, victimization, and violent episodes.' |
| Bellevue outcome study | 'The findings are conclusive... The study provides strong evidence that outpatient commitment has no intrinsic value.' | '[T]he authors acknowledged that a "limit on [the study's] ability to draw wide-ranging conclusions is the modest size of [the] study group." ... Additionally, nonadherence to a treatment order had no consequences.' |
| Duke outcome study | '[T]he Bazelon Center's analysis... find[s] weaknesses in the North Carolina study.' | '[T]he Duke Studies are the largest and most respected of the controlled examinations of assisted outpatient treatment (AOT). The Duke Studies proved the remarkable benefits of assisted outpatient treatment.' |
| Effect on hospital admissions | 'Statements that outpatient commitment reduces hospital admissions or hospital stays are often based on data from four published studies, all flawed.' | 'Several studies have clearly established the effectiveness of AOT in decreasing hospital admissions.' |
| Effect on treatment adherence | 'Statements that increased compliance with psychiatric treatment can be attributed solely to the effect of outpatient commitment are normally based on data from two studies – both flawed.' | 'AOT has also been shown to be extremely effective in increasing treatment compliance.' |

[a] The Treatment Advocacy Center refers to outpatient commitment as 'assisted outpatient treatment' (AOT).

### 3.1.5 An antidote to leverage

Usually, advance directives pertain to medical care at the end of life. But changes in American law have given impetus to patient advocates to promote the creation of advance directives for psychiatric treatment. These directives allow competent persons to declare their preferences for mental health treatment, or to appoint a surrogate to make decisions for them, in advance of a crisis during which they may lose capacity to make reliable health care decisions themselves [21]. Many patient advocates as well as clinicians see the use of a psychiatric advance directive as an antidote to, or at least an attenuation of, treatment mandated by others. As one commentator stated, 'The advent of advance directives for psychiatric care offers an unprecedented opportunity to reconcile, or at least accommodate, the opposing values represented by proponents of involuntary interventions, on the one hand, and by civil libertarians, on the other' [22].

## 3.2    The prevalence of mandated community treatment

How often are given forms of leverage – singly or in combination – imposed on people with mental disorder to get them to adhere to treatment in the community? Since the total amount of leverage used, and the distribution of different types of leverage, will vary across locations even within the same country, it is important to study people with mental disorder in a number of different sites. One study in the United States selected five sites that were diverse in terms of region, population and the density of mandated treatment programmes: San Francisco, CA; Chicago, IL; Tampa, FL; Worcester, MA; and Durham, NC. Over 1000 adults currently in outpatient treatment for a mental disorder with a publicly supported mental health service provider for at least six months were surveyed [23,24]. Amongst the key findings of this study were that approximately half of all outpatients – 44 to 59% across the five sites, with a mean of 51% – have experienced at least one form of leverage over the course of their lifetimes. Half of *these* patients have experienced two or more different forms of leverage. The most common forms of leverage were treatment in order to obtain subsidized housing (32% of all patients) and to avoid going to jail (23%), and the least prevalent forms of leverage were treatment to obtain disability benefits (12%), and to avoid inpatient mental hospitalization (i.e. outpatient commitment; 15%). A consistent picture emerged of leverage being used more frequently for patients – particularly younger males – with more severe, disabling and longer lasting psychopathology, with a pattern of multiple hospital readmissions, and with previous intensive outpatient service utilization. Substance abuse increased the likelihood of all forms of leverage except housing, since housing programmes often bar substance abusers.

In addition, recent American work has addressed the use of child custody as leverage to assure that parents with mental illness adhere to outpatient treatment [25], education as leverage to increase the likelihood that university students with mental illness will adhere to outpatient treatment [26], licences as leverage to induce professionals (e.g. physicians, lawyers and airline pilots) with mental illness to accept outpatient psychiatric services [27], and employment as leverage to secure the adherence of (non-licensed) employees with mental illness to outpatient treatment [28]. (For research mandating children with mental illness to adhere to treatment, see [29].)

In addition to providing data on the epidemiology of various forms of leverage, recent studies [23] also reported that 7% of all outpatients had completed a psychiatric advance directive, but two-thirds of all outpatients stated that they wanted to complete an advance directive, but did not know how to do so. Significantly higher demand for psychiatric advance directives was found amongst outpatients who were female and nonwhite, who had a history of self-harm, arrest and decreased personal autonomy, and who felt pressured by others to take medication [30].

## 3.3   The clinical and societal outcomes associated with mandated community treatment

What are the demonstrable impacts of mandated community treatment on individual patients subject to it, and on their communities? Regarding patients, hypothesized outcomes range from decreased symptoms of mental disorder as a result of improved treatment adherence, to decreased voluntary help-seeking because of patients' fears that treatment will be made involuntary [7]. Regarding the effects of given forms of mandated treatment on the community, one putative outcome of mandated treatment is its effect on reducing violence. Advocates of outpatient commitment have explicitly 'sold' the approach largely by playing on public fears of violence committed by people who have mental disorders [31–33]. As stated by Jaffe (quoted in [7]),

> Laws change for a single reason, in reaction to highly publicized incidents of violence. People care about public safety. I am not saying it is right, I am saying this is the reality. . . So if you're changing your laws in your state, you have to understand that. . . It means that you have to take the debate out of the mental health arena and put it in the criminal justice/public safety arena.

Much research to answer these questions is in progress, but the evidence to date is suggestive rather than conclusive. Whatever the measurable outcomes of mandated community treatment may be, the cost at which these outcomes are obtained is a crucial consideration for policy makers [34]. Initial substantive findings, from one American project, the MacArthur Research Network on Mandated Community Treatment, include the following:

### 3.3.1   Money as leverage

- Patients assigned a representative payee are more likely than other patients to experience 'financial coercion' to participate in outpatient treatment, and also more likely to adhere to outpatient treatment [35].

- Both consumers *and* their representative payees demonstrate deficiencies in the basic arithmetic abilities necessary to create a simple budget, and this often leads to conflict [36].
- Having a family member act as a representative payee doubles the likelihood of the patient engaging in family violence. The more a patient interacts with a family member who is a representative, the more likely the family violence [37].

### 3.3.2   Housing as leverage

- Housing is often used in combination with money as leverage, because it is usually property owners, rather than clinicians, who impose adherence to treatment as a requirement of obtaining housing, and the proprietors require that they be named representative payee in order to ensure that the rent gets paid [9].
- The use of housing as leverage often increases patients' perceived coercion [9].
- Housing programmes that do *not* require treatment as a condition of occupancy (called 'Housing-First' programmes) are becoming increasingly common and achieve a level of patient satisfaction with housing and with treatment comparable to that of programmes that use housing as leverage to obtain treatment adherence [38].

### 3.3.3   Jail as leverage

- Speciality probation agencies that have smaller and exclusively mental health caseloads, and that use problem-solving strategies rather than threats of incarceration, are more effective than traditional probation agencies in reducing the risk of probation violation [39]. New paradigms for reducing recidivism amongst probationers are emerging [40].
- When given a choice, 95% of mental ill defendants in one Florida county chose to have their cases heard in a mental health court rather than in a regular criminal court, and the defendants who chose a mental health court reported much less experience of coercion, and were much more satisfied with the court process, than were mentally ill defendants in the criminal court [41].
- In the 18 months following enrolment in a mental health court or in a usual criminal court, defendants with a mental illness whose cases were processed in the mental health court had fewer arrests and fewer days incarcerated than defendants in the usual court group. Defendants who 'graduated' from the mental health court had lower rearrest rates than defendants who failed to complete the mental health court process [42].

### 3.3.4    Hospitalization as leverage

- African Americans were more likely than whites to be involuntarily committed for outpatient psychiatric care in New York State. However, candidates for outpatient commitment are largely drawn from a population in which African Americans are overrepresented, that is, psychiatric patients with multiple past involuntary hospitalizations in public mental health facilities. Whether this overrepresentation under court-ordered outpatient treatment is racially discriminatory depends on one's view of whether outpatient commitment is best seen as providing increased access to treatment in a setting that is less restrictive than hospitalization, or whether it is best seen as a deprivation of personal liberty [43].
- While patients were under an outpatient commitment order, they experienced a substantial reduction in psychiatric hospitalizations and were more likely to consistently receive psychotropic medications. If the outpatient commitment order was in effect for one year or longer, these benefits continued after the order had expired [44].
- Patients on outpatient commitment felt neither more positive nor more negative about their experience with psychiatric treatment than did voluntary patients. More specifically, there were no significant differences between patients on outpatient commitment and voluntary patients in perceived coercion, the therapist–patient alliance, treatment satisfaction or life satisfaction [16].

### 3.3.5    Psychiatric advance directives

- Approximately half the mental health professionals in one survey agreed that psychiatric advance directives are helpful to patients. Clinicians have more positive attitudes about psychiatric advance directives when they correctly recognize that they are not required by law to honour a directive in which a person refuses appropriate psychiatric or psychological treatment. However, a majority of clinicians have practical concerns about getting access to psychiatric advance directives in a crisis. Other concerns include the problem of inappropriate treatment requests in psychiatric advance directives [45].
- There are important differences amongst patients, family members and clinicians on several aspects of psychiatric advance directives: 44% of patients (compared to only 14% of family members) believe that patients should be able to change an advance directive 'even when they are ill'. Three-quarters of patients believe that a psychiatric advance directive will help them avoid unwanted treatment, but only one-quarter of clinicians agree [46].
- Patients can complete a psychiatric advance directive with a one-hour facilitation session, but otherwise do not complete them: 79% of the patients randomly assigned

to have someone help them complete a psychiatric advance directives actually completed one, compared to only 6% of the subjects in the control group who had to complete the directive on their own [47]. The completion of a psychiatric advance directive is associated with significant reduction in the use of coercive interventions such as police transport, involuntary commitment, seclusion and restraints, and involuntary medications during mental health crises [48].

## 3.4  Controversial issues

Few issues in contemporary mental health policy are as contested as mandated community treatment. One argument often raised in opposition to the use of leverage to secure treatment adherence in the community posits that a person's freedom to 'choose' to enter a leveraged agreement to accept treatment is specious, given stark power imbalances between the individual on whom leverage is imposed and the social agency doing the imposition, and that mandated community treatment is therefore properly seen as coercive. A second and related argument often raised in international debates on mandated community treatment is that the findings of the existing research – even if those findings are empirically valid in the legal and social culture in which they were generated – may not be generalizable to other legal and social cultures.

Bonnie and Monahan [49], in response to the first of these two arguments, propose that framing the debate primarily in the vocabulary of 'coercion' has become counterproductive and that reframing it in the language of 'contract' may allow for new insights and invigorated discussion. They base their position on the work of Wertheimer [50], who has stated that the ability to obligate oneself by creating a binding contract is an important aspect of freedom. 'Voluntariness – and, in particular, the absence of coercion', according to Wertheimer, is 'a necessary condition of obligations grounded in agreement'. How is one to determine which contractual decisions are voluntary and which are the product of coercion? Wertheimer formulates the underlying issue as follows:

> The standard view of coercive proposals is that threats coerce but offers do not. And the crux of the distinction between threats and offers is that A makes a *threat* when B will be *worse off* than in some relevant baseline position if B does not accept A's proposal, but that A makes an *offer* when B will be *no worse off* than in some relevant baseline position if B does not accept A's proposal. On this view... the key to understanding what counts as a coercive proposal is to properly fix B's *baseline* [50].

Building on Wertheimer, Bonnie and Monahan [49] make distinctions amongst different types of leverage. They argue, for example, that that using jail as leverage for people who have pled or been found to be guilty of a crime is not properly seen as coercive at all. This is so because in treatment as a condition of probation (or in a mental health court) the legal baseline is going to jail to serve the sentence for the crime of which the person was convicted. In using jail as leverage, they argue:

> The key question. . . is whether the prosecutor's proposal is best construed as a "threat" to put the defendant in jail if he or she fails to adhere to treatment in the community, or as an "offer" of treatment in lieu of jail. According to Wertheimer, the prosecutor's proposal would be a "threat" if the defendant would be worse off than in his or her baseline position if the defendant does not accept the proposal, whereas it would be an "offer" (expanding choice) if the defendant would be no worse off than in his or her baseline position if the proposal is not accepted. [If] incarceration were an available sentencing option, as it is in the usual case, probation conditioned on medication compliance is properly regarded as an "offer," and the agreement is valid. [49]

On the other hand, using hospitalization as leverage in (preventive) outpatient commitment is 'unambiguously coercive'. Preventive outpatient commitment involves no choice at all. In preventive outpatient commitment, the person does *not* currently meet the statutory criteria for inpatient hospitalization, but rather is predicted to meet those criteria in the future if untreated in the community. In the use of jail as leverage, the individual's options are being *expanded* – from one option (jail) to two options (jail or treatment in the community). In preventive outpatient commitment, however, the individual's options are being *constrained*: before, the individual had two options (adhere to treatment or do not adhere to treatment in the community); now, the individual has only one option (adhere to treatment in the community). The individual is not being 'offered' anything in consideration for adhering to treatment in the community. In preventive outpatient commitment, therefore, the contract model does not apply.

A person's 'baseline' condition, however – from which one determines whether accepting outpatient treatment is in response to a coercive 'threat' or to a non-coercive 'offer' – is difficult to establish without taking into account cultural factors. This leads to the second controversy: are findings on mandated community treatment generated in one cultural context generalizable to other cultural contexts?

For example, one large and representative survey of attitudes toward outpatient commitment found the American public to be evenly split in their views – with 49.1% agreeing that people with schizophrenia 'should be forced by law to. . . get treatment at a clinic or from a doctor' and 50.9% disagreeing with this statement [51]. The researchers found that respondents' support of or opposition to outpatient commitment bore no significant relationship to self-rated political liberalism–conservatism.

Kahan *et al.* [52], in a large Web-based survey of American adults, tried to go beyond left–right political ideology to explain public views of mandated community treatment in cultural terms. Using Douglas' theory of 'cultural cognition'[53], they found that outpatient commitment was supported by people who are *hierarchical* and *communitarian* – that is, people who value authority, who trust experts, and who believe that securing conditions of societal wellbeing is a societal duty that takes priority over individual interests. People who are *egalitarian* and *individualistic* – that is, people who resent stratification, who distrust authority, and who place the prerogatives of individuals ahead of those of the collective – were more likely to oppose outpatient commitment. Because on many issues egalitarian and communitarian orientations converge on liberal policy stances, and hierarchical and individualistic orientations on conservative ones, they believe that it is not surprising that public opinion on outpatient commitment bears little relationship to conventional liberal and conservative ideological categories (see also [54]).

If such results can be found within one (American) culture, what are the prospects for generalizing research finding across cultures? In many cultures, the (competent) individual is taken to be the autonomous decision maker. In other cultures, the family plays a much stronger role in decision-making [55]. In some legal systems, housing or disability benefits are a matter of 'right' and cannot be used as leverage to promote treatment adherence. In other legal systems, housing or disability benefits are discretionary programmes that the government can provide or withhold, subject only to the political process [56]. Differences in the provision of mental health care itself – whether such care is publically available as part of a national health service, or is available if, and only if, one has private insurance – can make an enormous difference in the frequency and the manner in which outpatient treatment can be 'mandated' [34].

## 3.5  Conclusion

Unwanted institutional treatment for mental disorder remains a crucially important clinical, legal, moral and fiscal issue throughout the world. Early in the twenty-first century, however, unwanted treatment in the community is replacing unwanted institutional treatment as a growing object of controversy. Unwanted community treatment may take many forms, with negative events, such as incarceration or hospitalization being avoided, or positive events, such as placement in subsidized housing or the receipt of disability benefits, being obtained, contingent on whether a person adheres to outpatient treatment. A majority of patients in public-sector outpatient mental health treatment in the United States have experienced the application of at least one – and often more than one – of these forms of 'leverage'. Research on the outcomes associated with mandated community treatment is in its infancy, but there are suggestions that, if properly implemented, it may have value in increasing treatment adherence. Different forms of mandated community treatment may raise different legal and moral issues, and these issues are likely to vary greatly in different political and cultural contexts. One necessary but not sufficient prerequisite to the success of any form of mandated community treatment in any country is the ready availability of evidence-based mental health services. What the government of Scotland concluded when it recently initiated community treatment orders is true more broadly:

> Where society imposes an obligation on an individual to comply with a programme of treatment or care, a parallel obligation is imposed on health and social care services to provide safe and appropriate services and ongoing care. [57]

# References

1. Kahan, D., Braman, D., Monahan, J. *et al.* (2010) Cultural cognition and public policy: the case of outpatient commitment laws. *Law and Human Behavior*, **34**, 118–140.
2. Monahan, J. (2008) Mandated community treatment: applying leverage to achieve adherence. *Journal of the American Academy of Psychiatry and the Law*, **36**, 282–285.
3. Goffman, I. (1961) *Asylums: Essays on the Social Situation of Mental Patients and Other Inmates*, Doubleday, New York.
4. Monahan, J., Swartz, M. and Bonnie, R. (2003) Mandated treatment in the community for people with mental disorders. *Health Affairs*, **22**, 28–38.
5. Elbogen, E., Ferron, J., Swartz, M. *et al.* (2007) Characteristics of representative payeeship involving family of beneficiaries with psychiatric disabilities. *Psychiatric Services*, **58**, 1433–1440.
6. Appelbaum, P. and Redlich, A. (2006) Use of leverage over patients' money to promote adherence of psychiatric treatment. *Journal of Nervous and Mental Disease*, **194**, 294–302.
7. Monahan, J., Bonnie, R., Appelbaum, P. *et al.* (2001) Mandated community treatment: beyond outpatient commitment. *Psychiatric Services*, **52**, 1198–1205.
8. O'Hara, A., Cooper, E., Korman, H. *et al.* (2009) *Priced Out in 2008: The Housing Crisis for People with Disabilities*, Technical Assistance Collaborative, Boston.
9. Robbins, P., Petrila, J., LeMelle, S. *et al.* (2006) The use of housing as leverage to increase adherence to psychiatric treatment in the community. *Administration and Policy in Mental Health and Mental Health Services Research*, **33**, 226–236.
10. Skeem, J. and Eno-Louden, J. (2006) Toward evidence-based practice for probationers and parolees mandated to mental health treatment. *Psychiatric Services*, **57**, 333–342.
11. Steadman, H., Redlich, A., Griffin, P. *et al.* (2006) From referral to disposition: case processing in seven mental health courts. *Behavioral Sciences and Law*, **23**, 215–226.
12. Swartz, M., Swanson, J., Hiday, V. *et al.* (2001) Randomized controlled trial of outpatient commitment in North Carolina. *Psychiatric Services*, **52**, 325–329.
13. Steadman, H., Gounis, K., Dennis, D. *et al.* (2001) Assessing the New York City involuntary outpatient commitment pilot program. *Psychiatric Services*, **52**, 330–336.
14. Burns, T., Rugkasa, J. and Molodynski, A. (2008) The Oxford community treatment order evaluation trial (OCTET). *Psychiatric Bulletin*, **32**, 400.
15. Churchill, R., Owen, G., Singh, S. *et al.* (2007) *International Experiences of Using Community Treatment Orders*, UK Department of Health, London.
16. Swartz, M., Swanson, J., Steadman, H. *et al.* (2009) *New York State Assisted Outpatient Treatment Program Evaluation*, Duke University School of Medicine, Durham, NC.

17. Bazelon Center (2000) Position Statement on Involuntary Commitment. Available at http:// bazelon.org.gravitatehosting.com/Where-We-Stand/Self-Determination/Forced-Treatment/ Outpatient-and-Civil-Commitment/Resources.aspx (accessed 19 November 2010).
18. Bazelon Center (2001) Studies of Outpatient Commitment are Misused. Available at http:// bazelon.org.gravitatehosting.com/Where-We-Stand/Self-Determination/Forced-Treatment/ Outpatient-and-Civil-Commitment/Resources.aspx (accessed 19 November 2010).
19. Treatment Advocacy Center (2010) Briefing Paper: Assisted Outpatient Treatment (AOT). Available at http://www.treatmentadvocacycenter.org/storage/tac/documents/assisted_outpa- tient_treatment__aot_--2010.pdf (accessed 19 November 2010).
20. Treatment Advocacy Center (2008) A Benefit of Outpatient Commitment Often Overlooked – Preventing Victimization. Available at http://www.treatmentadvocacycenter.org/index.php? option=com_content&task=view&id=493&Itemid=97 (accessed 19 November 2010).
21. Swanson, J., Swartz, M., Hannon, M. *et al.* (2003) Psychiatric advance directives: a survey of persons with schizophrenia, family members, and treatment providers. *International Journal of Forensic Mental Health*, **2**, 73–86.
22. Gallagher, E. (1998) Advance directives for psychiatric care: a theoretical and practical overview for legal professionals. *Psychology, Public Policy, and Law*, **4**, 746–787.
23. Monahan, J., Redlich, A., Swanson, J. *et al.* (2005) Use of leverage to improve adherence to psychiatric treatment in the community. *Psychiatric Services*, **56**, 37–44.
24. Redlich, A. and Monahan, J. (2006) General pressures to adhere to psychiatric treatment in the community. *International Journal of Forensic Mental Health*, **5**, 126–131.
25. Busch, A. and Redlich, A. (2007) Patients' perception of possible child custody or visitation loss if not adherent to psychiatric treatment. *Psychiatric Services*, **58**, 999–1002.
26. Gallagher, R.P. (2008) *National Survey of Counseling Center Directors*, International Association of Counseling Services, Inc., Alexandria, VA. Available at http://iacsinc.org (accessed 19 November 2010).
27. Monahan, J. and Bonnie, R. (2004) License as leverage: mandating treatment for profes- sionals. *International Journal of Forensic Mental Health*, **3**, 131–138.
28. Weisner, C., Lu, Y., Hinman, A. *et al.* (2009) Substance use, symptom, and employment outcomes of persons with a workplace mandate for chemical dependency treatment. *Psychi- atric Services*, **60**, 646–654.
29. Pescosolido, B., Fettes, D., Martin, J. *et al.* (2007) Perceived dangerousness and support for coerced treatment for children with mental health problems. *Psychiatric Services*, **58**, 619–625.
30. Swanson, J., Swartz, M., Ferron, J. *et al.* (2006) Psychiatric advance directives among public mental health consumers in five U.S. cities: prevalence, demand, and correlates. *Journal of the American Academy of Psychiatry and Law*, **34**, 43–57.
31. Swanson, J., Borum, R., Swartz, M. *et al.* (2001) Can involuntary outpatient commitment reduce arrests among persons with severe mental illness? *Criminal Justice and Behavior*, **28**, 156–189.
32. Swanson, J., Van Dorn, R., Monahan, J. *et al.* (2006) Violence and leveraged community treatment for persons with mental disorder. *American Journal of Psychiatry*, **163**, 1404–1411.
33. Swartz, M. (2007) Can mandated outpatient treatment prevent tragedies? *Psychiatric Services*, **58**, 737.
34. Sinaiko, A. and McGuire, T. (2006) Patient inducement, provider priorities and resource allocation in public mental health systems. *Journal of Health Politics, Policy and Law*, **31**, 1075–1106.

35. Elbogen, E., Swanson, J. and Swartz, M. (2003) Effects of legal mechanisms on perceived coercion and treatment adherence in persons with severe mental illness. *Journal of Nervous and Mental Disease*, **191**, 629–637.

36. Elbogen, E., Ferron, J. and Swartz, M. (2007) Characteristics of representative payeeship involving family of beneficiaries with psychiatric disabilities. *Psychiatric Services*, **58**, 1433–1440.

37. Elbogen, E., Swanson, J. and Swartz, M. (2005) Family representative payeeship and violence risk in severe mental illness. *Law and Human Behavior*, **29**, 563–574.

38. Robbins, P., Callahan, L. and Monahan, J. (2009) Perceived coercion to treatment and housing satisfaction within two housing program models. *Psychiatric Services*, **60**, 1251–1253.

39. Skeem, J., Eno Louden, J., Polasheck, D. *et al.* (2007) Relationship quality in mandated treatment: blending care with control. *Psychological Assessment*, **19**, 397–410.

40. Skeem, J., Manchak, S. and Peterson, J. (2010) Correctional policy for offenders with mental illness: creating a new paradigm for recidivism reduction. *Law and Human Behavior*. doi: 10.1007/s10979-010-9223-7.

41. Christy, A., Poythress, N., Boothroyd, R. *et al.* (2005) Evaluating the efficiency and community safety goals of the Broward County Mental Health Court. *Behavioral Sciences and the Law*, **23**, 227–243.

42. Steadman, H., Redlich, A., Callahan, L. *et al.* (2010) Effect of mental health courts on arrests and jail days: a multisite study. *Archives of General Psychiatry*. doi: 10.1001/archgenpsychiatry.2010.134.

43. Swanson, J., Swartz, M., Van Dorn, R. *et al.* (2009) Racial disparities in involuntary outpatient commitment: are they real? *Health Affairs*, **28**, 816–826.

44. Swartz, M., Wilder, C., Swanson, J. *et al.* (2010) Assessing outcomes for consumers in New York's Assisted Outpatient Treatment Program. *Psychiatric Services*, **61**, 976–981.

45. Swanson, J., Swartz, M., Hannon, M. *et al.* (2003) Psychiatric advance directives: a survey of persons with schizophrenia, family members, and treatment providers. *International Journal of Forensic Mental Health*, **2**, 73–86.

46. Swartz, M., Swanson, J., Van Dorn, R. *et al.* (2006) Patient preferences for psychiatric advance directives. *International Journal of Forensic Mental Health*, **5**, 67–81.

47. Swanson, J., Swartz, J., Elbogen, E. *et al.* (2006) Facilitated psychiatric advance directives: a randomized trial of an intervention to foster advance treatment planning among persons with severe mental illness. *American Journal of Psychiatry*, **163**, 1943–1951.

48. Swanson, J., Swartz, M., Elbogen, E. *et al.* (2008) Psychiatric advance directives and reduction of coercive crisis interventions. *Journal of Mental Health*, **17**, 255–267.

49. Bonnie, R. and Monahan, J. (2005) From coercion to contract: reframing the debate on mandated community treatment for people with mental disorders. *Law and Human Behavior*, **29**, 487–505.

50. Wertheimer, A. (1987) *Coercion*, Princeton University Press, Princeton, NJ.

51. Pescosolido, B., Monahan, J., Link, B. *et al.* (1999) The public's view of the competence, dangerousness and need for legal coercion among persons with mental health problems. *American Journal of Public Health*, **89**, 1339–1345.

52. Kahan, D., Braman, D., Monahan, J. *et al.* (2010) Cultural cognition and public policy: the case of outpatient commitment laws. *Law and Human Behavior*, **34**, 118–140.

53. Douglas, M. (1970) *Natural Symbols: Explorations in Cosmology*, Barrie and Rockliff, London.

54. Swanson, J. (2010) What would Mary Douglas do? A commentary on Kahan *et al.*, "Cultural Cognition and Public Policy: The Case of Outpatient Commitment Laws." *Law and Human Behavior*, **34**, 176–185.

55. Gibbs, A., Dawson, J., Forsyth, H. *et al.* (2004) Maori experience of community treatment orders in Otago, New Zealand. *Australian and New Zealand Journal of Psychiatry*, **38**, 830–835.
56. Housing Rights, Inc. (2009) Universal Right to Housing. http://housingrights.org/yourrights/universalrighttohousing.htm. Housing Rights, Inc., Berkeley, CA (accessed 19 November 2010).
57. Ridley, J., Rosengard, A. and Hunter, S. *et al.* (2009) *Experiences of the Early Implementation of the Mental Health (Care and Treatment) (Scotland) Act, 2003: A Cohort Study*. Queens Printers of Scotland, Edinburgh. Available at http://www.scotland.gov.uk/Publications/2009/05/06155847/0 (accessed 19 November 2010).

# 4 Is it possible to define a best practice standard for coercive treatment in psychiatry?

## Tilman Steinert[1] and Peter Lepping[2]

*[1]Ulm University, Centre for Psychiatry Suedwuerttemberg, Ravensburg-Weissenau, Germany*
*[2]Betsi Cadwaladr University Health Board and Glyndŵr University, Wrexham Academic Unit, Wales, UK*

## 4.1  Introduction

All citizens of Europe who fall within the legislation of the European Convention on Human Rights have a right to be free from detention without judicial process (Article 5) and the right not to be tortured (Article 3; full details of convention available from http://conventions.coe.int). Coercive measures in psychiatric patients have therefore been high on the European agenda for quite some time. The other aspect is the notion of non-maleficence (do no harm), beneficence (do good),

*Coercive Treatment in Psychiatry: Clinical, Legal and Ethical Aspects*, First Edition.
Edited by Thomas W. Kallert, Juan E. Mezzich and John Monahan.
© 2011 John Wiley & Sons, Ltd. Published 2011 by John Wiley & Sons, Ltd.

autonomy and justice [1], which take into account the wider societal context of coercion in that they allow the consideration of other factors than the patient (staff, resources, societal priorities etc.). Ethically, treatment is only acceptable if a competent patient agrees to it, but what happens when the patient lacks capacity to agree? In that case the treating team (psychiatrists, nurses, social workers etc.) needs to come to a decision as to what is in the patient's best interest. This may be a coercive measure to reduce risk to the patient or others at that point in time. Obviously, any such measure has to be proportionate and as short as possible, as well as being designed to minimize the potential loss of dignity that the patient may experience. Therefore psychiatrists, other professionals, patients and their relatives would appreciate the abolition of coercive measures such as chemical, mechanical and physical restraint and seclusion more than a suggestion of best practice standards for these kinds of interventions. However, experts from many countries seem to agree that it is still not possible at this point in time to practice safe and just psychiatry completely without the use of coercive measures. This is particularly the case in the treatment of very agitated, aggressive or violent psychiatric inpatients. Thus it seems an acceptable approach to define at least quality standards for such interventions, which should be looked upon as means of providing safety and proportionality rather than something that has intrinsic therapeutic value. Within the last decade, research on the use of coercive measures of psychiatric inpatients in different countries has increased, and the research findings show that

- the kind of preferred intervention varies highly between different countries and even within countries; for example, physical restraint being nearly exclusively used in the UK, seclusion being preferred in the Netherlands and Switzerland, mechanical restraint in Germany, Italy or Norway, and net beds in some parts of Austria, the Czech Republic and Slovakia [2,3];
- the legal bases vary between countries [2];
- the duration of such measures varies hugely between countries [3];
- no broadly accepted ethical framework for the application of coercive measures has so far been accepted [4];
- evidence from randomized controlled studies is not available so far, though such studies are feasible [5];
- patients are becoming increasingly involved in the development of guidelines and recommendations [6,7].

According to their purpose, some national guidelines contain suggestions for best clinical practice for the process and practical application of coercive measures. The objective of this article is to critically examine how such standards can be achieved and whether they are of generalizable value. So far, as we can see, three approaches have been favoured: virtue ethics, evidence and consensus.

## 4.2   Virtue ethics

Virtue ethics may seem somewhat old-fashioned nowadays in its purest form, when ethics of care [8] or narratives [9] may be considered more appropriate to bring forward change. However, certainly this way of thinking about ethical problems with regard to coercion has historically been the most influential one in the history of psychiatry. The virtue theory, going back to Aristotle, suggests that a person has acquired so much wisdom and education linked with virtue in his or her character that he or she is able to find the best solutions for difficult ethical situations [4]. In many parts of the world this is still assumed of doctors or other experts whose advice will be followed on that basis. Virtue ethics was the basis on which Pinel and Esquirol in France, Chiarugi in Italy or somewhat later Conolly in England argued to literally remove the chains from mentally ill people in asylums. It has mostly been the ideals of such individually enlightened people which brought psychiatric treatment and mental health care forward to more humane conditions within the last two centuries. Even the requirements for involuntary treatment provided by the Steering Committee of Bioethics of the Council of Europe [10] and by the Committee for the Prevention of Torture and Inhumane or Degrading Treatment or Punishment (http://www.cpt .coe.int/en/) have been developed based on individual ideas of ideal practice, in combination with group consensus.

However, the definition of best practice standards by single wise experts is a rather paternalistic approach, is completely dependent on mostly unknown variables, and does not offer a clear idea of how to deal with conflicting values such as patient's autonomy and staff safety. Thus wise experts could come to quite different proposals, dependent on their personal experiences, their culture, religion, attitudes and so on. Furthermore, there is good reason to doubt whether the view of single experts can adequately reflect the different perspectives of all the actors in the field – doctors and other staff, patients, relatives, public authorities, courts, public opinion and so on. Thus the approach of virtue ethics can no longer be considered as sufficiently satisfying.

## 4.3   Evidence

Best practice standards are usually phrased in clinical guidelines, the number and quality of which has continuously been increasing over the past 20 years. The development of clinical guidelines is strongly linked to evidence-based medicine. Evidence has become the gold standard in reply to all medical questions. Basically, evidence-based medicine systematically uses available evidence from studies. In the development of clinical guidelines, the highest level of evidence is attributed to systematic meta-analyses from randomized controlled studies, whilst the lowest level is awarded to expert opinion, thus standing in stark contrast to virtue ethics where such opinion would have been ranked highest. It has been claimed that there is an urgent need to conduct randomized controlled trials (RCTs) on the use of coercive measures in psychiatry to improve the current level of evidence available to make suggestions on the use of coercion, as 'there is a surprising and shocking lack of published trials assessing the effects of secluding and restraining people with schizophrenia or similar psychotic illnesses' [11].

It has been shown that such studies are feasible and can evaluate comprehensive assessments by patients as primary outcome [5]. Such studies could provide some substantial evidence in the attempt to define the 'least restrictive alternative' [12] in any given cultural context; and probably it is not the same for all patients. However, we doubt whether this kind of approach is sufficient in order to produce definitive answers to the question of best practice standards. There are various reasons for this. What separates coercion from most other medical questions is that the objective of a coercive measure is not primarily therapy but safety, despite the fact that coercion is sometimes used to give therapeutic medication. The proposal to apply the approach of RCTs to issues of safety reminds us of the proposal to examine the use of parachutes in an RCT [13]. The authors ask ironically whether the supporters of evidence-based medicine would consider to be the control group [13]. In other words, some things are so obvious, they do not need to be further researched; yet others cannot be examined in RCTs because the alternative is too dangerous. Coercion to prevent danger to others is a typical example. Nobody would want to conduct a study examining the question of whether mentally ill sex offenders should be committed to a forensic psychiatric department or remain free. Evidence-based medicine has a rather narrow focus: patients, outcome and side effects. However, the ethical framework for many questions in psychiatry is much wider: effects are to be examined with respect not only to outcome and side effects, but also to issues such as autonomy, proportionality, fairness and law, and they do not refer only to patients but also to staff, relatives, other persons such as fellow patients and the society as a whole. Thus, only a minority of questions related to coercive measures can be addressed in RCTs. They lack the ability to look at outcome measures within wider society, and struggle to measure how they effect a person's subjective experience of potentially being restricted in their human rights, although this has been tried [14]. Further, the external validity and generalizability of RCTs frequently remains unclear. How far can we extrapolate certain results to a wider population? This is a never-ending discussion with RCTs because of their high rate of dropouts and exclusions. For example, a survey amongst British users of psychiatric inpatient services found that, amongst coercive measures which had been presented to them by pictures, physical restraint was considered to be the least restrictive and mechanical restraint and the use of net beds as being the most restrictive – in fact they were strongly rejected [15]. But can this be considered as an objective outcome regarding the question of which intervention is the least restrictive? Probably not, since in other countries the results could have been different, as British patients are not used to mechanical restraints and net beds. Only patients who would have been subjected to all three types of measures, delivered at a high standard, would have been able to comment on their preference fairly. And possibly, they would have still preferred the coercive measure they are acquainted with. The use of coercion in a particular way creates traditions amongst staff and expectations amongst patients that are not easy to change, even when everybody may subscribe to the general aim of a reduction of whatever coercive measure is used.

Another big problem is the notion that an absence of evidence does not prove an absence of efficacy. In other words, the fact that we have no trial results should not be seen as evidence that something does not work. The British National Institute for Health and Clinical Excellence (NICE) guidelines try to give guidance and technical appraisals on various illnesses, medications and procedures based entirely on the available evidence and, to a lesser degree, an analysis of cost effectiveness. This approach has had many positive effects as it allows providers of health care to argue for resources for approved medications and procedures. It also helps to standardize treatment at a high level (however, it also runs the risk of stifling innovations as doctors may not want to be seen to practise outside the approved norm). The guidelines for the treatment of aggression, and with it coercive measures, include many trials of recently developed drugs, but neglect older drugs and combinations that have been used successfully in day-to-day practice across Europe for decades. This is because of a lack of data about these treatments, which is primarily a consequence of the trial funding process. Whilst a lot of resource is available from the pharmaceutical industry to prove that their new drug works, little is available to examine whether cheap and traditionally used alternatives are effective as well. This creates an *evidence bias* towards newer treatments. Furthermore, evidence develops. The changes in the NICE schizophrenia guidelines exemplify this nicely, as they were changed to take into account newer evidence suggesting that some older (first generation) antipsychotics are equally good in many regards, and significantly cheaper [16].

Summarizing these aspects, evidence yields an important contribution to the definition of best practice standards. It is necessary, but not sufficient, due to biases and fundamental restrictions of the methods applied.

## 4.4  Consensus

One of the authors (T. Steinert) was responsible for the development of the German guideline for the treatment of aggressive behaviour [7]. The guideline development group applied the system of different levels of evidence which leads to different levels of recommendations, similarly to the method used in the NICE guideline from

2005 [6]. However, after having finished the guideline in this way, some doubts were raised about whether this method is really appropriate. A strong bias resulting from this method is that a high quality of studies nearly automatically leads to high levels of recommendations, mostly independent from study results. As a matter of fact, it happens rather frequently that more than one meta-analysis is available and they provide different results, such as in the case of second-generation neuroleptics [17–19], or effect sizes are only small (e.g. in the case of antidepressants), or results from several RCTs are inconsistent. On the other hand, the guideline development group felt that some of the achieved consensus on the procedure for coercive measures was very valuable and, in the opinion of the group, this consensus was undervalued with the lowest level of evidence (expert consensus) and, as a result, a low level of recommendation. In contrast, those interventions with the highest levels of recommendation – pharmacotherapy, due to available randomized controlled studies – could not achieve consensus with patients. Other than in evidence-based medicine, their value system is not primarily focused on outcome but on aspects such as autonomy, dignity and fairness.

A possible solution is to revalue consensus in relation to evidence. Such a procedure has recently been suggested in the GRADE workgroup's grid [20]. It is noticeable that the most recent published guidelines such as the NICE updated guideline on schizophrenia [16] and, to a lesser extent, the German guideline on unipolar depression [21] move in this direction by providing evidence summaries without division in levels of evidence and recommendations found by consensus. In a similar way the EUNOMIA study group, an EU-funded project, established recommendations by consensus for coercive procedures, based on the practice in different European countries [22]. However, even this method has some drawbacks: transparency in the step from the evidence to the recommendations is low, and results are probably strongly dependent on the composition of the group and the applied method for the consensus process. How can we ensure that members really represent the views of their respective group? This applies not only to patients and relatives but also to psychiatrists and other professionals. Which relative weight should each group have? Is an expert dominance justified? How is final consensus achieved? The latter can be achieved by majority voting or by methods such as the so-called Delphi method or a nominal group process, all of which strive for but do not guarantee a consensus between all members. Thus consensus is sometimes a question of policy rather than of evidence.

## 4.5 Conclusion

Suggestions for best practice standards of coercive measures will probably never contain objective answers but are always dependent on locations, traditions, historical contexts, attitudes and influences of stakeholder groups. All of the three approaches, wisdom and virtue, evidence and consensus, have some drawbacks. That does not mean, however, that we should abandon the suggestion of best practice standards for coercive treatment. They should comprise recommendations for involuntary admission, involuntary treatment and the use of freedom-restrictive measures such as seclusion, mechanical, chemical and physical restraint. Moreover, they should describe processes and possibilities of participation of the subjected persons, and mechanisms of external control and transparency. And, not least, such recommendations should be examined and revised regularly. Depending on the specific issues and cultural contexts in hand, a carefully balanced combination of all of the three approaches described above can currently be considered as appropriate.

# References

1. Beauchamp, T. and Childress, J. (2001) *Principles of Biomedical Ethics*, 5th edn, Oxford University Press, New York.
2. Steinert, T. and Lepping, P. (2009) Legal provisions and practice in the management of violent patients. A case vignette study in 16 European countries. *European Psychiatry*, **24**, 135–141.
3. Steinert, T., Lepping, P., Bernhardsgrütter, R. *et al.* (2010) Incidence of seclusion and restraint in psychiatric hospitals: a literature review and survey of international trends. *Social Psychiatry and Psychiatric Epidemiology*, **45**, 889–897.
4. Bloch, S. and Green, S.A. (2006) An ethical framework for psychiatry. *British Journal of Psychiatry*, **188**, 7–12.
5. Bergk, J., Einsiedler, B. and Steinert, T. (2008) Feasibility of randomized controlled trials on seclusion and mechanical restraint. *Clinical Trials*, **5**, 356–363.
6. National Institute for Clinical Excellence (NICE) (2005) *Violence – The Short-Term Management of Disturbed/Violent Behaviour in Psychiatric In-patient Settings and Emergency Departments*, NICE Clinical Guideline 25, Royal College of Nursing, London. Available at http://guidance.nice.org.uk/CG25/NICEGuidance/pdf/English (accessed 22 November 2010).
7. German Association for Psychiatry and Psychotherapy (DGPPN) (2009) *Therapeutische Maßnahmen bei aggressivem Verhalten in der Psychiatrie und Psychotherapie (S2 Praxisleitlinien in Psychiatrie und Psychotherapie)*, Steinkopff, Darmstadt.
8. Held, V. (2006) *Ethics of Care*, Oxford University Press, Oxford.
9. Carson, A.M. and Lepping, P. (2009) Ethical psychiatry in an uncertain world: conversations and parallel truths. *Philosophy, Ethics, and Humanities in Medicine*, **4**, 7. http://www.peh-med.com/content/4/1/7.
10. Council of Europe Steering Committee on Bioethics (CEBP) Working Party on Psychiatry (2000) "White Paper" on the Protection of the Human Rights and Dignity of People Suffering from Mental Disorder, Especially those Placed as Involuntary Patients in Psychiatric Establishment. DI R/JUR (2000) 2. Council of Europe, Strasbourg. http://www.coe.int/t/dg3/healthbioethic/Activities/08_Psychiatry_and_human_rights_en/DIR-JUR(2000)2WhitePaper.pdf (accessed 22 November 2010).
11. Sailas, E. and Fenton, M. (2000) Seclusion and restraint for people with serious mental illnesses. *Cochrane Database of Systematic Reviews*, 1 (Art. No.: CD001163). doi: 10.1002/14651858.CD001163.

12. Curie, C.G. (2005) SAMHSA's commitment to eliminating the use of seclusion and restraint. *Psychiatric Services*, **56**, 1139–1140.
13. Smith, G.C. and Pell, J.P. (2003) Parachute use to prevent death and major trauma related to gravitational challenge: systematic review of randomised controlled trials. *British Medical Journal*, **327**, 1459–1461.
14. Bergk, J., Flammer, E. and Steinert, T. (2010) Coercion Experience Scale (CES) – validation of a questionnaire on coercive measures. *BMC Psychiatry*, **10**, 5.
15. Whittington, R., Bowers, L., Nolan, P. *et al.* (2009) Approval ratings of inpatient coercive interventions in a national sample of mental health service users and staff in England. *Psychiatric Services*, **60**, 792–798.
16. National Collaborating Centre for Mental Health, commissioned by NICE (2009) *Schizophrenia. Core Interventions in the Treatment and Management of Schizophrenia in Adults in Primary and Secondary Sare. Updated Edition*. National Clinical Guideline Number 82. The British Psychological Society, Leicester and The Royal College of Psychiatrists, London. www.nice.org.uk/nicemedia/pdf/CG82FullGuideline.pdf (accessed 22 November 2010).
17. Geddes, J., Freemantle, N., Harrison, P. *et al.* (2000) Atypical antipsychotics in the treatment of schizophrenia: systematic overview and meta-regression analysis. *British Medical Journal*, **321**, 1371–1376.
18. Davis, J.M., Chen, N. and Glick, I.D. (2003) A meta-analysis of the efficacy of second-generation antipsychotics. *Archives of General Psychiatry*, **60**, 553–564.
19. Leucht, S., Corves, C., Arbter, D. *et al.* (2009) Second-generation versus first-generation antipsychotic drugs for schizophrenia: a meta-analysis. *Lancet*, **3**, 31–41.
20. Jaeschke, R., Guyatt, G.H., Dellinger, P. *et al.* (2008) Use of GRADE grid to reach decisions on clinical practice guidelines when consensus is elusive. *British Medical Journal*, **337**, a744.
21. Deutsche Gesellschaft für Psychiatrie, Psychotherapie und Nervenheilkunde (2009) *Nationale Versorgungsleitlinie unipolare Depression*. German Agency for Quality in Medicine, Berlin. Available at http://www.depression.versorgungsleitlinien.de/ (accessed 22 November 2010).
22. Kallert, T.W., Jurjanz, L., Schnall, K. *et al.* (2007) Practice recommendation for administering mechanical restraint during acute psychiatric hospitalization. *Psychiatrische Praxis*, **34** (Supplement 2), 233–240.

# 5 How to de-escalate a risk situation to avoid the use of coercion

## Dirk Richter

*Bern University of Applied Sciences, School of Health Sciences, Berne, Switzerland*

## 5.1 Introduction

It is well known that the use of coercion in psychiatry and other health care fields is very often the consequence of aggressive encounters between staff and patients, which in turn is the result of escalating situations. Data from several different countries have shown that up to 50% of aggressive incidents between patients and staff are followed by some kind of coercive intervention (physical or mechanical restraint, seclusion or forced medication) [1,2]. Depending upon the specific site and psychiatric sub-discipline (forensic psychiatry, acute psychiatry, geropsychiatry, child and adolescent psychiatry etc.), one can assume that up to two-thirds of all physically violent incidents in mental health care are preceded by an escalating interaction by at least two parties [2,3]. These figures justify the assumption that nonphysical interventions may reduce the number of aggressive incidents, which may then result in a lowered number of coercive measures.

*Coercive Treatment in Psychiatry: Clinical, Legal and Ethical Aspects*, First Edition.
Edited by Thomas W. Kallert, Juan E. Mezzich and John Monahan.
© 2011 John Wiley & Sons, Ltd. Published 2011 by John Wiley & Sons, Ltd.

Until recently however, the reaction of many mental health care workers towards aggressive patients resulted mainly in physical coercion. Over many decades, as the author is aware of from first-hand experience while working as a psychiatric nurse, the use of coercive measures was sometimes due to a 'tradition of toughness' [4]. This was quite prevalent in Western psychiatry, and still is in many parts of the world. At other times, physical coercion occurred due to mental health workers who were unskilled in nonphysical conflict-solving methods. However, the use of coercion was seldom questioned, and it frequently occurred that patient–staff conflicts were intentionally triggered by staff. Another 'conflict-solving method' was to just sit and wait while watching a patient attack a fellow patient (with the injection already prepared).

Luckily, the attitudes described above are today held by only a very small minority of mental health care workers, if not having entirely disappeared. After a considerable time lag that followed the psychiatric reforms in the Western world, discussions on violence spread through nearly all psychiatric hospitals and related institutions. This issue was brought to the attention of German and Swiss mental health care professionals during the 1990s, similarly to their counterparts in many other European countries. Surprisingly or not, the discussion itself was not so much triggered by notions of care for the patients being submitted to the coercive practices, but rather more by concerns regarding the physical and psychological health of staff. As many readers are aware, the notion of dangerousness in psychiatry had changed from dangerous and violent mental health care practice to dangerous and violent patients.

On the basis of concerns for the health of staff, many psychiatric institutions implemented courses for their employees, in which safe physical interventions were taught and trained. Hundreds of commercial companies, many of them coming from the security industry, became involved in health care, and designed defence and intervention courses for mental health care staff. Due to the background of the safety concerns of the staff, this development was understandable and welcomed by nearly all staff. Without doubt, these safety initiatives were, on a broad scale, quite successful, and did lead to safer coercion measures with less violence [6]. Thus, both sides of the conflict, staff and patients alike, benefited from the new development.

However, from a coercion and violence prevention perspective, the second step was completed before the first. Although physical violence was reduced during the application of coercion, staff training contained very limited information regarding prevention and avoidance of violent conflicts by means of de-escalation. The reasons for this are obvious: first, many courses taught a hands-on approach that was based on techniques normally administered by security personnel. Second, there was hardly any specific knowledge regarding nonphysical conflict-solving techniques available in the health care domain, with even less being available in psychiatry. It comes then as no surprise that the very early literature on de-escalation in psychiatry and other health care settings had not emerged before the 1990s [7–12].

The problem just mentioned is still currently an issue. Until recently, there was hardly any specific research and/or theoretical reasoning available related to nonphysical conflict-solving methods in psychiatry or other related health care fields. Interpersonal de-escalation is generally, with certain exceptions, quite a neglected research area, whereas efforts to de-escalate international conflicts or intergroup disputes are very well researched. The exceptions mentioned above are business negotiations, crisis intervention and hostage negotiations. Therefore, the outline of several nonphysical approaches to be discussed below stems largely from knowledge outside the core of mental health care and health care in general.

Although this situation in terms of evidence-based interventions is very unsatisfying, it is not impossible to transfer knowledge from other fields into psychiatry. As will be outlined below, aggressive situations in mental health care do not categorically differ from conflict situations elsewhere [13,14]. A basic approach to de-escalation in mental health care is an assumption that all physically aggressive situations result ultimately in an escalating interaction in which one party uses force to overthrow the other.

In the remainder of this chapter, firstly, empirical research on de-escalation efforts in health care will be reviewed. Secondly, a very brief theoretical sketch will be provided which will outline how situations in (mental) health care escalate. Thirdly, a general de-escalation approach will be adapted, from crisis intervention, business negotiation research and hostage negotiation experiences, to health care. Finally, specific interventions that have proven successful in several social conflict areas and that are recommended in research and textbooks from several related fields will be described.

## 5.2   Empirical research on the prevention of violence and coercion in mental health care – organizational approaches

Several reviews have been conducted which reported on the current evidence of the ingredients and the success of prevention strategies against violence and coercion [15–19]. Prevention strategies have often been triggered by legal provisions and other state level or even supra-state level interventions [20,21]. However, a recent vignette study has shown that, even within Europe, there is little harmonization of national laws, and consistent standards are lacking [22]. Empirical research, accordingly, is difficult to conduct and even more difficult to compare between countries. A general consensus, however, has emerged across several diverse psychiatric care systems. The general consensus is that coercive measures should be applied as little as possible.

Organizational policies on the safe use (and the reduction) of coercion in psychiatry have become more and more popular in recent years [23]. These policies aim at the security of staff as well as at the safety of patients. This dualistic approach quite often leads to dilemmas between clinical goals and safety goals (e.g. when patients' personal things are removed due to safety concerns). Based on experience, many conflicts between staff and patients result from these procedures. Related to organizational policies are changes in the organization and/or the care programme itself. Organizational changes aim sometimes at changing the wards' atmosphere (e.g. by separating or integrating potentially aggressive patients).

Training and support for staff is also regarded as helpful. As mentioned above, in many psychiatric institutions, aggression management training is mandatory for all clinical staff. Many of these training programmes contain approaches either to reduce and/or to safely apply coercive measures. A recent systematic review has revealed that the outcome of these programmes is not easy to obtain. Apparently due to methodological problems in the design of evaluation studies, some studies report increasing numbers of patient assaults and coercive measures following a training programme [5].

Along with training programmes, many institutions have established rules for reporting and/or for the external review of coercive measures. Reporting approaches need to have clear definitions concerning coercion because 'usual' clinical practice sometimes uses 'informal' or implicit coercion such as threats of coercion or applying oral medication with strong verbal pressure. Recent research has shown that comparing figures, policies and coercive practices between institutions might be a first step to transparency and to start questioning the practices in each individual institution [24]. Another interesting result from this study was that, although based on a small sample of psychiatric hospitals, written policies on the application of coercive measures were associated with lower rates of coercion.

A rather new approach for the acute psychiatric setting is the use of structured risk assessments and aggression prediction instruments. While these instruments are well known in forensic psychiatry in relation to medium or long-term violence prediction, short-term prediction seemed to be impossible due to the complexity of the current treatment situation. With short-term prediction of violence, clinical experience seemed to work as effectively as structured instruments [25]. Some new research, however, has shown that the regular use of a risk assessment instrument can predict not only aggressive situations, but can also lead to a reduction in the use of coercive measures [26,27].

## 5.3   Empirical research on preventing violence and coercion – situational and behavioural approaches

Apart from explicit organizational strategies to handle difficult and potentially aggressive situations, mental health care staff informally attempt to prevent violence and coercion on a day-to-day basis. This has been done for many decades to different extents by many clinicians. The studies that are reviewed in this section have 'exploited' the informal knowledge and strategies to gain insight into successful strategies. Nursing researcher Mary Johnson has conducted a series of qualitative studies on these practices in order to discover effective de-escalation strategies. According to this research, the baseline of de-escalation is the following pattern: noticing the patient; reading the situation and the patient; knowing where the patient is on the escalation continuum; understanding the patient's behaviour; knowing what the patient needs; connecting with the patient; and finally, matching the intervention to the situation and the patient [28].

Data from another grounded theory study indicates that the aim of achieving a safe environment for everybody on the ward is attainable utilizing strategies within the following four dimensions: ideology, space, time and people [29]. On many wards, a safety ideology has emerged to ensure that both staff and patients will try to solve disputes in a nonviolent manner. The main parts of this ideology were respect for the person and a non-confrontational style, when being confronted with aggressive behaviour. The space dimension of the ward was used to separate people from one another if necessary, but also to close certain rooms and locations in order to enhance visibility of the patients. The aim of the time dimension was to enhance the predictability of interactions and reactions. A thoroughly structured day on the ward, according to staff, is able to give orientation to otherwise more or less disoriented subjects. Data on the people dimension revealed that it was not only the staff-to-patient ratio that ensured a calm atmosphere, but also the appropriate mix of certain staff to certain patients. The 'keeping the unit safe' approach aimed at a milieu that was able to ensure safety for everybody on the ward.

A related study tried to explore the different skills that staff would require in order to fulfil the task of keeping the unit safe [30]. The skills that were revealed clustered around four aspects: being there and becoming aware, caring and connecting, balancing, and deciding how to respond. Being there and becoming aware means that staff have to show visibility and become aware of what is happening on the ward. The next aspect was to explicitly demonstrate to patients that they were being cared for by the nurses, which was accomplished primarily by connecting with certain patients. Decisions on how to respond to behaviours and challenges were made by balancing the need for control of the patient versus the need for control of the situation.

Utilizing a similar methodology, an Australian study has attempted to answer the question of what strategies nurses would use after having come to the prediction that a patient is likely to become increasingly aggressive [31]. Generally, nurses tried to minimize the stress of patients and to preserve the patients' dignity. By applying a non-aversive approach, nurses utilized the following de-escalation techniques: paying attention, planning interventions and non-interventions, calming techniques (mainly by avoiding confrontational communication), allowing time for responding, ensuring safety, addressing the fundamental problems and working with and for the patient.

The only existing quantitative study regarding this topic questioned nurses regarding the frequency of strategies utilized in the management of 'difficult' clinician–patient situations [32]. The 10 most frequently utilized strategies were: respecting the patient's dignity; approaching the patient with respect, openness, and sincerity; showing respect explicitly; focusing on the problem at hand; paying attention to the nonverbal communication, being patient, acting empathetically; asking for the patient's needs and complaints; sharing information with the patient and trying to understand the patient's perspective.

In summary, these studies have demonstrated that the implicit de-escalation knowledge and behaviour can best be described as a problem-centred approach which aims at preserving the patient's dignity and autonomy while trying to communicate in a calming manner. This approach is very similar to the recommendations from relevant textbooks that will be reviewed in detail below.

## 5.4    Aggressive situations in mental health care – situational dynamics and escalation

One of the most important aspects of the development of de-escalation interventions is a thorough understanding of the aggressive situation and its causes. Therefore, an appropriate model of the causes of violence in mental health care is essential [13,14,33]. When only the patient and his or her psychopathology are regarded as the sole cause of violence, de-escalation efforts are seemingly fruitless and inefficient. A patient's psychopathology cannot be changed by behavioural interventions, at least not within a short time period. De-escalation interventions rely very much on an understanding in which staff behaviour and the whole environment is part of the escalating situation. This notion does not blame staff for increasing tensions on the ward or in other locations, but attempts to acknowledge and to raise awareness that certain environmental and behavioural features may contribute to the patient's aggression.

Empirical research on the constituents of aggression situations in mental health care has revealed that prior to the ultimate physical assault, certain events and behavioural features of the 'aggressor' can usually be identified [3,34,35]. In many incidents, patients who ultimately become physically violent previously reveal angry or agitated behaviour, often shouting or using abusive language or other verbal aggression. In many cases, violence against staff or fellow patients is preceded by aggression against objects.

While an escalation curve is an oversimplification of many incidents, it is quite useful to think of it as an increase in the input of force that is applied. Escalation is, thus, defined as the application of ever-increasing forceful methods and interventions [36].

This notion of an escalating interaction coincides very well with the dominating current psychological aggression model, the General Aggression Model, GAM [37]. The GAM favours a social psychological perspective which highlights the embedding of an aggressive person (including his/her biological makeup) within a certain situation. Within the GAM, personal and situational inputs interact with present affective, cognitive and arousal states of the individual. Following an appraisal and decision-making process, either a thoughtful action or an impulsive action will occur, with the impulsive action possibly leading to a violent incident [38].

As indicated before, another important feature of the GAM is that there are at least two parties with escalating interaction involved in the aggressive situation. After having experienced a trigger stimulus, the cycle of escalations is initiated, and every retaliation mounts to a higher level of force input. Inherent in this escalation is a clash of perspectives in which every one of a person's own actions is regarded as justified, and every action by the other party is seen as inappropriate, and is thus answered by more force. Scholars from several disciplines have empirically demonstrated how social interaction in many diverse areas finally leads to physical violence (e.g. street crime, prison aggression or domestic violence) [39–41].

The same is true for most aggressive situations in mental health care. Empirical research has shown that, prior to many violent incidents, certain behavioural features such as shouting or damaging property can be identified [3,42]. A prototypical situation usually starts with what is regarded by staff as rule violence (e.g. noncompliance to ward rules or to therapeutic regimens), after which staff try to implement verbal and sometimes later physical measures, in order to ensure the patients' compliance. The following typical situations are well known: applying medications against the patient's will, hindering patients from absconding, settling disputes between patients or maintaining the hygienic standard on the ward. Henk Nijman and colleagues [43] demonstrated, utilizing a simple map of a locked psychiatric ward in which violent incidents had occurred over a one-year period, that most of the assaults on staff occurred in the nurses' office, in front of the locked door, and, to a lesser degree, in the living room. It is in these locations that most of the daily interactions between staff and patients occur.

It is also well known that patients and staff very often attribute the causes of violence to different features. While staff regard the patient's mental disorder as the main factor of the later violent incident, patients usually identify staff behaviour as the most important trigger [44–47]. Prior to the occurrence of violent incidents, patients have reported feeling provoked, abused or threatened. They felt that often their needs were being denied.

Staff behaviour and other environmental features such as a locked door, can, from a patient's perspective, be regarded as aversive stimuli (which usually precede aggressive incidents) [48]. Apart from the very few psychopathologically motivated violent incidents with a background of a personality disorder, violence is usually not committed out of a stable and positive emotion. In nearly all cases, violence is committed by persons who feel provoked, frustrated and otherwise aversively stimulated. An important mediator between aversive stimulation and severe aggression or violence is the emergence of anger [49]. Anger is mainly generated by aversive stimuli but it is also a general personality feature. Some people can more readily be angered by external stimuli than others; thus, anger is being addressed more and more as a contributor to aggression which can be managed by cognitive and/or behavioural interventions [50].

In regards to the emergence of violence via an escalating interaction which triggers anger and aggression, certain psychological and psychopathological factors serve as mediating contributors (e.g. the present psychopathological state (psychosis etc.), drug and alcohol intoxication and impulse control or empathy skills). However, in regards to de-escalation efforts, these contributors have to be conceptualized as working in the background only. The main intervention point of de-escalation approaches is to avoid aversive stimuli as much as possible. However, it may be possible to tailor the intervention to the disorder in question (ideas on this issue are available in regards to hostage-taking experiences) [51].

## 5.5   De-escalation basics for mental health care – being prepared on an organizational level

As reviewed above, there is some empirical evidence that organizational aspects may contribute to aggressive situations in psychiatric institutions [46]. Unfortunately, there is only little research on these topics, but one can assume that it is not unimportant. On the basis of this research, some recommendations concerning the minimization of aggression and coercion can be made:

- All staff should be trained in aggression management and in the application of coercive measures.
- A warm and cooperative ward atmosphere should be created by all staff.
- Reliable inter-professional cooperation should be present.
- Policies on aggression management and the use of coercive measures should be implemented.
- Reporting systems and prediction scales should be used (according to the ward's necessity).

Preparations on an organizational level, as well as on a personal level, as described below, can be regarded as primary prevention efforts in avoiding aggression and coercion. Very often, these preventative measures work indirectly towards a low level of aggression and coercion. Aggression management is a complex social intervention, and the significance of each single component is often difficult to measure.

Although the mechanisms of efficacy remain unknown, there is some evidence that organization-wide and multidimensional interventions reduce the use of coercion in mental health settings [19,52].

## 5.6   De-escalation basics for mental health care – being prepared on a personal level

As mentioned previously, the escalation process in aggressive situations is similar across various social settings. Therefore, de-escalation approaches in mental health care can benefit from basic elements utilized in other fields. There is much to be gained from fields such as crisis intervention research, negotiation research and crisis negotiation research (e.g. in hostage-taking situations).

One of the most well researched areas from other fields is interpersonal or intergroup negotiations. Although this literature refers mainly to conflicts within business relations and organizations, the basics can easily be transferred to psychiatric care situations. According to this research, interpersonal conflicts often emerge because of 'natural' reactions and emotions of the parties involved. Relying on theory and research from Harvard Law School's negotiation programme, Ury has identified five main barriers to constructive conflict solving [53]:

- natural reactions during an increasingly tense interaction (e.g. becoming angry);
- negative emotions on both sides of the conflict (e.g. fear, suspicion or hostility);
- sticking to one's position (inflexibility regarding the content of the conflict);
- objective conflicts of interest;
- refusal to cooperate.

These natural reactions are physiologically mediated and triggered. We all know the typical physiological reactions to aversive, anger- or fear-provoking stimuli, such as perspiration or an increasing heartbeat frequency. Related to such a state of heightened arousal, are specific emotional and cognitive features which may trigger further adverse outcomes and may lead to aggressive behaviour.

De-escalation, thus, is mainly an effort to deal with these 'natural' reactions and emotions. De-escalation also focuses on the obvious conflicts of interests. In other words, a major ingredient of de-escalation is not to react as one would like to. Immediate verbal reactions very frequently function as communication barriers that are likely to escalate the level of aggression. The following response modes frequently occur and are well known as barriers to communication [54–56]:

- threatening
- ordering
- warning

- moralizing
- (logically) arguing
- blaming
- shaming
- judging
- name-calling
- analysing
- probing
- irony/sarcasm
- evaluative praising
- belittling
- excessive questioning.

A skilled and competent mental health professional must look beyond verbal reactions, and learn to recognize, acknowledge and manage the following stress reactions and conflict styles:

- emotions (e.g. anger, fear, hostility);
- cognitions (e.g. expectations, mistrust, attributions);
- status vulnerability (e.g. being belittled, professional competence being questioned);
- verbal and nonverbal communication style (e.g. argumentativeness, assertiveness, body language);
- individual conflict styles (e.g. being avoidant or proactive).

The more one is informed about the personal features of conflict communication beforehand, and the more one is prepared to be challenged in this regard, the better one is able to adapt to difficult and diverse situations and people. Everybody has psychological critical points, and it is advantageous to know about them and how to handle attacks on these points. If somebody's weak point is, for example, an attack on the professional competence or on the body height, one should have neutralizing responses prepared in advance. A general point concerning verbal attacks is to expect them during an aggressive encounter, and not to take them personally [53].

Stress management and anger management are key features of personal readiness for conflict management [55]. A key step to manage one's own emotions is self-awareness [50]. Mental health professionals need to be aware of their own individual response styles, their personal vulnerabilities and about the options to deal with these issues. According to research, one option is to use self-talk to prepare for provocation, such as, 'this may upset me, but I know how to deal with it'. Another option is to know about one's personal physiological reactions to aggressive encounters and how to handle the effects ('My muscles are getting tight. This is my signal for a deep and relaxing breath').

Another similar important aspect of de-escalation in psychiatric settings is to be prepared for the obvious ambiguous role of professionals [57]. On one hand, staff are committed to aggression management and minimization of coercion. On the other hand, clinical routines, institutional guidelines and ward rules have to be applied. Every mental health clinician has surely experienced the discussions within a ward regarding the often-conflicting goals, priorities and coercive interventions. Clinicians have to keep a delicate balance between individualization of treatment and maintenance of ward rules.

Conflict solving skills and styles can be judged from two related dimensions that must be kept in balance: effectiveness and appropriateness [58]. Effectiveness indicates whether the goals of the conflict strategy were attained, and appropriateness indicates whether the strategy was suitable for the conflict and the setting in question. Of course, one can be effective in attaining one's own goals while being inappropriate in the communication style. However, being only appropriate does not ensure attainment of the goals.

## 5.7  Nonverbal communication skills

In the current communication society, we rely heavily upon the written and spoken word. Nonphysical communication approaches do also stress the contents and techniques of verbal exchanges (e.g. active listening). While this is undoubtedly of high importance (as will be outlined below), nonverbal behaviour is largely underrated regarding its consequences on communication in general, and especially regarding escalation/de-escalation of aggressive situations.

In order to be effective in nonphysical interventions during aggressive situations, one has to be sensitive to the nonverbal communication of the involved parties. Current nonverbal behaviour research deals with issues such as facial expression, vocal expression, proxemics (spatial behaviour, e.g. interpersonal distance), kinesics and gaze [59]. One task is to 'read' the emotional display of the other party using clues from the issues just mentioned. Experts in this field especially recommend taking notice of changes in an individual's body language. Behavioural changes often reveal what a person is about to do, and provide the observer with time to prepare his or her own reaction [60].

The other task related to nonverbal communication is to be aware of and to control one's own body language. Inappropriate nonverbal behaviour might serve as an aversive stimulus that triggers aggressive reactions from the other party. Body language develops more or less automatically and is difficult, without training in advance, to control. One has to be aware that the body 'speaks' our emotions.

Role-playing stressful situations, combined with video recordings may provide hints as to what our behaviour and body language reveals to others.

In general, there are two main nonverbal strategies. One is a pacifying approach and the other is an aggressive approach. It must always be remembered that these approaches are highly culturally sensitive. Pacifying behaviour aims at minimizing threats and giving a signal of openness to the patient's concerns. Lowered and uncrossed arms with a relaxed body posture that is turned toward the other party may signal that we are not in a defensive position and are interested in the perspective of the other party. This body language should be accompanied by a soft voice, head nodding and a relaxed gaze. Aggressive behaviour, in contrast, aims at making the body appear to be larger. A body posture that often is used to demonstrate superiority is known as 'arms akimbo'. This is when one places the hands on the hips and so bows the elbows outwardly. The higher the arms are held, the more it appears that we are prepared to defend or to attack.

## 5.8    Strategic options for de-escalation in mental health settings

Psychological research has revealed that interpersonal conflict strategies can be subsumed under the following three main approaches [58]:

- the distributive strategy which aims at defending oneself, including against threats, hostility, and demands;
- the avoidance strategy which denies that there is any relevant conflict and aims at withdrawal and acquiescing to the demands;
- the integrative strategy which reflects cooperation, mutuality, negotiation and support.

It is clear that the distributive or confronting approach is, apart from its inherent dangerousness to all persons involved, not usually compatible with the therapeutic goals of psychiatric settings. The avoidance strategy is not rare, especially in long-term care settings, where staff attempt to cope with the daily challenging behaviour of certain patients. The 'soft' avoidance approach has a similar likelihood of leading to an escalation as the 'tough' approach. The avoidance strategy quite often results in 'complementary' escalation, where the submission or avoidance of staff will reinforce the patient's unwelcome challenging and aggressive behaviour [61].

Therefore, the integrative de-escalation strategy is the only approach that is reasonable due to its simultaneous compatibility with the therapeutic goals. Throughout the literature on de-escalation, crisis intervention and conflict solving, similar topics have emerged that are regarded as successful parts of the strategy. In an earlier publication, the author of this chapter has proposed the following basic rules for de-escalation of aggressive encounters in psychiatric settings [55]:

- A de-escalation intervention functions best as an early intervention.
- A key tool for de-escalation is gaining time for responses.
- Conduct a risk assessment and have realistic expectations concerning a nonviolent outcome of the situation.
- Share risk assessment, responsibilities and decision-making with fellow colleagues.
- Demonstrate an attitude of empathy, concern, sincerity and fairness while communicating caring and therapeutic intentions.
- Attempt not to control the patient, but the situation.
- Consider spatial aspects and keep distance.
- Apply interventions with apparent self-confidence and certainty, without being provocative.
- Avoid power plays between staff and patients.
- Be aware of general safety issues related to other patients and inexperienced staff.

Within the crisis intervention context, Roberts has developed an intervention model [62] which has been adapted in the literature [63]. With some minor modifications for psychiatric settings, this strategic intervention model can be adapted based on the following components:

- safety and security assessment of the whole situation;
- establishing a rapport and a working relationship with the 'aggressor';
- identification of and dealing with the substantive problems of the 'aggressor';
- dealing with feelings and emotions (including active listening) of the 'aggressor';
- generation and exploration of options and alternatives.

It is important to note that these elements are usually not applied in a sequential order, but simultaneously. Establishing a rapport without dealing with the emotions of the 'aggressor' is practically impossible. An approach that attempts to match the escalating situation with related interventions, integrating many of the strategies, has been developed by Paterson and Leadbetter [64].

It may also occur that only a few points of Robert's model need to be used while solving a conflict without coercion. In the remainder of this chapter, the single components of this intervention model will be outlined briefly. It should be understood that the given examples of de-escalating behaviours are only to illustrate the argument and the recommendations, and cannot be transferred one-to-one into real-life psychiatric situations.

## 5.9    Safety and security assessment

A very important issue within de-escalation concerns thorough decision-making. The options for de-escalation interventions depend upon several aspects within the whole situation. The notion of an escalating interaction indicates that the intensity of aggression is likely to increase. Therefore, the interventions should be matched to the level of aggression that is obvious at that certain moment in time. The more aggression is observed, the less likely is the chance of success for a nonviolent or nonphysical intervention. Other characteristics that have to be taken into account are architectural features such as available flight ways or the ability to raise the alarm with fellow staff members. Obviously, the different options do depend on the skills of the health care professionals regarding nonphysical techniques. While balancing the demands and the individual possibilities, very often a quick decision has to be taken. Objective indicators and recommendations cannot be given in most situations, and expert professionals rely mainly on their intuition in making decisions.

The safety of other patients as well as the safety of less experienced and trained staff has to also be considered. De-escalation interventions of a higher level demand highly skilled individuals who are convinced and confident about their competencies. Nonphysical interventions cannot be implemented in an ordered and prearranged manner, but instead have to be applied in a very flexible and sometimes counterintuitive way.

In cases where professionals are unsure regarding their strategic options and the efficiency of a nonphysical intervention, an alternate plan should then be quickly followed. That usually involves receiving assistance and support from colleagues. If one is not confident with the application of a nonphysical intervention, it should not be undertaken. The risk is high that there will be incongruence between the verbal and nonverbal behaviour, and that it will appear implausible and not authentic.

## 5.10    Building a working relationship

Aggressive situations between patients and staff are very often characterized by the patients mistrusting the professionals. By addressing emotions such as anger and fear, and by dealing with substantive demands, health care professionals have a chance to decrease this mistrust. Building rapport between the professional and the aggressive patient is, strategically, the most important goal. When this professional relationship cannot be established, any nonphysical intervention is unlikely to succeed. The building of a working relationship may be seen as the primary prevention goal. Upon admission to the ward, the priority of staff should be to as quickly as possible establish rapport and a relationship with the patient. There is some empirical evidence that primary nurses are less frequently assaulted than other staff [42]. Well-known and trusted staff can be assumed to be less frequently involved in aggressive situations with patients.

A central point concerning the working relationship is identification of the sometimes hidden needs behind the emotional outburst. A core strategy is to address the needs behind the emotion [65]. Emotions, however, are not to be neglected. As will be outlined below, emotions should be dealt with specifically. Needs that may be hidden behind emotions are: acknowledgement of the person and the person's point of view, attachment, autonomy, status and role [65]. Practically, what meaning do these demands have for a de-escalation intervention? Firstly, acknowledgement means that the person is valued, and this evaluation will be communicated. For health professionals, it is necessary to be honestly interested into the 'aggressor's' point of view ('I see what you mean and I see that this is very important to you'.). Secondly, attachment is especially important in long-term settings. Over time, staff and patients develop an emotional relationship that might be disturbed by staff behaviour. When staff become emotionally important persons for the patient, a disturbed attachment might lead to aggressive responses. Thirdly, autonomy refers to the requirement that all persons involved have the feeling that they are free from the control or influence of others. One way to enhance autonomy is to negotiate different options ('Could you please think about doing . . .'; 'Would it be possible for you to. . .'). Fourthly, status implies that all persons involved are not put down or belittled by other persons. Finally, the roles of all persons involved must be clearly defined. This recommendation is especially valid for the mental health professional, as not all patients are aware that nurses and doctors in psychiatric hospitals have both the key authority as well as the aim of providing support.

## 5.11  Identification of and dealing with substantive demands

Behind almost all aggressive acts lie one or more substantive problems that may or may not coincide with the main needs described above. Aggressive acts are usually executed because needs, demands and expectations are perceived by the 'aggressor' as not being met by the other party (i.e. by the psychiatric clinicians) [45]. For example, often patients feel threatened by locked doors or by the behaviour of individual staff members. Sometimes patients also do not want to take part in diagnostic or therapeutic activities, and would rather be left alone and not be disturbed. A de-escalation perspective tries to identify and to deal with these demands. If a patient complains about ward doors being locked ('It's ridiculous to keep me on a closed ward!'), the staff member could respond with a confirming and neutral reply ('People often feel scared about locked doors, but locked doors support safety and security'.) [56]. Put this way, the clinician shares the patient's position while explaining the necessity to have doors locked. If a patient refuses to attend occupational therapy ('I'll never again go to this absurd handicraft thing'), the staff member could respond to that position in a similar manner ('In the beginning patients often do not see the value of such occupational therapies').

Whereas emotional issues are not negotiable, demands and needs are. From a de-escalation position, clinicians should adopt a problem-solving stance [63]. When there are too many demands to be met, it might be efficient to separate them. If a patient wants to be discharged from a locked ward, which is not possible, it may be useful to help him with phoning his wife. After having established a working relationship it may be possible to shift the patient's goals towards common goals ('How can we solve this problem together? What can we both do to avoid any further escalation?').

## 5.12    Dealing with feelings and emotions

When aggressive situations escalate, there are emotions involved. Anger, fear, hurt or guilt constitute the necessary components of a conflict situation [66]. Emotional conflicts do occur when the goals of the involved parties are incompatible and when expectations are violated. Viewed psychologically, emotions serve as appraisals of a situation. The other party does not react as one has assumed or expected and the appraisal process is started. As already indicated above, anger seems to be the prototypical appraisal outcome during aggressive encounters. It can be stimulated by nearly any aversive event such as: identity threats, aggression, frustration, unfairness, incompetence, attachment threats, etc.

In regards to emotions, de-escalation aims at targeting the 'aggressor's', as well as the staff members' emotional regulation. Emotions cannot and must not be ignored, because they may unwillingly overwhelm one's behaviour. The higher the emotional arousal, the less possible it is to act rationally. A very high anger arousal makes it difficult to control one's own aggression, attributions and empathy. As neuropsychologist Simon Baron-Cohen has nicely put it, 'Aggression, even in normal quantities, can only occur because of reduced empathizing. You just can't set out to hurt someone if you care how they feel. . . During aggression you are focused on how *you* feel, more than on how *the other person* feels.' [37,67] Strong negative emotions evoke a mental tunnel that makes it difficult to react flexibly and rationally. Simultaneously, it increases one's vulnerability because small gestures or verbal expressions are likely to be interpreted as aggressive acts.

Therefore, one of the first tasks is to check the emotional states of everybody involved in the conflict: is it manageable, risky or out of control [65, p. 148]? Indicators for high arousal are deviations from the 'normal' state (e.g. loud voice, facial expressions and the entire body language). Although the emotional state of all involved parties is of high importance, it may be, however, only the clinician who is able to control his/her own state of arousal. The arousal state of the other party in the conflict may only then be influenced, by indirect adaption to the less aroused state of the clinician.

If patients are highly aroused and cannot be reached by a 'normal' loudness, it may be necessary to match the state artificially by shouting: 'Stop!' In cases where somebody is out of control, synchronizing is the measure of choice [53,56]. However, the next immediate step should aim at two goals: decreasing the emotional state and building a working relationship. This can be done by lowering the volume and trying to listen actively to the patient's problems and complaints. The main active listening techniques are [53,55,57]:

- to encourage the patient to talk about problems and positions;
- to demonstrate that you are paying attention;
- to listen for both content and meaning;
- to respond to the emotional message;
- to respond honestly;
- to paraphrase the patient's message to show your understanding;
- to not interrupt while the patient is talking;
- to not give advice;
- to not discount the patient's feelings;
- to indicate a clear interest in the patient's opinion and acknowledge his/her position ('I see what you mean'; 'I'd like to hear more about it').

Active listening also refers to reduction of the other's tension by acknowledgement of the other's emotional state ('I see that you're upset. After what you've been through, it is quite understandable.'). However, one must be aware that to acknowledge the other's point of view and emotions does not necessarily denote that one concedes to anything.

When the 'aggressor' is approachable again, a method founded on much evidence in research can be used. This method is based on the evidence that emotions are contagious [65]. This is not only true for increased anger on both sides of the conflict, but also for less aroused states. Related to emotional contagion is the other rule that communicative interaction is a feedback loop [56]. Therefore, favourable emotional states on the other side of the conflict should be reinforced, while less favourable states should be worked on. This is accomplished by breaking the circle of actions and counteractions that correspond to the increasing anger and aggression. How can this be done? A key option in defusing the other's negative emotions is the use of time. Negotiation textbooks give the recommendation 'Go to the balcony!' for situations that are likely to escalate [53]. In an aggressive encounter with a patient, a similar way could be to look out of a window for several seconds. The idea behind this recommendation is not to react directly to an accusation or a verbal threat with an aggressive response. Gaining time decreases emotionality and increases the chance for rationality. Another advantage of gaining time is a heightened chance to look for support from fellow staff members [57].

## 5.13   Generation and exploration of options and alternatives

After and parallel to having dealt with demands and emotions and after having established a working relationship, the final task of de-escalation is to find a way out of the dangerous situation. Before one can explore and negotiate options and alternatives, it is absolutely necessary that the other party is receptive. It is futile to negotiate with somebody who is unable to listen or understand [53, p. 53]. When exploring the demands, it should be possible to explore options for both parties involved in the conflict. The key question is: is there a satisfying solution for both sides? Only in this final stage of the intervention is it suitable for staff to express their own positions and interests. The previous time period should be utilized to establish rapport and to deal with the issues mentioned above.

Previously learnt from negotiation research and from textbooks is the importance of having a plan B. It is a comfortable negotiation position if one can take a step backwards from the initial point. One must, however, determine the different possible options and have a bottom line. The Best Alternative To A Negotiated Agreement (BATNA) should be the evaluative point, before any further steps in the de-escalation effort are taken [53]. Thought-provoking questions around BATNA are: Which goal do you want to attain? Which outcome would be satisfying? Which solution can you live with?

A key strategy at this point is to integrate the other party as a partner: 'Do you have any ideas of how to get out of this situation?'; 'We have a common interest to solve this conflict in a nonviolent manner.' Cooperation can also be initiated by using the reciprocity rule of (nearly) all human communication. The rule of reciprocity is that if a favour is done for the other side, the other side then feels obligated to repay the favour [57, p. 239]. Thus, if one is generous in relation to minor issues, one can then ask the other side for a cooperative step.

## 5.14   Conclusions and disclaimers

Although the de-escalation approach in mental health care is still lacking an evidence base, it is clear from the sections above that there is already some knowledge which is available and waiting for implementation. The author is convinced that the application of such nonphysical techniques has the ability to, at the very least, significantly minimize the need for physical interventions. Several educational and training approaches have adopted the previously outlined basics. By utilizing video feedback techniques, role-playing and/or aggressive simulation patients, it is possible to develop professional expertise in nonphysical techniques.

De-escalation techniques cannot, however, be learned and applied in an ordered and prearranged manner. Efficacy and outcome of a nonphysical intervention depend upon the situation in general, and also upon the mental state of the 'aggressor'. Receptiveness is a key prerequisite, and, therefore, a high level of flexibility is required. One can also not assume that the same successfully applied intervention for the same patient will be effective several days later. A successfully applied verbal intervention depends on the personality of the clinician who applies it. Experienced mental health professionals are likely to develop individualized strategies which match their personality characteristics. If one wants to convince someone of something, one must first be convinced oneself regarding the options, strategies and argumentativeness or assertiveness.

In order to achieve safer, more humane and less restrictive mental health care, de-escalation training should be mandatory for all staff. It may be true that a few aggressive situations cannot be managed without coercion. However, coercive interventions should only be applied by those clinicians who have been trained in alternative nonphysical approaches. A further advantage that follows from this postulation would be that coercive interventions, if necessary at all, would be applied utilizing a de-escalation approach. One could expect that after such training, coercion would not be used with brute force, but with the aim to maintain contact with the patient, and as much as possible to provide information and transparency.

For more humane psychiatry it is also mandatory that the research base for nonphysical interventions be developed. Recent guidelines on aggression management and coercion have made clear that the current state of knowledge is not acceptable. The UK National Institute for Health and Clinical Excellence (NICE) guideline on short-term aggression management has stated that '... despite the emphasis that is often placed on the importance of de-escalation, little research has been carried out into the effectiveness of any given approach, leaving nurses [and other clinicians, D. R.] to contend with conflicting advice and theories.' [68, p. 50] The very recent German guideline on therapeutic measures for aggressive behaviour has noted that 'A scientific basis for interpersonal de-escalation techniques is missing up to now.' ([69, p. 46]; my translation, D. R.) The fact that the field of aggression and coercion prevention is so severely lacking in research does not reflect positively upon the discipline of psychiatry as a whole.

## Acknowledgement

This chapter was prepared while working on an empirical research project on verbal aggression in health care settings. The financial support by the Public Occupational Accident Insurance North Rhine-Westphalia, Germany, is kindly acknowledged.

The author would like to thank Tannys Helfer, BSc, for providing language editing.

## References

1. Nijman, H.L.I., Palmstierna, T., Almvik, R. and Stolker, J.J. (2005) Fifteen years of research with the Staff Observation Aggression Scale: a review. *Acta Psychiatrica Scandinavica*, **111**, 12–21.
2. Richter, D. and Berger, K. (2001) Patientenübergriffe auf Mitarbeiter – Eine prospektive Untersuchung der Häufigkeit. *Situationen und Folgen. Nervenarzt*, **72**, 693–699.
3. Whittington, R. and Patterson, R. (1996) Verbal and non-verbal behaviour immediately prior to aggression by mentally disordered people: enhancing the assessment of risk. *Journal of Psychiatric and Mental Health Nursing*, **3**, 47–54.
4. Morrison, E.F. (1990) The tradition of toughness: a study of nonprofessional nursing care in psychiatric settings. *Image: Journal of Nursing Scholarship*, **22**, 32–38.
5. Richter, D., Needham, I. and Kunz, S. (2006) The effects of aggression management trainings for mental health care and disability care staff: a systematic review, in *Violence in Mental Health Settings: Causes, Consequences, Management* (eds D. Richter and R. Whittington), Springer, New York, pp. 211–227.
6. Needham, I., Abderhalden, C., Meer, R. *et al.* (2004) The effectiveness of two interventions in the management of patient violence in acute mental inpatient settings. *Journal of Psychiatric and Mental Health Nursing*, **11**, 595–601.
7. Turnbull, J., Aitken, I., Laura, B. and Paterson, B. (1990) Turn it around: short-term management for aggression and anger. *Journal of Psychosocial Nursing and Mental Health Services*, **28**, 6–13.
8. Stevenson, S. (1991) Heading off violence with verbal de-escalation. *Journal of Psychosocial Nursing and Mental Health Services*, **29**, 6–10.
9. Maier, G.J. (1996) Managing threatening behaviour: the role of talk down and talk up. *Journal of Psychosocial Nursing and Mental Health Services*, **34**, 25–30.
10. Harris, D. and Morrison, E.F. (1995) Managing violence without coercion. *Archives of Psychiatric Nursing*, **9**, 203–210.
11. Smith, B.J. and Cantrell, P.J. (1988) Distance in nurse-patient encounters. *Journal of Psychosocial Nursing and Mental Health Services*, **26**, 22–26.
12. Leadbetter, D. and Paterson, B. (1995) De-escalating aggressive behaviour, in *Management of Violence and Aggression in Health Care* (eds B. Kidd and C. Stark), Gaskell, London, pp. 49–84.
13. Whittington, R. and Richter, D. (2005) Interactional aspects of violent behaviour on acute psychiatric wards. *Psychology, Crime, and the Law*, **11**, 377–388.
14. Whittington, R. and Richter, D. (2006) From the individual to the interpersonal: environment and interaction in the escalation of violence in mental health settings, in *Violence in Mental*

*Health Settings: Causes, Consequences, Management* (eds D. Richter and R. Whittington), Springer, New York, pp. 47–68.

15. Sailas, E. and Wahlbeck, K. (2005) Restraint and seclusion in psychiatric inpatient wards. *Current Opinion in Psychiatry*, **18**, 555–559.

16. Scanlan, J.N. (2009) Interventions to reduce the use of seclusion and restraint in inpatient psychiatric settings: what we know so far – a review of the literature. *International Journal of Social Psychiatry*. doi: 10.1177/0020764009106630.

17. Gaskin, C.J., Elsom, S.J. and Happell, B. (2007) Interventions for reducing the use of seclusion in psychiatric facilities: review of the literature. *British Journal of Psychiatry*, **191**, 298–303.

18. Johnson, M.E. (2010) Violence and restraint reduction efforts on inpatient psychiatric units. *Issues in Mental Health Nursing*, **31**, 181–197.

19. Delaney, K.R. (2006) Evidence base for practice: reduction of restraint and seclusion use during child and adolescent psychiatric inpatient treatment. *Worldviews on Evidence-Based Nursing*, **3**, 19–30.

20. Jones, R. and Kingdon, D. (2005) Council of Europe recommendations on human rights and psychiatry: a major opportunity for mental health services. *European Psychiatry*, **20**, 461–464.

21. Keski-Valkama, A., Sailas, E., Eronen, M. *et al.* (2007) A 15-year national follow-up: legislation is not enough to reduce the use of seclusion and restraint. *Social Psychiatry and Psychiatric Epidemiology*, **42**, 747–752.

22. Steinert, T. and Lepping, P. (2008) Legal provisions and practice in the management of violent patients: a case vignette study in 16 European countries. *European Psychiatry*, **24**, 135–141.

23. Cowman, S. (2006) Safety and security in psychiatric clinical environments, in *Violence in Mental Health Settings: Causes, Consequences, Management* (eds D. Richter and R. Whittington), Springer, New York, pp. 253–271.

24. Steinert, T., Martin, V., Baur, M. *et al.* (2007) Diagnosis-related frequency of compulsory measures in 10 German psychiatric hospitals and correlates with hospital characteristics. *Social Psychiatry and Psychiatric Epidemiology*, **42**, 140–145.

25. Steinert, T. (2006) Prediction of violence in inpatient settings, in *Violence in Mental Health Settings: Causes, Consequences, Management* (eds D. Richter and R. Whittington), Springer, New York, pp. 111–123.

26. Abderhalden, C., Needham, I., Dassen, T. *et al.* (2008) Structured risk assessment and violence in acute psychiatric wards: randomised controlled trial. *British Journal of Psychiatry*, **193**, 44–50.

27. Björkdahl, A., Olsson, D. and Palmstierna, T. (2006) Nurses' short-term prediction of violence in acute psychiatric intensive care. *Acta Psychiatrica Scandinavica*, **113**, 224–229.

28. Johnson, M.E. and Hauser, P.M. (2001) The practices of expert psychiatric nurses: accompanying the patient to a calmer personal space. *Issues in Mental Health Nursing*, **22**, 651–668.

29. Johnson, M.E. and Delaney, K.R. (2006) Keeping the unit safe: a grounded theory study. *Journal of the American Psychiatric Nurses Association*, **12**, 13–21.

30. Delaney, K.R. and Johnson, M.E. (2006) Keeping the unit safe: mapping psychiatric nursing skills. *Journal of the American Psychiatric Nurses Association*, **12**, 198–207.

31. Pryor, J. (2006) What do nurses do in response to their predictions of aggression? *Journal of Neuroscience Nursing*, **38**, 177–182.

32. Robinson Wolf, Z. and Robinson-Smith, G. (2007) Strategies used by clinical nurse specialists in 'difficult' clinician-patient situations. *Clinical Nurse Specialist*, **21**, 74–84.

33. Richter, D. (in press) Aggressives und gewalttätiges Verhalten gegen Mitarbeiter im Ge-sundheitswesen – Ein Erklärungsmodell, in *Aggression im Gesundheitswesen* (eds G. Walter, N. Oud and J. Nau), Huber, Bern.

34. Aiken, G.J.M. (1984) Assaults on staff in a locked ward: prediction and consequences. *Medicine, Science and the Law*, **24**, 199–207.

35. Powell, G., Caan, W. and Crowe, M. (1994) What events precede violent incidents in psychiatric hospitals? *British Journal of Psychiatry*, **165**, 107–112.

36. Pruitt, D.G. and Kim, S.H. (2004) *Social Conflict: Escalation, Stalemate, and Settlement*, 3rd edn, McGraw-Hill, Boston.

37. Anderson, C.A. and Bushman, B.J. (2002) Human aggression. *Annual Review of Psychology*, **53**, 27–51.

38. Anderson, C.A. and Carnagey, N.L. (2004) Violent evil and the general aggression model, in *The Social Psychology of Good and Evil* (ed. A.G. Miller), Guilford Press, New York, pp. 168–192.

39. Miethe, T.D. and Regoeczi, W.C. (2004) *Rethinking Homicide: Exploring the Structure and Process Underlying Deadly Situations*, Cambridge University Press, Cambridge.

40. Winstok, Z. (2007) Toward an interactional perspective on intimate partner violence. *Aggression and Violent Behaviour*, **12**, 348–363.

41. Edgar, K., O'Donnell, I. and Martin, C. (2003) Tracking pathways to violence in prison, in *Researching Violence: Essays on Methodology and Measurement* (eds R.M. Lee and E.A. Stanko), Routledge, London, pp. 69–87.

42. Richter, D. (1999) *Patientenübergriffe auf Mitarbeiter Psychiatrischer Kliniken. Häufigkeit, Folgen, Präventionsmöglichkeiten*, Lambertus, Freiburg.

43. Nijman, H.L.I., Allertz, W.F.F., Merckelbach, H.L.G.J. *et al.* (1997) Aggressive behaviour on an acute psychiatric admission ward. *European Psychiatry*, **11**, 106–114.

44. Nolan, K.A., Shope, C.B., Citrome, L. and Volavka, J. (2009) Staff and patient views of the reasons for aggressive incidents: a prospective, incident-based study. *Psychiatric Quarterly*, **80**, 167–172.

45. Ilkiw-Lavalle, O. and Grenyer, B.F.S. (2003) Differences between patient and staff perceptions of aggression in mental health units. *Psychiatric Services*, **54**, 389–393.

46. Abderhalden, C., Hahn, S., Bonner, Y.D.B. and Galeazzi, G.M. (2006) Users' perceptions and views on violence and coercion in mental health, in *Violence in Mental Health Settings: Causes, Consequences, Management* (eds D. Richter and R. Whittington), Springer, New York, pp. 69–92.

47. Duxbury, J. and Whittington, R. (2005) Causes and management of patient aggression and violence: staff and patient perspectives. *Journal of Advanced Nursing*, **50**, 469–478.

48. Berkowitz, L. (1993) *Aggression: Causes, Consequences and Control*, McGraw Hill, New York.

49. Novaco, R.W. (2007) Anger dysregulation, in *Anger, Aggression, and Interventions for Interpersonal Violence* (eds T.A. Cavell and K.T. Malcolm), Erlbaum, Mahwaj, NJ, pp. 3–54.

50. Nay, W.R. (2004) *Taking Charge of Anger: How to Resolve Conflict, Sustain Relationships, and Express Yourself Without Losing Control*, Guilford Press, New York.

51. Miller, L. (2007) Negotiating with mentally disordered hostage takers: guiding principles and practical strategies. *Journal of Police Crisis Negotiations*, **7**, 63–83.

52. Paterson, B. (in press) Restraint, seclusion and compulsory medication. Still valid after all these years? in *Mental Health Nursing Ethics* (ed. P. Barker), Macmillan, London.

53. Ury, W. (1991) *Getting Past No: Negotiating in Difficult Situations*, Bantam, New York.

54. Dutschmann, A. (2003) *Aggressionen und Konflikte unter emotionaler Erregung: Deeskalation und Problemlösung (Das Aggressions-Bewältigungs-Programm ABPro)*, 2nd edn, DGVT-Verlag, Tübingen.
55. Richter, D. (2006) Non-physical conflict management and de-escalation, in *Violence in Mental Health Settings: Causes, Consequences, Management* (eds D. Richter and R. Whittington), Springer, New York, pp. 125–144.
56. Elgin, S.H. (1999) *Language in Emergency Medicine*, XLibris, Bloomington, IN.
57. McMains, M.J. and Mullins, W.C. (2006) *Crisis Negotiations: Managing Critical Incidents and Hostage Situations in Law Enforcement and Corrections*, 3rd edn, LexisNexis, Albany, NY.
58. Cupach, W.R., Canary, D.J. and Spitzberg, B.H. (2010) *Competence in Interpersonal Conflict*, Waveland Press, Long Grove, IL.
59. Harrigan, J.A., Rosenthal, R. and Scherer, K.R. (eds) (2008) *The New Handbook of Methods in Nonverbal Behavior Research*, Oxford University Press, New York.
60. Navarro, J. and Karlins, M. (2008) *What Every Body is Saying: An Ex-FBI Agent's Guide to Speed-Reading People*, Harper Collins, New York.
61. Omer, H. (2004) *Non-Violent Resistance: A New Approach to Violent and Self-Destructive Children*, Cambridge University Press, Cambridge.
62. Roberts, A.R. (2005) Bridging the past and present to the future of crisis intervention and crisis management, in *Crisis Intervention Handbook: Assessment, Treatment, and Research*, 3rd edn (ed. A.R. Roberts), Oxford University Press, New York, pp. 3–34.
63. Hammer, M.R. (2007) *Saving Lives: The S.A.F.E. Model for Resolving Hostage and Crisis Incidents*, Praeger, Westport, CT.
64. Paterson, B. and Leadbetter, D. (1999) De-escalation in the management of aggression and violence: towards evidence-based practice, in *Aggression and Violence: Approaches to Effective Management* (eds J. Turnbull and B. Paterson), Palgrave Macmillan, Basingstoke, pp. 95–123.
65. Fisher, R. and Shapiro, D. (2005) *Beyond Reason: Using Emotions as You Negotiate*, Penguin, New York.
66. Guerrero, L.K. and La Valley, A.G. (2006) Conflict, emotion, and communication, in *The SAGE Handbook of Conflict Communication: Integrating Theory, Research, and Practice* (eds J.G. Oetzel and S. Ting-Toomey), Sage, Thousand Oaks, CA, pp. 69–96.
67. Baron-Cohen, S. (2003) *The Essential Difference: Men, Women and the Extreme Male Brain*, Allen Lane, London.
68. National Institute for Health and Clinical Excellence (2005) *Violence: The Short-Term Management of Disturbed/Violent Behaviour in Psychiatric In-patient Settings and Emergency Departments*, NICE Clinical Guideline 25, Royal College of Nursing, London.
69. Steinert, T., Bergk, J., Bosch, S. et al. (2010) *Therapeutische Massnahmen bei aggressivem Verhalten – DGPPN S2-Behandlungsleitlinie*, Springer, Berlin.

# Section 2

## Legal aspects of coercive treatment

# 6 Psychiatry and the law – do the fields agree in their views on coercive treatment?

## Julio Arboleda-Flórez

*Queen's University, Department of Psychiatry and Department
of Community Health and Epidemiology, Kingston, ON, Canada*

## 6.1 Introduction

Coercion is an essential element of psychiatric treatment and interventions. Legislation in many jurisdictions contemplates it as a legitimate form of patient management through clearly specified parameters for involuntary admission and specifications for the use of restrictive treatments. A trend in the past years has been to widen the parameters required for commitment, thus extending coercive elements of psychiatric treatments to less immediate situations not necessarily leading to admission to a psychiatric facility, such as in assertive community treatment strategies and, most pointedly, as in community treatment orders. Elements of coercion may be observed at all levels of psychiatric interventions from 'voluntary' acceptance of treatment when this is more or less forced by expectations from others, usually the relatives, to psychological pressures, or in the outright use of physical force to submit to treatment. Coercion is an integral part of psychiatry, so much so that it could even be used as its defining element. Szasz, for example, rather

*Coercive Treatment in Psychiatry: Clinical, Legal and Ethical Aspects*, First Edition.
Edited by Thomas W. Kallert, Juan E. Mezzich and John Monahan.
© 2011 John Wiley & Sons, Ltd. Published 2011 by John Wiley & Sons, Ltd.

hyperbolically stated that 'psychiatry is the theory and practice of coercion' [1]. More to the point, he added that the diagnoses of mental conditions are rationalizations of coercion so as to justify medical treatments and interventions supposedly aimed at protecting the patient from him or herself, and society from the patient. For Szasz, therefore, coercion is the essence of psychiatry.

In this chapter, coercive interventions will be considered from the point of view of legal mandates and a balance, between the needs for protection of the individual and the public, and the preservation of individuality and autonomy. The ethics of coercion will be reviewed from a point of view of human and civil rights, both negative and positive rights of mental patients. This chapter is, therefore, dedicated to a review of the theory of coercion and its applications, with a special section on the case of coercive intervention in forensic psychiatric practices.

## 6.2   Definition

Coercion is the act of exercising power, defined as an agent intentionally influencing the behaviour of others. The agent could do this by persuasion, but if this fails, the agent can make the other person do it against their will, by trickery, intimidation, threats, force or extortion. It may involve infliction of physical or psychological pain in order to enhance the credibility of the threat, as in the extreme case of torture. The aim of coercion is to seek cooperation or obedience in the coerced as well as to send a message to those who support them. Coercion is closely related to the exercise of power. In fact, power can be exercised in a threefold fashion – either immanently as a felt essence that is used to overcome resistances; by implying the possible use of persuasion, manipulations, coercion, compulsion, pressures, constraints; or by resorting to the actual use of duress, force and violence.

Coercion theory resulted from the larger behavioural perspective of social learning theory. Sidman reminds us that we use coercion almost exclusively to control each other [2], and he traces the origins of coercion theory to Patterson, who developed it to explain interactions in family dyads in which aversive action affects either the performance of the other person or the performance of the target subject. Patterson insisted that for a behaviour to be labelled 'coercive' it must not only be aversive, but should consistently follow specific behaviours, and should produce a consistent reaction in the victim that ultimately serves the aggressor [3].

Coercion is, then, an overt manipulation of behaviour whose main characteristics are the intention of the coercer to coerce and the simultaneous presentation of an offer and a threat. That is, coercion works via a bi-conditional proposition composed of making, at the same time, a threat and an offer with motivation and intentionality to coerce being a *sine qua non* in the coercer. On the other hand, the coerced has freedom to choose a course of action between the threat and the offer, but in this situation, whichever way the person chooses, he or she will come out the loser [4]. An example of this situation is the simple proposition 'you can go and play after you do your homework', which carries the offer of permission to play, but also the implied threat that this will be denied if homework is not done. If the child goes to play without doing the homework, there will be repercussions and the child will be the loser; if, on the other hand, he does the homework first, the child is denying himself the enjoyment of his preferred choice, so the child again is the loser.

The field of action for the coerced is limited within the dyadic relationship as described by Patterson. However, the relationship is, rather, a triadic one, in which the coerced is caught between him or herself as agent, the object of the person's choice, and all other agents, many of whom may be intent on exercising power through threats to prevent the coerced from making his or her choice of objects. It follows that, in any situation, a set of feasible choices can be obtained by the presence of two elements: an *initial endowment* or original state of the world which the person wishes to change, and *transformation rules*, which is the action that could be undertaken to effectuate the desired change or which others could apply to prevent the change. Coercion, then, may take place by manipulating either of these elements.

Within a hypothetical continuous set of social circumstances, coercion would be found at the opposite end to freedom, as the latter is a state of not being constrained and of being able to act with free will. In a state of complete freedom, there would not be political forces that intimidate, threaten or use force to prevent such expression of free will. However, if freedom is defined in positive terms as 'consisting of being one's own master', then, by following orders, freedom is coerced. If, on the other hand, freedom is defined in negative terms as consisting of 'not being prevented from choosing as others do' [5], then, again, orders to abstain from doing what one desires are coercive.

While the expression of free will and the use of freedom are usually factors of state policies in democratic nations, unfortunately, their expression also depends to a large extent on entitlements and other social determinants such as social and economic arrangements that include education, shelter and health care [6]. If the full expression of life is constrained by such social calamities as abject poverty, disease and short life spans, the person may just be subsisting instead of living. Thus, referring to people living in extremely impoverished countries, Farmer reflects on how difficult it would be to imagine how restricted the lives of many human beings are and what little living they would be able to manage in such circumstances [7].

Yet, abject poverty and extremely trying situations to eke out a living are not seen only in impoverished countries, for those conditions are not attached solely to geography, but to levels of income. In all countries, including those in the developed world, pockets of subpopulations go hungry, have no shelter and lack proper health care, as happens often in the case of the mentally ill, whose vulnerabilities span the spectrum of distress [8]. In these cases, vulnerability is defined as the characteristic displayed by an individual or group of persons when judgement and decision-making capacity have been compromised, and cannot be exercised, by virtue of some incapacity or position in life. More specifically, vulnerability is '. . .a substantial incapacity to protect one's own interests owing to such impediments as lack of capability to give informed consent, lack of alternative means of obtaining medical care or other expensive necessities, or being a junior or subordinate member of a hierarchical group.' [9] The Law Commission of the United Kingdom proposed that a person is vulnerable if 'by reason of old age, infirmity or disability (including mental disorder) the person is unable to take care of himself or to protect himself from others.' [10] Many individuals or groups of persons could be considered vulnerable, but the mentally ill, as a group, easily stand out amongst them both because of the vulnerability resulting from their condition, the related effects of unemployment and poverty, and the social distancing imposed by others in the form of stigma and discrimination [11]. Under these conditions it would not only be difficult to manage the exercise of free will and to enjoy fully the experience of freedom, but also the circumstances would expose the person to being the victim of extortions, manipulations and coercion.

Coercion could be used for beneficial reasons, as in education, in which case it has an altruistic reason, but it may also be a response to selfish interests on the part of the teacher–coercer. Coercive tactics may also be seen at work in religious and political indoctrinations. Coercion might be imposed via psychological means through the use of manipulations, by physical means via force and torture, or by economical means via deprivations.

In Law, being coerced is akin to acting 'under duress' or because of 'undue influence' and, of late, coercion is equivalent to a crime of 'extortion'. In the case of a victim, if the threat is substantial, coercion can be used as a defence with two possible meanings – when the victim was compelled by force of authority to do something, or when actual force was used on the victim to cause him or her to do something (compulsion) the person would not otherwise do.

Coercion could also be conceived as a form of exercising social influence via the use of intentional power exercised either through authoritative requests, persuasion, inducements, threats, offers, or actual use of force.

## 6.3   On rights

Coercion is an intrinsic element in human relations. Those at a certain level of authority seek to explain their commands and seek the support of the others, but there is no doubt amongst the others that if orders are not followed or requests are not acquiesced to, or obeyed, there will be negative consequences. Thus, coercion works either through persuasion or through imposition, and it is the opposite of freedom, however defined, whether in positive or negative terms.

In psychiatry, even when the patient enters into treatment voluntarily, there is always the open or veiled threat that imposition of coercive measures is a possibility and, sometimes, even a probability. Coercion is an ever-present characteristic of psychiatric interventions. The limitation on the freedom to choose has impacts on the person's ability to exercise his or her individual rights, whether these are negative or positive rights.

Negative rights are those held by the individual on a guarantee that the state, at least in well-developed democracies, has no right to prevent the person from their enjoyment, to interfere with them in any way or form, or to abrogate them unless there are good legal reasons; those rights are inalienable. To the contrary, positive rights are those that the state provides as perks of citizenship and according to circumstances and the financial ability to pay for them. Negative rights go to the issue of liberty, while positive rights pertain to aspects of living as comfortably as possible.

A more comprehensive list of these rights would include the classical negative rights (autonomy, bodily integrity, liberty and property) along with equality and non-discrimination, freedom from inhuman and degrading treatment and a least-restrictive environment. Such a list will also include positive rights such as adequate food and shelter; health together with timely access to quality mental and physical health care and services; the right to involvement in planning and decision-making and policy and management within the health system; the right to treatment and to refuse treatment; voting rights; driving rights; rights to own and use property; right to expression of sexuality, marriage and reproduction; right to social inclusion and community integration; right to housing or shelter, to employment and safe working conditions; right to education and training; right to control of personal and financial affairs and to insurance and social security; right to information and participation; right to legal counsel and access to courts, and appropriate protection, care and treatment of mentally ill offenders [12].

## 6.4   Coercion in psychiatry

There is inevitably a relationship between the freedoms and rights as listed above and the extent of the use of powers, especially powers to restrict, and policies and procedures of a coercive nature as seemingly needed in psychiatric institutions and forensic psychiatry facilities.

Coercion has been a constant of psychiatric interventions since antiquity where, according to prevailing beliefs about the nature of mental illness [13], mental patients were usually placed at the mercy of the state, in person and their properties, or were sent to dungeons, placed in chains or banished from their homes and towns [14].

In more modern times, mental health reform efforts have been successful at substituting a deinstitutionalization model for the custodial model of imprisonment in asylums, sometimes for life, that was originally developed to manage the mentally ill. More recently, the deinstitutionalization model has also given way to a recovery model in which it is expected that the person will return to a previous, higher functioning level and different station in life. The recovery model, however, has already been implicated in coercive practices because it is prone to placing expectations and demands to perform on the threat that if the person does not meet the expectations, he or she will be cut off, for example from social welfare benefits, that is to say from enjoyment of his or her positive rights.

Historically, the mental health system has had variable levels of coercion ever since its inception in the 1800s. The system, however, and its associated coercion, has gone through multiple stages of reform as it has expanded and become more entrenched in the social dynamics. Easier access to services and the community relocation of the mentally ill have made deinstitutionalization a reality in many communities, but not without some misgivings. Citizens often complain about the mentally ill sleeping in the streets or begging, and neighbourhoods have objected to halfway houses being constructed in their midst, a social phenomenon sometimes referred to as NIMBY – Not in My Backyard.

The mental health system from the late 1800s to the 1970s was based on a basic bipolarity of options, consisting only of either jail or mental hospital. Such a situation was captured pointedly by Penrose, who in 1939 was able to demonstrate that, in European countries, criminality rates and numbers of psychiatric facilities were inversely related (Penrose Law). His 'balloon theory' proposed that, as the number of mental hospital beds increased, beds in prisons decreased and vice versa [15]. Note that Penrose was simply stating a statistical relationship and that he did not enter into speculations of the aetiological relationship between criminality and mental illness. However, conditions in his time may have been more humane at the jails than at the old asylums, where coercive measures ranged from mind games and psychological warfare to outright sexual and physical abuse and even treatment abuse via electroshock therapy. Such abuses were also made easier by the location of these institutions in remote, far-away rural communities that produced major life dis-locations for patients who were removed from their families, friends, jobs and surroundings. In time, the institutions became veritable *snake pits* [16]; patients became disenfranchised and 'institutionalized' as a response to the bureaucratic structures and as a psychological defence against the suffering usually inflicted by the very staff that had been hired to look after them and to protect them [17]. The appalling conditions of old asylums and the sadistic characteristics of some of the staff in them have been well depicted in books and in memorable movies [18]. Some of these books and films are part of the record of one of the darkest moments in the history of psychiatry.

Originally in America, the asylums were a solution as a response to the abuses that chronically ill insane persons suffered in the county poorhouses. The inhumane conditions in such places led Dorothea Dix to mount a crusade for the development of the asylums [19]. It did not take long for these new structures, unsupervised and away from public scrutiny, to become places also where abuses of every kind were rampant. This situation gave impetus to the movement for community psychiatry in the 1960s and to a call to close the asylums and replace them with a more open and responsive system where patients came first, not the staff. Alas, sadly this has not happened, to judge by every kind of reported abuse even to our day, both in formal institutions and in community agencies.[1]

The problem seems to relate to the closed nature of these mental health agencies, to a lack of supervision by government departments and to a lack of outside public surveillance of the practices of the staff in agencies charged with the care of vulnerable persons who, by definition, do not have the ability to speak for themselves, or to physically protect themselves. Children in orphan homes, the mentally disabled, the physically handicapped, the elderly and the mentally ill are the groups most vulnerable to these depredations.

The beginning of deinstitutionalization in the 1960s led to the hospital initiatives such as development of open door psychiatric units to work in close cooperation with community-based mental health agencies and services. Concomitantly, these developments led to an increase in the involvement of legal and correction agencies which, then, became part and parcel of the mental health system. Deinstitutionalization has been credited with the transmigration or returning of large numbers of mental patients to prisons through specialized court hearings, which, in turn, has contributed to the emergence of forensic psychiatry as a major subspecialty. Forensic psychiatrists, unlike other psychiatrists that tend to stay as far away as possible from these systems, have become the systems brokers – superspecialists that feel comfortable either in the hospital forensic units, in a court of law or at the psychiatric infirmary at the prison.

Although the high level of mental and physical abuse of patients has moderated considerably, coercion in the era of admissions to psychiatric units in general hospitals has remained a concern. General hospital psychiatric units were designed with the purpose of making psychiatric hospitalizations easier to access in the patient's own community, and to take a more holistic approach to the health of the patient because of easy access to medical support from other departments and specialties to provide consultations on request. General hospital psychiatric units were also conceived as a way to minimize the stigma associated with mental hospitals, with their long periods of internments and commitments. In these units, however, in line with its paralegal functions, coercion would be imposed 'under duress', via civil commitment that impacts on the negative rights to liberty, freedom of expression, freedom from fear and inviolability of the person, in case forced injectable medications are required to calm down the person. In many jurisdictions, committed persons temporarily lose their rights to manage their own financial affairs.

Coercion is experienced even on entrance at the emergency department. Emergentologists perform the first screening on seriously and severely disturbed suicidal or violent patients before calling in the psychiatrist. An initial approach with these patients would be to negotiate admission on a voluntary basis – a persuasion definition of coercion – on the unstated premise, however, that if the patient does not come in voluntarily, commitment powers would be invoked.

In community psychiatry, while working with patients who do come in voluntarily to receive medications and psychotherapy, the veil of coercion does not pale, but is always present in the form of 'throffers' [20], defined by Steiner as a mix of 'threats' and 'offers'. These are manipulations whereby patients accept 'arrangements' for housing, finances, or other social services in exchange for cooperation on where to live and with whom they may associate; they also have to acquiesce to report every two weeks for injectable, long-acting, antipsychotic medications. Assertive community treatment teams and mobile crisis teams often use 'throffers' as bartering chips to develop or increase compliance with treatment. 'Throffers' have multiple implications in regard to coercive mechanisms from implicit curtailments of freedom to ascription of vulnerability. The former would include threats to personal autonomy, instilling fear in regard to a potential loss of freedom, an increase of dependency with mistrust of one's own capabilities to manage the business of living and, hence, an increase of feelings and attitudes of helplessness. The ascription of vulnerability overrides the principle of equality between the partners, constitutes an invasion of privacy and impacts on the positive rights of individuals.

'Throffers' are a form of social engineering, without which deinstitutionalization, the *sine qua non* theoretical foundation for community psychiatry, would have not worked. Even so, deinstitutionalization requires an array of community agencies working in close liaison with a multitude of other agencies, many of which relate to forensic psychiatry and whose *raison d'être* is social control, hence coercion.

Psychiatry is well known for its interest in shackling the minds if thoughts and expressed ideas do not fall well within the orthodox political or religious constructions of the time. Rhoda Roe, Virginia Wolf, Louis Riel[2] and Ezra Pound are just some names that quickly come to mind as having been 'railroaded'. In the process, creativity could be mangled. Would van Gogh have produced *Starry Night* if he had been given electroconvulsive therapy?

However, if diagnostic manoeuvres carry a large potential for coercion, no less is to be found in treatment and therapeutic interventions. For many patients, just the threat of being subjected to electroconvulsive therapy is therapeutic enough to at least make them behave better. This treatment is worse if it is without anaesthesia, as still happens in many countries, or for the purpose of 'depatterning'[3] the mind. Often, psychiatric hospitalization is tantamount to imprisonment, especially if the hospitalization is via commitment. Isolation, sometimes in a padded cell, carries a major threat of coercion, whether it is for therapeutic or for punishment reasons. Shackling

of the mind may come in the form of rattling the brain via electroconvulsive therapy
or through attempts at putting it to sleep as in sleep therapy. But sometimes it would
be better to simply disconnect the brain by cutting one centre from the others as
in lobotomy, or severing the thinking brain from its 'animalistic tendencies' by
extirpating the amygdalae in the hypothalamus. Sadly, psychotropic drugs also carry
a heavy potential for coercion as when used for punishment reasons or during
dubious attempts at putting the mind at rest via massive doses of these medications,
as in sleep therapy and insulin shock therapy. In many cases, consent to treatment is
no more than a perfunctory function, as often the patient lacks full appreciation of
what is being consented to.

## 6.5   Forensic psychiatry

Coercion is the tie that binds psychiatry and the law. As deinstitutionalization
became the favourite model for the social management of the mentally ill, restraints
had to be devised and put in place to protect society, a role that in the past had been
fulfilled by the mental hospital. As such, forensic psychiatry systems were necessary
and, as a result, they encroached further into general psychiatry activities. Because
of its legal clout, forensic psychiatry often dictates the parameters of action, many of
which are based on coercion. For if coercion has been a constant of psychiatric
interventions since antiquity, in forensic psychiatry it is a constitutive element.
Forensic psychiatry is by definition coercive. Patients do not come on their own to
seek help from a forensic psychiatrist, but are usually referred by a legal or quasilegal
agency with the specific purpose of conducting an assessment or evaluation and
preparing a psychiatric-legal report. While, in any other medical visitation, patients
expect the physician to offer help and to be there for them in health or disease,
patients who come to forensic psychiatrists are not usually sick in medical terms, but
afflicted in their legal management of their particular situation. The inherent
coerciveness in forensic psychiatry has made it necessary to attempt to regulate
such interventions in ethical codes and guidelines, such as in the Ten Principles of the
World Health Organization, the Declaration of Caracas of the Pan American Health
Organization or the Declaration of Madrid of the World Psychiatric Association.
Forensic psychiatrists are usually expected on first visit to provide a *caveat* to their
clients in the sense that their interventions may not result in any benefit to them and
may actually be harmful to their interests if the findings are negative. Thus, a forensic
client may lose some rights and some may even lose their freedom as a result of the
forensic intervention.

   Forensic psychiatry, defined as the interface between psychiatry and the law, is
a direct offshoot of the legal system and is the quintessential coercive system.
Forensic psychiatry is also the repository of the failures of the mental health system

and, in many ways, the last port of call for many patients. As an offshoot of the legal system, forensic psychiatry deals with problems originating in civil and in penal law. In civil law, forensic psychiatrists are frequently requested to provide assessments for controversial decisions on civil commitment regarding whether a patient represents a danger to him or herself or others, or is in need of protection that they cannot provide for themselves at the moment. In penal law, forensic psychiatrists are usually involved in the assessment of persons with severe personality disorders, dangerous offenders and dangerous sexual predators and in decisions regarding indeterminate detentions. Forensic psychiatrists and epidemiologists have carved a niche in the understanding of violence amongst the mentally ill and in the assessment, treatment (or management) of violent mentally ill individuals [21]. For these functions, forensic specialists rely on the use of risk assessments and, sometimes, profiling techniques. Risk assessments entail an in-depth review of all the materials collected on a mentally ill offender including results from specialized psychological and neuropsychological tests, medical and neurological investigations as well as social relationships. From this review a picture of the criminal emerges that could give an idea of probabilities of recidivism that could justify loosening or tightening the social controls the system believes it should exercise on the person.

A large portion of the work of forensic psychiatrists is conducted in prisons, usually in the role of evaluating defendants kept in prison (jails) while awaiting trial, for the purposes of determinations on fitness to stand trial or insanity decisions. Part of the work of forensic psychiatrists is also to look after the mental health needs of prisoners, where they provide treatment for inmates in need. However, even this medical function is tinged with elements of coercion as clinical notes are usually part of the prisoner's dossier and are of relevance when parole decisions on release are made. Treatment functions, however, are essential in prisons, given the large number of prisoners who suffer from mental conditions.

The large prevalence of mental illness amongst prisoners makes prison infirmaries appear as veritable mental hospitals [22]. Pathology amongst prisoners may predate incarceration when the mental condition was not considered a factor severe enough to have granted a finding of insanity, or it might develop *de novo* in prison as a result of the rigours of prison life. Mentally ill offenders carry a double layer of stigma and discrimination as criminals and mentally ill, and are treated differentially in the system to the point that, on exit at the end of the sentence, they might be shunted to a forensic unit at a mental hospital. Mental illness justifies further encroachments on the rights to liberty of the person, while the person is in prison and after the person has already served his dues to society. While in prison, mental patients are usually placed in solitary confinement, which increases their vulnerability to further mental deterioration and is a step-up version of coercion. On the outside, forensic psychiatry has brought an extra clout to the coercive-paternalistic traditional psychiatric approach of protecting the patient from him or herself and the public from the patient, in order to answer questions about the nature of the threat and its import; that is, what the threat is and how big it is. The threat flows from the public perception that the mentally ill are unpredictable and dangerous, and hence violent. Studies on this issue, however, have failed to prove that there is a significant risk of violence amongst the mentally ill compared to the population at large. Studies that show a moderate increase in risk amongst persons with schizophrenia have also pointed out that the risk seems to flow from the comorbidity of schizophrenia with personality disorder or the association between schizophrenia and substance abuse disorder as opposed to just schizophrenia alone [23]. If that is the case, then, the problem is more related to stigma and discrimination than to the actual need for protection against the mentally ill.

## 6.6   The ethics of coercion

Coercion is an integral part of the treatment and management techniques available in psychiatry and in law for purposes of controlling human behaviour when it runs contrary to social expectations or openly afoul of the law. The key concept is human behaviour, which when acceptable causes no problems. However, if the behaviour is not acceptable, problems develop. Human problems are usually the reason persons come on their own or are brought to see the psychiatrist, either voluntarily or under some kind of constraint. Human problems are the business of psychiatry. Understanding the reason for the misbehaviour is seldom a concern for the law, whose main function is to uphold group standards and to apply sanctions when these are breached. However, in the interplay between psychiatry and the law, courts of law have become used to looking for and seeking explanations from the psychiatrist in order to exculpate from guilt, mitigate possible sentences, or weigh factors not ordinarily brought before the court at trial. It is the role of psychiatry to provide such explanations. High-principled psychiatrists, as most profess to be, and there are always rotten apples in any basket, are not the 'whores of the courts', ready to sell their opinion to the higher bidder [24]. They are there to provide factual evidence about the mental condition of a defendant so that he or she will not be coerced into admitting guilt when there is none, denying it when there is, or using his or her mental condition as an alibi to coerce the system into letting them go with minor sanctions. However, while the mentally ill need to be protected from the abuses and the coercive manipulations of others, coercion in itself may be justified and legitimized as needed to protect the person from him or herself when severely affected by mental problems, and to protect others if the mental condition causes them to believe in a state of affairs that is not based on external, factual and confirmed evidence. In these circumstances the person may become dangerous either to themselves or to others and/or may be in need of protection. These, in fact, are the usual parameters for commitment in many jurisdictions and the reason or justification for coercive measures that may include involuntary and forced treatment.

Human problems are seldom limited to one person; they tend to impact on others, especially the family. Eventually human problems involve issues of personal responsibility and individual rights including liberty. When personal responsibility has been missing, and invoking freedom of action has been pushed to the extent of affecting others, most others claim for justice. Any recourse to justice, however, is an invitation to use coercive measures of control. It is submitted that invocation of those measures not too infrequently signals social intolerance against any type of behaviour that does not fall into the mould; as well, calling them into action does not only affect the person they are to be applied to, but they may 'boomerang' and in turn come to affect those who call on their application. In regard to coercive measures against the mentally ill, one factor that has to be considered is the frequency of these conditions. Their high prevalence is such that nobody can claim exception from mental illness until days before death, or exception for anybody in the family. Consequently, any call for coercive measures against somebody else, and for any reasons, could potentially create a precedent for legal action that could be applied to anybody later on. Yet, the paradox is that not calling for coercive measures when they are needed could be construed as a dereliction of legal duty at worst, or at least, a lack of human compassion and moral turpitude. Thus, coercion has elements of both moral ugliness and of sublime instances of human decorum. If there can never be a blanket prohibition of coercive measures in psychiatry, an open acceptance of coercion powers at the whim of anybody in charge of a group of psychiatric patients will also be unacceptable.

Soft forms of coercion such as negotiation, education and persuasion are a common thread in human interactions and in psychiatric work. They should be favoured over extreme forms, especially those that use manipulation, intimidation or force. Respect for the autonomy and human rights of persons as free moral agents should be the leading considerations before undertaking coercive measures to obtain compliance to directives. These values, however, are usually trampled upon in the hustle and bustle of busy psychiatric emergencies or at times of violent behaviours in psychiatric units. Many times these abuses result not from the problems in the immediate situation, but due to a lack of sophistication and ignorance of the issues amongst psychiatric staff. Sadly, teaching of biomedical ethics is absent in the curriculum of many medical schools for medical students or for residents, and concerns about human rights of patients seldom become a matter of rounds at any Department of Psychiatry. Would that these flaws were remedied before further outrages are perpetrated to the autonomy and personal freedoms of mental patients.

# Notes

1 Dorothy Dixon, a mentally disabled pregnant woman, died on 30 January 2008 after unspeakable abuse at the hands of Michelle Riley, coordinator at a regional centre for the developmentally disabled in Alton, Illinois; http://www.crimerant.com/?p=1548. Riley has been sentenced to 45 years in prison (8 February 2010).

2 This leader of the Métis people in Canada was affected by mental illness. Historians argue that his mental condition was used to render him ineffectual politically at the time of the expansion of English Canada into the West. His illness was used to avoid a political confrontation between Québec and Ontario at the beginning of the Canadian Confederation.

3 This is a controversial therapeutic technique in which patients are administered a large number of successive electroshock treatments supposedly for purposes of rearranging memories and 'reconstructing' the mind.

# References

1. Szasz, T. (2007) *Coercion as Cure*, Transaction Publishers, London.
2. Sidman, M. (2001) *Coercion and its Fallout*, Authors Cooperative, Boston.
3. Patterson, G. (1993) Coercion as a basis for early age of onset for arrest, in *Coercion and Punishment in Long-Term Perspective* (ed J. McCord), Cambridge University Press, New York, pp. 124–138.
4. Gorr, M.J. (1989) *Coercion, Freedom and Exploitation*, Peter Lang Publishing Inc., New York.
5. Berlin, I. (1969) *Four Essays on Liberty*, Oxford University Press, Oxford.
6. Sen, A. (1999) *Development as Freedom*, Anchor Books, New York.
7. Farmer, P. (2003) *Pathologies of Power*, University of California Press, Berkeley.
8. Arboleda-Flórez, J. and Weisstub, D.N. (1998) Ethical research with vulnerable populations, in *Research on Human Subjects: Ethics, Law and Social Policy* (ed D.N. Weisstub), Pergamon, Oxford, pp. 433–450.
9. Council for International Organizations of Medical Sciences (CIOMS) (2002) *International Ethical Guidelines for Biomedical Research Involving Human Subjects*, CIOMS, Geneva.
10. The Law Commission of the United Kingdom (1993) Mentally-Incapacitated and Other Vulnerable Adults: Public Law Protection (Consultation Paper No. 130), HMSO, London, at Section 2.29.
11. Arboleda-Flórez, J. (2005) Stigma and discrimination: an overview. *World Psychiatry*, **4** (Supplement 1), 8–10.
12. Weisstub, D.N. and Diaz Pinto, G. (2008) *Autonomy and Human Rights in Health Care*, Springer, Dordrecht.
13. Neaman, J.S. (1975) *Suggestion of the Devil*, Anchor Books, Garden City.
14. Porter, R. (2002) *Madness, a Brief History*, Oxford University Press, Oxford.
15. Penrose, L.S. (1939) Mental disease and crime: outline of a comparative study of European statistics. *British Journal of Medical Psychology*, **18**, 1–15.
16. Litvak, A. (1948) The Snake Pit (movie – Olivia de Havilland as patient Virginia Stuart Cunningham). 20th Century Fox, Hollywood.

17. Goffman, I. (1961) *Asylums: Essays on the Social Situation of Mental Patients and Other Inmates*, Doubleday, New York.
18. Forman, M. (1975) One Flew Over the Cuckoo's Nest (movie – Jack Nicholson as patient Randle Patrick McMurphy). United Artists, Hollywood.
19. Mora, G. (1967) History of psychiatry, in *Comprehensive Textbook of Psychiatry* (eds H. Freedman, L. Kaplan and H.C. Kaplan) The Williams & Wilkins Company, Baltimore.
20. Steiner, H. (1975) Individual liberty. *Proceedings of the Aristotelian Society*, **75**, 33–50.
21. Stuart, H.L. (2003) Violence and mental illness: an overview. *World Psychiatry*, **2**(2), 121–124.
22. Arboleda-Flórez, J. (2009) Mental patients in prisons. *World Psychiatry*, **8**, 1–3.
23. Stuart, H.L. and Arboleda-Flórez, J. (2001) Mental illness and violence: are the public at risk? *Psychiatric Services*, **52** (5), 654–659.
24. Hagen, M.A. (1997) *Whores of the Court*, Regan Books, New York.

# 7 Reducing discrimination in mental health law – the 'fusion' of incapacity and mental health legislation

George Szmukler[1] and John Dawson[2]

[1]*King's College London, Institute of Psychiatry, London, UK*
[2]*University of Otago, Faculty of Law, Dunedin, New Zealand*

## 7.1  Introduction

In many jurisdictions, the circumstances in which medical treatment may be provided without the consent of the patient are governed not by one uniform set of legal principles, but by several distinct legal regimes. These different legal regimes tend to operate in parallel, and a patient may be eligible for involuntary treatment under more than one at the same time, but different legal standards govern their use, and they draw upon different sources of law.

Moreover, it is also common for different legal regimes to cover the involuntary treatment of different medical conditions. Notably, different regimes may cover the involuntary treatment of so-called 'physical' and 'mental' conditions. In the common law world, as in England for instance, mental health legislation (or civil

*Coercive Treatment in Psychiatry: Clinical, Legal and Ethical Aspects*, First Edition.
Edited by Thomas W. Kallert, Juan E. Mezzich and John Monahan.
© 2011 John Wiley & Sons, Ltd. Published 2011 by John Wiley & Sons, Ltd.

commitment) tends to be the preferred regime covering the involuntary treatment of psychiatric disorders, whereas an adult guardianship (or incapacity) scheme, or general judge-made principles governing situations of medical 'emergency' or 'necessity', tend to be the preferred legal vehicle for authorizing involuntary treatment of general medical conditions. Different legal criteria apply to use of the different schemes. The criteria governing involuntary treatment under mental health legislation will usually incorporate some concept of 'mental disorder' or 'mental illness', plus some notion of 'dangerousness' or 'risk' (to the patient or others), while the law governing involuntary treatment of general medical conditions usually relies mainly on the concept of the 'incapacity' or 'incompetence' of the patient to make necessary treatment decisions, plus the notion of the 'best interests' of the patient.

The aim of our 'fusion' proposal, discussed in this chapter, is to question the adequacy of this general legal situation. We argue that these arrangements discriminate unfairly against people with mental disorders, by subjecting them to less favourable treatment under the law, and that this situation should be remedied by fusing together a number of these separate legal regimes into a single, comprehensive involuntary treatment statute. This would apply to all people who lack decision-making capacity, regardless of its cause or setting. We will examine the general legal context in which such fusion must be considered and then describe in some detail the key potential provisions of such a fused statute. Finally we discuss some possible objections to the fusion proposal.

## 7.2   How does mental health legislation discriminate?

A patient with a 'physical disorder' such as cancer may refuse treatment even if the disease is life threatening. UK courts, and other common-law jurisdictions in Western countries, set a very high value on the 'autonomy' of the individual (in the sense of being able to determine what shall be done to one's body). The courts have ruled that a mentally competent patient has an absolute right to refuse to consent to medical treatment for any reason even where the decision may lead to his or her own death. We accept the individual's decision unless there is reason to believe that the patient's decision-making capacity is impaired. Paternalistic interventions in medicine (with the notable exception of psychiatry) that override the individual's autonomy are only allowed when (i) a patient lacks the mental capacity to make treatment decisions for himself or herself, and (ii) treatment is in the person's 'best interests' [1] .

Capacity involves the patient's ability to understand and retain information about the nature of the treatment and the consequences of accepting it or not, and to use and weigh up that information so as to arrive at a choice. 'Best interests' attempts to determine what the patient might have chosen in this situation if he or she had capacity, based on past statements (as in an advance statement) or according to those who know the patient well. When a future period of incapacity is predictable, a patient may also appoint a person to take health care decisions on his or her behalf according to stated preferences or principles. The patient's values are thus given weight, important in a multicultural society.

### 7.2.1 The anomalous position of mental illness

In contrast to impairment in decision-making by patients with 'physical disorder', under the mental health legislation of many jurisdictions (such as the Mental Health Act 1983 (MHA) in England and Wales), which permits the detention and non-consensual treatment of those with 'mental disorder', capacity plays little role in decisions to initiate psychiatric treatment against a patient's wishes.[1] The MHA allows involuntary treatment if the person is suffering from a mental disorder (very broadly defined); the disorder is of 'a nature or degree which makes it appropriate... to receive medical treatment'; and, treatment is 'necessary in the interests of the health or safety of the patient or for the protection of other persons' (Section 7.3).

Staying with the health or safety of the patient for the moment, compared with the tests for those with 'physical disorders', the criteria for the involuntary treatment of 'mental disorders' fail to respect the autonomy of the patient. The patient's reasons for rejecting the treatment are not required to be explored (as they must be in determining capacity), nor is the question of whether treatment is in the best interests of the patient. The key considerations are the presence of a mental disorder and risks to the patient's 'health or safety', presumably from the perspective of the clinician or treatment team (or other representatives of society), not the patient's. But we accept that patients with physical disorders, provided they have capacity, can make decisions that may be seriously detrimental to their health or safety. For persons with capacity, their personal values are given dominion. Those with mental disorder are not accorded this privilege.

There seems to be an underlying assumption in legislation of this kind that 'mental disorder' necessarily entails mental incapacity, so the question does not need to be asked, and that the values espoused by a person with a disordered mind are not to be taken seriously in determining where their best interests lie. By failing to respect the mentally disordered patient's autonomy; by not presuming capacity unless there is reason for doubt; by assuming that mental disorder entails incapacity; and by enshrining these prejudices in legislation which applies uniquely to those with 'mental disorder', current mental health legislation discriminates against those with mental disorders and serves to stigmatize them.

### 7.2.2 Treatment for the protection of others

Just as discriminatory as those aspects of mental health legislation that refer to the safety of the patient are those referring to the 'protection of other persons'. People

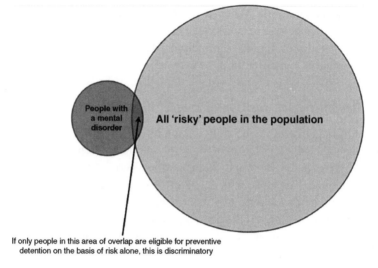

People with a mental disorder

All 'risky' people in the population

If only people in this area of overlap are eligible for preventive
detention on the basis of risk alone, this is discriminatory

**Figure 7.1**    The relationship between mental disorder, risk and liability to preventive detention.

with mental disorders are unusual in being liable to detention (in hospital) because they are assessed as presenting a risk of harm to others, but before they have actually committed an offending act. This is best illustrated diagrammatically in Figure 7.1. Those people in the area of overlap between the circles, representing those with mental disorders and those who are judged 'risky', can be detained under legislation such as the MHA on the basis of risk, not on the basis of an offence. This constitutes a form of preventive detention to which our society, in other contexts, has had an aversion on civil liberty grounds. Such hospital disposals are available both under civil and forensic provisions of the legislation.

Mental health legislation often confuses paternalism and the protection of others. They are quite separate ends; the former is concerned with the health interests of the patient and empowers others to act when the patient lacks the capacity to act in his or her best health interests, while protection of others turns on the risk of harm. This risk may not have much to do with a patient's capacity to make treatment decisions. If a patient lacks capacity and treatment is in his or her 'best interests', non-consensual treatment is, on our account, justified. Whether there is a danger to others or not would have no relevance if the person has capacity. For the person without capacity it would be taken into account in 'best interests' considerations and might prompt particularly urgent action to ensure the safety of the patient and others.

Let us assume for the moment that dangerousness is reliably linked to an individual's mental disorder and further that some form of 'treatment' will reduce the risk. If the patient *has* capacity, can we say that danger to others provides an ethically acceptable reason for compulsory treatment? Our argument would suggest that if involuntary 'treatment' is to be imposed under these circumstances, no health interest for the patient may be served – the person with capacity is usually regarded as the best judge of what is in their best interests. Protection of the public would thus be the sole interest.

Figure 7.1 shows an overlap between two populations – people with a mental disorder and people who present a risk to others. Let us imagine that everyone in the larger circle of Figure 7.1 presents an equal level of judged risk. Why, as is commonly the case, should the person with a mental disorder (who has capacity) be more liable to be detained on the basis of that risk than the person without a mental disorder? If preventive detention is to be allowed for the mentally disordered solely on account of their risk to others, if we are to avoid discrimination, so should it be for all of us. Thus fairness demands that all those presenting an equal level of risk to others (that is, all those in the larger circle in Figure 7.1) should be equally liable to detention.

This of course amounts to a generic dangerousness or preventive detention provision against which many will recoil. But the principle of non-discrimination requires that either we have generic legislation applicable to all of us; or that we have no preventive detention for anyone, including those with mental disorder.

Why has this prejudicial situation arisen and why is it so rarely challenged? It presumably reflects deeply ingrained fears of the mentally ill and stereotypes of dangerousness that are so inherent in 'folk' notions of mental illness that their uncoupling is not even thought about.

But this is a dangerous situation. There is a tendency for societies to try to expand the 'mental disorder' circle to include people with various socially undesirable behaviours. This potential is clearly demonstrated in proposals under which the application of a state-defined 'diagnosis' ('dangerous severe personality disorder') and an ascription of risk has been argued to be sufficient to detain someone, even in the absence of a previous violent offence or the possibility of effective treatment [2]. Persons with mental disorder do not receive the protections from preventive detention that the rest of us do. Mental health legislation denies such protection, thus reinforcing an underlying stereotype that the mentally ill are inherently dangerous. It is therefore stigmatizing.

### 7.2.3   Compulsory treatment in the community

As the locus of treatment has shifted from hospital to community and concerns about non-adherence to treatment have grown, many jurisdictions have introduced involuntary treatment in the community. This has been a controversial measure. If a patient lacks capacity and treatment is in his or her best interests (and can be given effectively and safely), our analysis suggests no ethical objection to the treatment being given in the community rather than in a hospital. But non-consensual treatment should end when the patient recovers capacity. This is especially important in the use of outpatient commitment to prevent relapse in patients with a history of persistent noncompliance. Such orders may be prolonged, for months if not years. Clear criteria for terminating the order are essential. In our framework, the criteria for termination of the order would be based on recovery of capacity to make treatment decisions (or, if incapacity continues, the compulsory treatment no longer being in the best interests of the patient).

Following on from the earlier discussion of 'protection of others', involuntary treatment in the community for patients with capacity, for the protection of others, is unjustified on any health interest basis. This is especially important given increasing expectations from the public that they should be protected from disturbing persons whom they see as threatening.

### 7.2.4    The need for a generic approach

Thus we conclude that conventional mental health legislation, as in England, discriminates against people with mental disorders. It reflects stigmatizing stereotypes. Autonomy is not respected; preventive detention is unfairly applied to this group. The 'two-track' approach, one set of rules for the mentally disordered and another for the rest of medicine, is inconsistent with the principles of health care ethics and with basic notions of human rights, especially freedom from unnecessary discrimination in the law. Some other form of legislation is thus required.

It is for these reasons that we propose a single comprehensive statute that 'fuses' the strengths of capacity-based regimes with those of civil commitment regimes. In this statute, there would be no need for specific reference to 'mental disorder'. Nor would there be any need for a separate legal regime focused solely on involuntary psychiatric treatment. We could operate one comprehensive involuntary treatment regime based on a functional capacity test, like the one found in Section 7.2 of the Mental Capacity Act 2005 for England and Wales, that requires us to assess the ability of a person to understand, recall, process and weigh relevant treatment information, and their ability to communicate treatment decisions.

In our view, there is little evidence that impairment of patients' capacity differs in any essential respect in mental and physical disorders. In both cases, some impairment or disturbance of mental functioning is the cause of the patient's incapacity, and we believe legal criteria that are sufficiently inclusive to cover the full range of situations can be devised. We have therefore made proposals for the design of such a comprehensive involuntary treatment statute for England and Wales based on a general incapacity test [3], and (with Rowena Daw) we have now drafted a full model law to show that those proposals can be given practical expression [4,5].

However, before proceeding to a description of its provisions, a number of contextual considerations are necessary, particularly for the reader who may not be familiar with UK law.

## 7.3    The 'fusion' law proposal in context

A model law such as we are proposing must, of course, be designed in a manner that would permit its proper integration, or fit, with wider features of the legal system in the jurisdiction in which it would operate. Thus, any model, comprehensive, involuntary treatment statute would have to mesh with the surrounding legal matrix governing regulation of the health professions, the operation of forensic mental health care, the structure and procedures of the courts or tribunals through which involuntary treatment decisions would be reviewed, ruling conceptions of human (or civil) rights, and so on. All these features of the legal system will have their own history and may be undergoing simultaneously their own process of development and review.

Designing a comprehensive involuntary treatment statute within this shifting environment is a challenging task, yet any model law must be designed for a particular jurisdiction, with a particular legal fabric and history. So our proposals have been designed for England (and Wales), but they have been influenced by significant developments that have taken place in recent decades that have altered the shape of English medical law.

Since the mid 1980s, many important developments have occurred in England in the law governing treatment without consent, and we have had to take these into account. Firstly, during this period, greater judicial attention was paid to the common law doctrine of 'necessity' as a justification for the treatment of patients who lack the capacity to consent.[2] Then, in the mid 1990s, the Law Commission issued its proposals for the enactment of comprehensive legislation governing the treatment of incapacitated patients [6]. These developments focused attention, in many fields of medical care, on the need to assess patients' capacity to consent, and led eventually to the enactment by the UK Parliament of the Mental Capacity Act 2005 (MCA). This Act provides a general legal regime governing substitute decision-making for patients who lack the capacity to consent (a regime which might be called an adult guardianship or conservatorship scheme in other jurisdictions). It also incorporates into legislation (in Part 1) the common law doctrine of 'necessity' (or emergency) as a justification for treatment without consent, which had been under exploration by the courts.

Secondly, from the late 1990s, attention began to turn to the need to reform the mental health legislation for England and Wales: the Mental Health Act 1983 (UK) (MHA) [7]. Two prominent issues in this law reform process were the proper scope of the definition of 'mental disorder' in the legislation, and whether involuntary psychiatric treatment should ever be authorized when the patient retains the capacity to consent.

By the early 2000s, therefore, proposals for both new incapacity and new mental health legislation were proceeding in tandem, and reform was being contemplated of the law governing the involuntary treatment of both physical and mental conditions. Discussion therefore began about the possibilities for rationalizing or integrating the provisions of these two legal regimes. Was there really a need for two separate legal regimes? Why should different legal criteria apply to the compulsory psychiatric treatment of patients who objected to their care than would apply to the treatment without consent of other medical conditions? Should not the autonomous treatment choices of all patients who retain their capacity receive equal respect under the law?

All these debates have been greatly sharpened, from the mid 1990s, by the increasing emphasis given to compliance with European human rights principles within UK law. This trend culminated in direct incorporation of the European human rights regime into the law of the UK, through passage by the UK Parliament of the Human Rights Act 1998. This Act permits complaints concerning breach of European human rights to be directly adjudicated in the courts of the UK. This development produced a significant stream of mental health litigation based on human rights grounds [8].

In a collateral human rights development, the European Court of Human Rights ruled in 2004 that it was contrary to the right to liberty protected by the European Convention on Human Rights for the staff of hospitals or rest homes to maintain complete control over the freedom of patients who lacked the capacity to consent, *even if the patient did not object* to that situation, without providing a proper process for reviewing the propriety of that aspect of their care.[3] This decision had major implications for care of the elderly and of people with learning disabilities, and the response of the UK Parliament was to enact a further legal regime, named the *Deprivation of Liberty Safeguards*, which was added to the MCA. This regime extended limited procedural protections to persons in this situation, such as the requirement that a second opinion be obtained, from an independent clinician, concerning the need for that person's liberty to be deprived.

Revised mental health legislation was also ultimately passed for England and Wales, in the form of the Mental Health Act 2007 (UK), which significantly amended (but did not replace) the Mental Health Act 1983. No general incapacity test was added, however, to the legal criteria governing compulsory psychiatric care. Some new capacity-based rules were introduced to English mental health law. The new regime of Community Treatment Orders (CTOs) that has been introduced, for instance, does not authorize the treatment without consent of outpatients who retain their capacity. But patients on CTOs may still be treated without their consent if they are recalled to hospital, regardless of their capacity, as may other sectioned inpatients under English law [9]. In the revised Scottish mental health legislation, by contrast, a modified incapacity test – one that requires significantly impaired capacity to consent on the part of the patient – has become a general legal standard governing both detention and involuntary treatment under mental health law.[4]

These legal developments as a whole have therefore significantly altered the structure of the law governing involuntary treatment in England and Wales. Nevertheless, some aspects of the law have remained stable. Many features of the mental health legislation, in particular, remain largely unchanged since 1983: notably the powers of emergency intervention and compulsory hospitalization; review of patients' compulsory status by a multidisciplinary tribunal; the need for a second medical opinion to be obtained to authorize certain intrusive forms of treatment, including the use of ECT and the long-term use of psychotropic medication without consent; and the established pathways between the criminal justice and the mental health systems that permit persons charged with or convicted of crimes to be directed into forensic care [10].

It is this total structure of the law governing involuntary treatment in England that we therefore had to take into account when designing our proposals for legislation that would have the effect of 'fusing' the MCA and the MHA into a single, comprehensive involuntary treatment scheme. This scheme would govern the treatment without consent of all medical conditions, avoiding the problematic distinction between 'physical' and 'mental' illness. These proposals recognize that many people with mental disorders retain their capacity to consent to treatment, and that the law already requires the capacity of people with mental disorders to be assessed for many purposes, including their capacity to manage property, make a will, drive a car, stand trial and so on. Our aim is to reduce discrimination against people with mental disorders, by not making psychiatric treatment, unnecessarily, the subject of special legislation, and, instead, to apply consistent principles concerning involuntary treatment across all fields of medical law.

It is not our intention in these proposals to contest many specific aspects of the current legal arrangements. We accept that many aspects of both the MCA and the MHA are valid. Our proposals are designed instead to make the different point: that these two regimes could be successfully fused into a single, comprehensive involuntary treatment scheme. That scheme could be based squarely on a test of incapacity to consent to treatment, on the part of the patient. That incapacity test could apply both to a person's *detention* for treatment purposes, and to their *treatment* without consent, and it could apply to the treatment of both 'physical' and 'mental' conditions.

## 7.4   Overview of the 'fusion' model law

The fusion proposal builds on the strengths of the two existing regimes. The MCA's strength in giving due weight to the patient's autonomy when capacity is retained is counterbalanced by a number of weaknesses. These lie in the lack of sufficient attention to powers governing emergency treatment, forced treatment and detention in hospital. But these are exactly those areas in which civil commitment schemes, such as the MHA, are strong. The use of force, and the detention and involuntary treatment of objecting patients, is clearly authorized and regulated by mental health legislation. The lack of clarity in these areas in capacity-based legislation poses a problem for the treatment of patients with 'physical disorders', as it would for those with mental disorders, who object to treatment. Patients who object to treatment but who do not suffer from a 'mental disorder' (as defined under the MHA) are not uncommonly treated under the MHA – inappropriately – because of a reluctance of clinicians to use force unless they can rely on clear statutory authority of this kind. Or perhaps, even worse, they are not treated at all even though treatment would have been in their best interests. We therefore advocate a legal regime that retains the strengths of both incapacity and mental health legislation, but still relies squarely on the incapacity of the person to make necessary care or treatment decisions as the primary justification for intervention in their life.

The model law operates on a number of levels, and is divided into several Parts. In all cases, the patient must lack capacity to consent, to be covered by the regime, but other features of the situation then determine precisely which Parts of the model law apply. These distinguishing features include whether the patient: objects to their treatment or care; is effectively detained for treatment purposes, even if they do not object; or requires 'serious medical treatment', of a kind already subject to special regulation under English law. In addition, certain provisions cover aspects of forensic mental health care.

The first level of the model law, then, provides a 'general authority' to give care and treatment to an incapacitated patient, when that patient does not object, or when emergency intervention is required. These rules cover much the same ground as the older common law justification of necessity that has been incorporated into the MCA.

The second level covers patients who lack capacity, and are effectively detained in an institutional setting, but do not appear to object. Here our model law provides procedural safeguards required in response to the decision of the European Court of Human Rights.

A third part of the model law then regulates certain 'serious medical treatments', such as the use of ECT and the long-term use of psychotropic medication without consent, which are already regulated in a similar manner by English mental health law. This Part also regulates some other medical decisions for people who lack capacity, such as withdrawal of life support and non-therapeutic sterilization, for which special forms of approval are already required by the English courts. Much of the detail here, concerning the precise forms of treatment that would be subject to special forms of approval under this Part (such as a requirement for confirmation by a second, independent medical opinion), are left to be handled through delegated legislation, that would be issued by the executive branch of government (subject to parliamentary scrutiny).

The fourth Part of the model law then establishes a regime for the compulsory treatment of objecting patients who lack the capacity to consent, regardless of the cause of their incapacity. This regime is not based on criteria of mental disorder and dangerousness, but on the patient's incapacity and best interests. It would cover all forms of compulsory treatment of such patients: that is, treatment of both 'physical' and 'mental' disorders. This Part includes many familiar features of a civil commitment regime, including powers of entry and immediate detention of the person; compulsory examination and certification of the person by qualified health professionals; a period of compulsory assessment; mandatory consultation with the patient's family and other carers; and automatic access to independent review of compulsory status before a tribunal. The process would culminate in the patient being placed under a Compulsory Treatment Order, with an initial life of six months, based on a prepared treatment plan.

The final Part concerns the special position of forensic patients, and indicates how they would be managed under a regime based principally on the concepts of incapacity and best interests, not mental disorder and dangerousness. We recognize that a limited compromise of pure incapacity principles may be required in this area, to promote the safety of other people, and that some limited reliance on the concepts of mental disorder and dangerousness may still be required in this difficult area of law. Nevertheless, we take the position that incapacity principles can still be applied through most of the forensic field.

Those are therefore the central elements of our 'fusion' proposals mapped out in our model law. These proposals are not intended, however, to provide an exhaustive regime governing the detention or involuntary treatment of people whose medical condition may produce a situation that causes others concern. In most legal systems, a range of other powers or justifications for intervention would also be available that would supplement any comprehensive involuntary treatment scheme. These might include general justifications for the use of reasonable force in self-defence, or in defence of property, or to prevent suicide or serious self-harm. They might include use of the criminal law, including laws that ban stalking, and threatening to kill, and those that permit intervention when one person *attempts* to inflict serious harm on another.

We do not intend to suggest that general legal provisions of that kind would be abrogated, or would not continue to apply, in appropriate cases, to people whose condition may – simultaneously – deserve medical attention. It is our argument, however, that the combination of such general legal regimes and a comprehensive involuntary treatment statute, based on incapacity criteria, of the kind we have described, could (with some minor exceptions for forensic patients) handle the full range of situations where treatment without consent is required, without the need for reference to 'mental disorder' in the criteria for intervention set by law.

For a more detailed overview the reader is referred to Dawson and Szmukler [3]. We have now drafted a 'model law' to demonstrate that it is possible to give practical expression to the principles underlying the fusion concept and its applicability across all patient groups and settings [4].[5]

## 7.5   Some key provisions of the model law

We provide here some details of the most important provisions of the model law – the principles, general provisions, compulsory treatment, and forensic provisions.

### 7.5.1   The principles

#### Principles of the Act

The following principles apply for the purposes of the Act:

1. A person must be assumed to have capacity unless lack of capacity is established.
2. A person is not to be treated as unable to make a decision unless all practicable steps to help the person to do so have been taken without success.
3. A person is not to be treated as unable to make a decision merely because the person makes an unwise decision.
4. An act done, or decision made, under the Act for or on behalf of a person who lacks capacity must be done, or made, in his or her best interests, except as otherwise specified. Before the act is done, or the decision is made, regard must be taken as to whether the purpose for which it is needed can be as effectively achieved in a way that is less restrictive of the person's rights and freedom of action.
5. All powers shall be exercised, and all services provided without any direct or indirect discrimination on the grounds of disability, age, gender, sexual orien- tation, race, colour, language, religion or national, ethnic or social origin, and any differences on these grounds should be respected.
6. Any compulsory detention or treatment of a person under the Act should be matched by a reciprocal duty to provide treatment and support that is likely to provide a health benefit to that person.
7. Family members, friends or partners, who provide care to patients on an informal basis, should receive respect for their role and experience and have their views and needs taken into account.

### 7.5.2   General provisions

The general provisions include a definition of 'capacity' and 'best interests', largely based on those in the MCA. However, the definition of capacity that we offer is broader, explicitly including the ability to 'appreciate' the necessary information. A person may be able to use information for some purposes yet still not be able to appreciate how the information is relevant to their predicament (this is discussed further in the final section of this chapter).

In defining the scope of the model law, reference is made to persons with 'an impairment or disturbance in the functioning of the mind'. This reference is included to ensure that the legislation is consistent with the European Convention on Human Rights. The Convention does not explicitly authorize the detention of persons who lack capacity, though it does authorize the lawful detention of persons of 'unsound mind' (Article 5(e)). We do not use the term 'mental disorder', however, because this may be interpreted as referring only to 'psychiatric' disorders.

## Scope of the Act

Except as otherwise provided, the Act applies to persons who because of an impairment or disturbance in the functioning of the mind lack the capacity at the material time to make a decision relating to their care or treatment.

## Definition of capacity

1. For the purposes of the Act a person ('P') is unable to make a decision and lacks capacity if unable:

   a. to understand the information relevant to the decision;
   b. to retain that information;
   c. to use, weigh or appreciate that information as part of the process of making the decision; or
   d. to communicate the decision (whether by talking, using sign language or any other means).

2. The fact that P is able to retain the relevant information for a short period only does not prevent P from being regarded as able to make the decision.

## Definition of best interests

1. In determining what is in the best interests of a person ('P'), the decision-maker must consider all the relevant circumstances including whether it is likely that P will at some time have capacity in relation to the matter, and if so when that is likely to be.

2. He or she must, so far as reasonably practicable, permit and encourage P to participate, or to improve P's ability to participate, as fully as possible in any act done, and any decision made, affecting P.
3. The decision-maker must consider, so far as is reasonably ascertainable:
   a. P's past and present wishes and feelings (and, in particular, any relevant written statement made by P with capacity);
   b. the beliefs and values that would be likely to influence P's decision if he or she had capacity; and
   c. the other factors that P would be likely to consider if able to do so.
4. The decision-maker must take into account, if it is practicable and appropriate to consult them, the views of:
   a. anyone named by P as someone to be consulted on the matter in question or on matters of that kind;
   b. anyone engaged in caring for P or interested in P's welfare;
   c. any substitute decision-maker appointed by the person or appointed for the person by the Tribunal;

   as to what would be in P's best interests.
5. Notwithstanding (4) above, if a clause of this Act requires the agreement of any person, that provision shall apply.
6. The principle of best interests applies to all decisions and to those participating as carers (or advocates) in decisions made on behalf of P, unless otherwise specified.
7. For the purpose of this Act a substitute decision-maker is a person who has been appointed by the person ('P') or by the Tribunal to act on behalf of P for the purposes of making decisions in relation to the care or treatment of P.
8. If all the other factors above are met, a decision may be in P's best interests although it is not in accordance with P's present expression of wishes and feelings, and although P objects to the treatment.

A 'General Authority' is then provided that permits people caring for a person who lacks capacity to do certain routine acts without requiring specific authority under other provisions. A proportionate degree of restraint of the person in their best interests is permitted under this section. Generally, where medication is to be administered over the person's objection, or to prevent harm to others, the compulsory treatment process should be initiated. Medication may only be administered using force under the 'General Authority' if it is immediately necessary to prevent serious harm to the patient.

A general requirement for consultation concerning a person's best interests applies throughout the model law, but is supplemented in different clauses by specific additional requirements.

### *7.5.3  Compulsory treatment*

Before a person is placed under compulsory care and treatment over their objection, a set of conditions must be met. These provide a proper legal basis for a person to be treated involuntarily and to be detained, if necessary, for treatment to occur.

### *Compulsory provision of care and treatment*

Application of this Part

1. This Part applies to a person ('P') if the following conditions are met:
   a. P has an impairment or dysfunction of the mind.
   b. P lacks capacity to make a decision about his or her care or treatment.
   c. P needs care or treatment in his or her best interests.
   d. P objects to the decision or act that is proposed in relation to his or her care or treatment and that decision or act is not authorized by Clause 6. [That is, the General Authority.]
   e. The proposed objective cannot be achieved in an alternative, less restrictive fashion.
   f. Treatment is available that is likely to alleviate or prevent a deterioration in P's condition.
   g. The exercise of compulsory powers is a necessary and proportionate response to the risk of harm posed to P or any other person, and to the seriousness of that harm, if the care or treatment is not provided.

2. If any of these conditions are no longer met, P shall be discharged from compulsory powers.

Illustrating the value of the 'fusion' approach, impaired capacity is a necessary condition, but the processes of emergency assessment and treatment, detention, the use of force, and compulsory treatment, are clearly regulated.

In emergency circumstances, a 'reasonable belief' that the patient lacks capacity in this sense is sufficient to authorize intervention. Suitably qualified professionals can then intervene, using similar powers to those provided by a civil commitment scheme: that is, powers of entry, detention of the person, transportation to assessment, use of reasonable force and so on.

The patient then enters a staggered compulsory assessment process, during which immediately necessary treatment can be authorized. A more structured assessment of the patient's capacity can then take place requiring a second opinion, and if involuntary treatment is to continue beyond 28 days, authorization by a tribunal. Downstream decisions about the details of treatment are required: decisions, for instance, concerning the need for their detention for treatment purposes, the appropriate place of treatment – which includes the community – the contents of the treatment plan, and the value of any continuing care.

Comprehensive review and accountability mechanisms also apply. All involuntary patients must have ready access to rights advice and to independent review of their status before a court or tribunal. A substitute decision-maker for treatment is appointed (and parameters for the patient's treatment set).

In our proposed scheme, with two minor exceptions (see below), involuntary treatment is restricted to patients who lack capacity. This does not preclude involuntary treatment for the protection of others, which is permitted in two sets of circumstances; first, where treatment for the protection of others is in the patient's best interests, and, second, where in the course of providing treatment in the best interests of the patient, there arises a risk of harm to others.

### 7.5.4   Forensic provisions

Applying capacity principles to forensic care may appear problematic since it might be seen that protection of the public may suffer as a consequence. Most of the problems are soluble if the following principles are applied. First, any mentally impaired offender with capacity who consents to their treatment could be treated in an appropriate facility (while any sentence they were under could continue to run). Second, any mentally impaired offender who lacks capacity could be treated involuntarily like any other incapacitated patient if treatment is in their best interests. Provisions for those on remand, or already in prison, usually follow these principles already.

We recognize, however, that protecting the autonomy over treatment of patients with capacity is not the only important ethical principle in this field. So some limited modification of pure capacity principles may be required in the forensic field in exceptional circumstances.

We propose two options for a person with a mental impairment or disturbance of mind who has been convicted of a *serious criminal offence*.

1. The person can be sentenced to the usual period of imprisonment, but if they were found to lack capacity and need treatment, they could be transferred to hospital for necessary care. If capacity is regained in hospital, the person has the choice of continuing treatment with consent; if not, the person would be transferred to prison for the remainder of their sentence. A person with a mental impairment sentenced in this way, who retains capacity and who would benefit from treatment in hospital, could be offered treatment, but would need to accept it voluntarily.
2. We retain the option of disposal to a compulsory treatment order without a concurrent sentence, which would deem the person to be subject to an equivalent

civil order and which would be terminated by the responsible clinician when the necessary conditions for civil patients were no longer met.

A special problem is presented by criminal defendants found 'unfit to plead' or 'not guilty by reason of insanity' who are ordered to be detained in hospital but are subsequently assessed to have capacity and refuse voluntary treatment. We propose that they might still be treated without their consent, even if they retain or regain their capacity, if certain conditions apply:

- the person has committed acts or omissions constituting a serious offence; and
- a serious mental impairment or disturbance of functioning has contributed significantly to that conduct; and
- an effective treatment can be offered that could be expected to reduce the risk of that disorder's reoccurrence.

This exception to the capacity-based principle is accepted in the model law in these narrowly defined circumstances in order to prevent harm to others. Why this inconsistency in the model law? It is almost inevitable that at some points of intersection, the different perspectives on human conduct from health care and criminal justice viewpoints will not allow tidy reconciliation. The problem arises currently where a person with a mental impairment, who has been found to have committed a serious offence (on a 'trial of the facts'), is judged dangerous, but has capacity and therefore cannot be subject under the model law to an involuntary treatment order. At the same time, such persons cannot be placed under a sentence under the criminal justice system if not convicted. The problem of forensic patients who have been found 'not guilty by reason of insanity' is of this kind. How does one deal with a person who was 'insane' at the time of the offence, has been found not guilty as a consequence, and has been directed into forensic care without the possibility of transfer to prison, but who is now assessed to have capacity, refuses treatment, and is deemed dangerous? We consider their involuntary treatment may be justified under the conditions described above.

In this manner, capacity principles can still be followed in most forms of forensic care, subject to some limited modifications of that kind that are required to respect the competing ethical principle of preventing serious harm to others.

## 7.6  Some potential objections to the model law

We have presented an outline of the rationale for, and the main features of, the fusion proposal. We have now also had the benefit of detailed commentaries on its principles and on some of the details [5]. Some of these are usefully discussed at this point.

Four major lines of criticism have been raised: the practical difficulties of using a capacity criterion; the 'exceptionalism' of mental disorders; the adequacy of protections for the public despite the forensic provisions; and, the potential regulatory burden on patients in general medical settings.

### 7.6.1   Capacity in practice

It has been questioned whether capacity criteria can be readily or reliably applied, especially in three sets of circumstances:

1. **In emergencies**
   In an emergency situation, the model law requires that the assessor determine as a first step whether there is a reasonable likelihood that the person lacks capacity. This will turn largely on whether a person behaving abnormally is able to give a coherent account of their reasons for doing so. We see no reason to believe that this assessment would be any more difficult than one that determines the person has a 'mental disorder'. Indeed we argue that such an assessment examines what is intuitively of most interest when we confront someone who is acting bizarrely – what account could they give that would make it understandable?

2. **Cognitive bias**
   An area of current debate involves treatment decisions entailing a serious risk to the patient, but where a 'cognitive' bias in the conventional criteria for capacity might lead to a mistaken conclusion that capacity is retained. It has been argued that the assessment may not pay adequate regard to emotional influences and questions of 'value' [11]. We agree that there is still work to be done on the meaning of capacity, especially in relation to what appear to be imprudent choices. Hence we propose that an 'appreciation' criterion be added to the definition which would point to a need to examine the influence of emotions and what have been termed 'pathological values'. Otherwise, despite current limitations, the evidence suggests that capacity can be assessed shortly after admission to a psychiatric ward no less reliably than following admission to a general medical ward [12,13].

3. **Fluctuating capacity**
   There are concerns that fluctuating capacity in 'mental disorders' may make capacity-based legislation problematic. In a series of studies of capacity in psychiatric patients recently admitted to hospital in which one of us was an investigator, this did not emerge as a significant observation [14]. Fluctuation of conscious level, even over the course of a day, is a well-recognized clinical feature in acute confusional states and can be taken into account in determining when capacity is stably restored. Psychoses, unless caused by an acute, organic disturbance of brain function, do not fluctuate in this manner – recovery is generally progressive. How long a period of restoration of capacity would be

required before it could be judged 'stable'? This would depend on the trajectory of recovery and involve the same kind of reasoning as in determining under current legislation how long a person should no longer present an apparent risk to their health or safety for it to be judged that such a risk is no longer substantial enough to merit ongoing involuntary treatment.

### 7.6.2   The 'exceptionalism' of mental disorder

Two types of 'exceptionalism' have been suggested, questioning the applicability of capacity-based law in respect of those with a 'mental' or 'psychiatric' disorder.

1. **The associated risk of violence**
   Some suggest that the association of mental disorder with violence makes mental illness not comparable to physical illness. Some specific points are considered below under forensic issues, but at this stage we draw attention to a more general point. Dangerousness is not a necessary condition of having a mental illness. It may be a consequence in a small minority of patients having a mental illness. The risk, in the absence of alcohol or substance misuse, or of an antisocial personality, is modestly, if at all, raised [15–17]. People with severe mental disorder perpetrate only a small fraction of serious violence in our society [18]. We must avoid the damaging stereotype of mental illness, as we discussed in the introductory section to this chapter, as somehow necessarily entailing a risk to others.

2. **Autonomy may not be the highest value in the treatment of mental disorder: beneficence may be more important**
   In this objection, the idea that, somehow, despite apparently having capacity, people with mental disorders cannot be relied upon to be fully autonomous or capable of deciding what is in their best interests, is often present in a more or less muted form. For example, it may be stated that since prison is a non-therapeutic environment for persons with a mental disorder, they should be in a hospital, even if they have capacity and choose prison over hospital.

   As discussed in our introduction to this chapter, this notion rests on the stereotype of the person with mental illness as being incapable of normal agency, and is inconsistent with the respect for autonomy shown to all other patients in medical practice. The record of doctors acting 'beneficently' in the past offers some important lessons. Patients have been subjected 'for their own good' and in good faith to what are later discovered to be damaging treatments – lobotomy, insulin coma therapy, removal of organs for 'focal sepsis'. We cannot see why persons who are capable of making decisions for themselves should be denied the privilege of doing so. They are the best judges of what is in their best interests.

   It should also be noted that the 'best interests' determination, engaged when capacity is absent, is primarily concerned with beneficence. In the model law, as in the MCA, the patient's best interests is also defined in a way that is an important advance on the notion that best interests should be based on what the doctor considers it to be. Moreover, to determine best interests, the decision-maker must take account of the medical, psychological and welfare aspects of an intervention.

It is noteworthy, therefore, that these two appeals to the 'exceptionalism' of mental disorder both rest on the negative stereotypes of the mentally ill we considered earlier – that they are dangerous and that they do not merit the respect we accord full persons.

### 7.6.3   Protection of the public

Others have asked whether the protections for the public in the model law are really adequate. In particular, the model law provides no equivalent of a 'restriction' order for a convicted person who is considered to be mentally disordered, to ensure they can be supervised and treated without consent as long as necessary, which would usually extend well beyond the period of treatment in hospital. Some see that kind of medical disposal as therapeutically beneficent since it removes the mentally disturbed person from the aggravating effects that imprisonment (or some other criminal sentence) may have on their illness.

We have outlined above the two options under the model law for the mentally impaired person who has committed a serious offence:

1. A compulsory treatment order based on capacity principles under the health care system, with no long-term option of a restriction order.
2. A criminal sentence, the duration of which is determined by the seriousness of the offence, with the additional option of:
   a. involuntary hospital treatment for the person who lacks capacity until he or she regains it, when they might continue as a voluntary patient, or, if they decide against treatment, transfer to prison for the rest of the sentence; or
   b. if the person has capacity but has a mental disorder which might benefit from treatment, voluntary treatment with consent.

But this does not mean that a person with a mental disorder deemed potentially dangerous will be discharged with no more than a referral to a community mental health service. Under the second option, the sentence might be a life sentence or one of the 'extended sentences' for persons convicted of a serious offence who are deemed to pose a risk beyond the term of a normal sentence.[6] An example, in England, is an indeterminate 'sentence for public protection'. If so, the person will subsequently be under some form of supervision in the community following discharge: for example, on a licence for life following release from a sentence of life imprisonment. Assuming that supervision does not compel treatment as one of its conditions, at the very least, the person with capacity who might be a risk to others will be regularly monitored and appropriate action could be taken if there is a relapse of illness. Involuntary treatment could be initiated if the conditions are met, or the person could be returned to court if they breach the conditions of their supervision, and then perhaps be imprisoned. In effect, this permits a person to be placed on a restriction order, but one that is non-discriminatory, as it applies to all offenders with capacity, whether or not they have a mental disorder. The objection that this form of restriction order uses the non-therapeutic framework of the criminal justice system must be set against the fact that restriction orders under mental health legislation, in England, already operate at least partly on criminal justice principles, as, in effect, a form of tariff system operates, the order's duration being influenced by the nature of the offence. Restriction orders may not therefore be as therapeutic as they may initially appear, and we maintain that the authority they provide for the indeterminate involuntary treatment of persons with capacity cannot be justified.

### 7.6.4    *The burden of new regulations in general medical settings*

Concern has been expressed that the model law imposes a set of burdensome regulations governing informal patients who lack capacity, especially those on general hospital wards, some of whom will now require an involuntary treatment order.

We argue that the model law recognizes the relevant domains that should be covered for all patients, wherever they are treated, and establishes the right principles. While in most, but not all, places the model law has followed the MCA, we agree that in the real world there are resource limitations that may need to be taken into account. The challenge is to formulate a law that is practicable so that all cases with impaired capacity can be covered by the same principles.

The domains covered in the model law can be governed by variations in a range of requirements: as to second opinions, consultation with others, advocacy, reviews, appeals and time intervals for their implementation. We believe that a combination of these requirements can be found that will be applicable across the whole range of services. If necessary, a 'lighter touch' can be adopted at some points in the original version of the model law.[7] An important contextual factor is the accreditation and inspection of health and social care institutions and our confidence in these procedures.

## 7.7    Conclusions

Mental health legislation, as currently conceived in most jurisdictions, discriminates against people with a mental illness. It carries underlying assumptions that people with such illnesses are not fully autonomous and that they are dangerous to others. Thus such legislation reinforces damaging stereotypes of people with a mental illness. By building on the complementary strengths of capacity-based and civil commitment legislation, we propose a 'fusion' of legal principles into a model law which has decision-making capacity at its centre, but which clearly defines how the use of detention and force are to be governed. This comprehensive law is designed to apply to all persons who lack capacity, from whatever cause and in whatever health care setting. We have drafted a model law which demonstrates that these principles can be given practical expression.

## Notes

1 In some jurisdictions, mental health legislation allows a mentally ill or disordered patient with capacity to refuse treatment, but such a patient may nevertheless be involuntarily admitted to hospital. In such cases it is the liability to detention that is discriminatory.
2 In re F [1989] 2 WLR 1025; R v. Bournewood Community and Mental Health NHS Trust, ex parte L [1999] 1 AC 458.
3 *HL v. UK* (2004) 40 EHRR 761.
4 Mental Health (Care and Treatment) (Scotland) Act 2003, Section 64(5).
5 The presentation of the model law is accompanied by a series of commentaries and a response to these by the authors. As a result of some of the points raised in the commentaries, a number of amendments are proposed in an addendum.
6 The Criminal Justice Act 2003 (UK) introduced extended sentences, beyond the normal tariff, for persons convicted of a range of serious offences who are judged to continue to present a high risk.
7 We have proposed some amendments along these lines in an addendum to the model law.

## References

1. UK General Medical Council (2008) *Consent: Patients and Doctors Making Decisions Together*, GMC, London.
2. Maden, T. and Tyrer, P. (2003) Dangerous and severe personality disorders: a new personality concept from the United Kingdom. *Journal of Personality Disorders*, **17**, 489–496.
3. Dawson, J. and Szmukler, G. (2006) Fusion of mental health and incapacity legislation. *British Journal of Psychiatry*, **188**, 504–509.
4. Szmukler, G., Daw, R. and Dawson, J. (2010) A model law fusing incapacity and mental health legislation. *Journal of Mental Health Law, Special Issue*, **20**, 11–22, and 101–126.
5. Szmukler, G., Daw, R. and Dawson, J. (2010) Response to the commentaries. *Journal of Mental Health Law, Special Issue*, **20**, 91–98.
6. The Law Commission (1995) *Mental Incapacity*, HMSO, London.
7. Department of Health (1999) *Report of the Expert Committee (Richardson Report): Review of the Mental Health Act*, HMSO, London.

8. Bartlett, P., Lewis, O. and Thorold, O. (2007) *Mental Disability and the European Convention on Human Rights*, Martinus Nijhoff, Leiden.

9. Dawson, J. (2010) Community treatment orders, in *Principles of Mental Health Law and Policy* (eds L. Gostin, P. Bartlett, P. Fennell *et al.*), Oxford University Press, Oxford, pp. 513–554.

10. Gostin, L., Bartlett, P., Fennell, P. *et al.* (eds) (2010) *Principles of Mental Health Law and Policy*, Oxford University Press, Oxford.

11. Tan, D.J., Hope, P.T., Stewart, D.A. and Fitzpatrick, P.R. (2006) Competence to make treatment decisions in anorexia nervosa: thinking processes and values. *Philosophy, Psychiatry & Psychology*, **13**, 267–282.

12. Cairns, R., Maddock, C., Buchanan, A. *et al.* (2005) Reliability of mental capacity assessments in psychiatric in-patients. *British Journal of Psychiatry*, **187**, 372–378.

13. Raymont, V., Buchanan, A., David, A.S. *et al.* (2007) The inter-rater reliability of mental capacity assessments. *International Journal of Law and Psychiatry*, **30**, 112–117.

14. Owen, G.S., Szmukler, G., Richardson, G. *et al.* (2009) Mental capacity and psychiatric in-patients: implications for the new mental health law in England and Wales. *British Journal of Psychiatry*, **195**, 257–263.

15. Coid, J., Yang, M., Roberts, A. *et al.* (2006) Violence and psychiatric morbidity in a national household population – a report from the British Household Survey. *American Journal of Epidemiology*, **164**, 1199–1208.

16. Elbogen, E.B. and Johnson, S.C. (2009) The intricate link between violence and mental disorder: results from the National Epidemiologic Survey on Alcohol and Related Conditions. *Archives of General Psychiatry*, **66**, 152–161.

17. Fazel, S., Gulati, G., Linsell, L. *et al.* (2009) Schizophrenia and violence: systematic review and meta-analysis. *PLoS Medicine*, **6**, e1000120.

18. Fazel, S. and Grann, M. (2006) The population impact of severe mental illness on violent crime. *American Journal of Psychiatry*, **163**, 1397–1403.

# 8 Mental health care and patients' rights – are these two fields currently compatible?

**Thomas W. Kallert**[1,2,3]

[1]*Park Hospital Leipzig, Department of Psychiatry, Psychosomatic Medicine and Psychotherapy, Leipzig, Germany*
[2]*Soteria Hospital Leipzig, Leipzig, Germany*
[3]*Dresden University of Technology, Faculty of Medicine, Dresden, Germany*

## 8.1 Introduction

Within the last three to four decades, the provision of mental health care has changed dramatically. Community-orientated services could be seen as the main conceptual framework of restructuring care for people with chronic mental illness [1]. Guided by this concept and driven by underlying intentions such as deinstitutionalization and avoiding or shortening periods of hospitalization, a broad range of new services was established. Examples include supported housing and sheltered employment in various forms, day care and drop-in centres, the diversification of outpatient departments attached to psychiatric hospitals addressing the therapeutic needs of specific disorders (e.g. schizophrenic, bipolar, obsessive-compulsive, substance

*Coercive Treatment in Psychiatry: Clinical, Legal and Ethical Aspects*, First Edition.
Edited by Thomas W. Kallert, Juan E. Mezzich and John Monahan.
© 2011 John Wiley & Sons, Ltd. Published 2011 by John Wiley & Sons, Ltd.

abuse or personality), the increasing availability of psychotherapeutic treatments, crisis intervention and self-help initiatives, and the establishment of care concepts provided in the patients' own apartments [2–6]. It must be emphasized, however, that these changes are mostly concentrated at the institutional level, and that responsibilities and staffing of these types of services, as well as their general availability, do not follow clear standards of health care planning, financing and implementation, thus leading to significant variation on a cross-regional as well as cross-national level [2,6].

These institutional innovations are accompanied by increasing scientific activities in the field of national and international mental health services research. Stimulated by the general aim in medicine of providing services or treatments guided by the highest possible level of scientific evidence, more and more randomized controlled trials (RCTs) assessing the effectiveness of complex interventions or services [7] have been conducted within the last decade. Examples of services assessed are: acute day hospital care [8], clinical case management [9], assertive community treatment [10–12], home treatment [13–15], and placement and training of people with mental illness into regular employment [16]. Results of such research are and will be increasingly integrated into regional or national mental health care plans. They also play a role in the development of best practice guidelines – a process no longer restricted to the highly important fields of innovative pharmacological and psychotherapeutic treatments, but now also including the field of psychosocial and complex interventions provided primarily in the community [15,17,18].

Further, mental health care is now also influenced by efforts to strengthen the position of the individual patients and the protection of their autonomy while being treated. This includes increasing or restoring the patients' competencies in such a way that they can act as responsible and reliable partners in the care process. One innovative development focusing on the content of best clinical practice of mental health care is the availability of a best practice standard for facilitating and structuring diagnostic evaluations in psychiatry as defined in the International Guidelines for Diagnostic Assessment [19]. This standard demonstrates a clear focus on individualization and person-centeredness (note: the importance of the last two conceptual terms for all professional activities in the field of mental health can be seen most prominently in the Psychiatry for the Person concept of the World Psychiatric Association (see Chapter 1). Other examples include the rise of the empowerment movement, the increasing importance of the concept of recovery [20], and the establishment of psychiatric advance directives [21]).

Finally, two other recent developments are influencing trends in mental health care provision at this time. Firstly, many European countries currently face an era of so-called reinstitutionalization, indicated by a rising number of forensic beds, increased long-stay placements in homes, and more involuntary hospital admissions [22]. The atmosphere of decreasing commitment to deinstitutionalization and community orientation enforces the need to monitor meticulously the potential infringement of patients' rights.

The second development, the focus on the association between health care including mental health and human rights, underscores this conclusion. A 2007 article series in *The Lancet* [23–26] demonstrates the importance of this issue for medicine in general. Using case studies from India and South Africa with a focus on HIV/AIDS patients, researchers studied the impact of including the right to health care, food, water and social security in individual state constitutions. By making these rights enforceable and binding to the state, significant public health benefits were achieved [24]. Another important issue within the Lancet series concerns the governments' responsibilities beyond the provision of essential health services to addressing the determinants of physical and mental health such as the provision of adequate education, housing, food and favourable working conditions [23]. It further demonstrates that integration of human rights in international health systems is increasingly driven by the recognition that the respect, protection and fulfilment of human rights are essential drivers for the improvement of the health status of individuals and populations. Finally, the series emphasizes that civil and political rights, such as those relating to life, autonomy, information, free movement, association, equality and participation, are as relevant to health as economic, social and cultural rights, such as education and food. Three areas in urgent need of further research were presented [23]: first, developing adequate monitoring instruments that measure both health and human rights concerns or violations; second, heeding the mounting evidence of the effects of application of health and human rights frameworks to health practice; and third, creating a research agenda to advance the understanding of the associations between health and human rights.

The field of psychiatry has also started to analyse the special importance of human rights for mental health care [27,28], in accord with the conclusions listed above. In psychiatry, at least two concerns drive the interest in human rights issues: the current trend in general medicine, and the need for in-depth historical analyses of previous severe human rights abuses in mental health care (see Chapter 10).

Within this context, this chapter addresses the following five issues concerning the intersection of mental health care and patients' rights. The chapter aims to answer the following five questions from a European perspective:

1. Are the human rights of mental health patients sufficiently guaranteed and respected? The European Convention on Human Rights, the UN Convention

on the Rights of Persons with Disabilities, and the practice of the European Court of Human Rights serve as examples to analyse if and how these rights are taken into account.

2. Do new approaches in the field of mental health care endanger patients' rights? Outpatient commitment and laws on mental health care reporting are taken as examples to answer this question.

3. Can promising initiatives for improving patients' rights be identified? Revisions of national mental health laws, the elaboration of best practice guidelines for the use of coercive measures, and the formulation of psychiatric advance directives are analysed regarding their potential to improve patients' rights.

4. Is autonomy still the supreme principle guiding recent socio-legal developments with regard to mental health care? The right of the individual patient to choose a so-called personal (financial) health care budget for chronic mental illness (as defined in the German socio-legal system) and the concept of leverage from the social welfare system are two examples examined on this issue.

5. Are there legal areas that need clearer definitions in order to respect patients' rights? The patient's freedom to choose a psychiatric hospital for inpatient care, and involuntary placement and treatment in long-stay care homes are two examples from Germany of such areas of concern.

## 8.2   Are the human rights of mental health patients sufficiently guaranteed and respected?

The analysis of this question must start with the historically important [29] Universal Declaration of Human Rights, adopted and proclaimed by the General Assembly of the United Nations on December 10, 1948 [30]. This document, constructed in the post-war era and a reference document for all subsequent Conventions of Human Rights [31–36], contains several articles of outstanding importance for clinical behaviour and practice in the field of psychiatry, as well as for the quality of mental health care and for the general position of people with mental illness in society. These include:

Article 3: Everyone has the right to life, liberty and security of person.

Article 5: No one shall be subjected to torture or to cruel, inhuman or degrading treatment or punishment.

Article 7: All are equal before the law and are entitled without any discrimination to equal protection of the law. All are entitled to equal protection against any discrimination. . .

Article 8: Everyone has the right to an effective remedy by the competent national tribunals for acts violating the fundamental rights granted him by the constitution or by law.

Article 22: Everyone, as a member of society, has the right to social security and is entitled to realization, through national effort and international co-operation and in accordance with the organization and resources of each State, of the economic, social and cultural rights indispensable for his dignity and the free development of his personality.

Article 23 (1): Everyone has the right to work, to free choice of employment, to just and favourable conditions of work and to protection against unemployment.

Article 25 (1): Everyone has the right to a standard of living adequate for the health and well-being of himself and of his family, including food, clothing, housing and medical care and necessary social services, and the right to security in the event of unemployment, sickness, disability, widowhood, old age or other lack of livelihood in circumstances beyond his control.

Article 29 (2): In the exercise of his rights and freedoms, everyone shall be subject only to such limitations as are determined by law solely for the purpose of securing due recognition and respect for the rights and freedoms of others and of meeting the just requirements of morality, public order and the general welfare in a democratic society.

The European Convention of Human Rights (04 November 1950) [31] closely refers in its content to the Universal Declaration of Human Rights. A recent analysis of the potential of this Convention to secure the human rights of people with mental disorders and disabilities concluded [37] that the European Convention is better at protecting them from unwanted or unnecessary treatment or care than it is at securing for them equal access to the treatment and care they want or need.

The UN Convention on the Rights of Persons with Disabilities (13 December 2006) [36] may be seen as the most advanced document in the series of Conventions of Human Rights in terms of the rights of people with chronic mental illness. In its preamble, this Convention expresses the concern that

despite various instruments and undertakings, persons with disabilities continue to face barriers in their participation as equal members of society and violations of their human rights in all parts of the world.

Further, the document emphasizes that

a comprehensive and integral international convention to promote and protect the rights and dignity of persons with disabilities will make a significant contribution to redressing the profound social disadvantage of persons with disabilities and promote their participation in the civil, political, economic, social and cultural spheres with equal opportunities, in both developing and developed countries.

The Convention's definition of persons with disabilities (Article 1) clearly states that this includes 'those who have long-term physical, *mental, intellectual,* or sensory impairments which in interaction with various barriers may hinder their full and effective participation in society on an equal basis with others.' Focusing on health-related issues of these persons, the following regulations in this Convention deserve special attention because they have to be guaranteed by States Parties: '. . . the identification and elimination of obstacles and barriers to accessibility, shall apply to, *inter alia*, buildings, roads, transportation and other indoor and outdoor facilities, including schools, housing, medical facilities and workplaces' (Article 9 a); further, 'States Parties shall ensure that persons with disabilities, on an equal basis with others: a) Enjoy the right to liberty and security of person; b) Are not deprived of their liberty unlawfully or arbitrarily, and that any deprivation of liberty is in conformity with the law, and that the existence of a disability shall in no case justify a deprivation of liberty' (Article 14); Article 15 outlines that

1. No one shall be subjected to torture or to cruel, inhuman or degrading treatment or punishment. In particular, no one shall be subjected without his or her free consent to medical or scientific experimentation.

2. States Parties shall take all effective legislative, administrative, judicial or other measures to prevent persons with disabilities, on an equal basis with others, from being subjected to torture or cruel, inhuman or degrading treatment or punishment

and, Article 16(4) defines that

States Parties shall take all appropriate measures to promote the physical, cognitive and psychological recovery, rehabilitation and social reintegration of persons with disabilities who become victims of any form of exploitation, violence or abuse, including through the provision of protection services. Such recovery and reintegration shall take place in an environment that fosters the health, welfare, self-respect, dignity and autonomy of the person and takes into account gender- and age-specific needs

further, 'persons with disabilities have access to a range of in-home, residential and other community support services, including personal assistance necessary to support living and inclusion in the community, and to prevent isolation or segregation from the community' (Article 19 b); and, 'States Parties recognize that persons with disabilities have the right to the enjoyment of the highest attainable standard of health without discrimination on the basis of disability. States Parties shall take all appropriate measures to ensure access for persons with disabilities to health services that are gender-sensitive, including health-related rehabilitation' (Article 25); and finally,

1. States Parties shall take effective and appropriate measures, including through peer support, to enable persons with disabilities to attain and maintain maximum independence, full physical, mental, social and vocational ability, and full inclusion and participation in all aspects of life. To that end, States Parties shall organize, strengthen and extend comprehensive habilitation and rehabilitation services and programmes, particularly in the areas of health, employment, education and social services, in such a way that these services and programmes: a) Begin at the earliest possible stage, and are based on the multidisciplinary assessment of individual needs and strengths; b) Support participation and inclusion in the community and all aspects of society, are voluntary, and are available to persons with disabilities as close as possible to their own communities, including in rural areas.

2. States Parties shall promote the development of initial and continuing training for professionals and staff working in habilitation and rehabilitation services

(Article 26).

As will be shown by several arguments, the field of psychiatry in its current state should be deeply concerned that these rights – in their complexity and comprehensiveness that clearly exceeds the issue of coercive treatments – are, at least, inadequately addressed and respected, and might even be severely endangered. Firstly, current international health policy recommendations for mental health care frameworks, while emphasizing the importance of mental health in general [38], are not as clearly orientated to respecting these rights comprehensively as they could or should be. Secondly, recent research demonstrates significant variation of legal regulations in the area of mental health laws. Thirdly, determining if and how the protection of human rights can be measured in the field of mental health care remains a work in progress. Fourthly, institutions or bodies tasked with ensuring that these rights are respected are not well known, have a low-key profile or can be difficult to access. And fifthly, authorities responsible for clinical governance are not established following a clear standard, and the impact of their reports on clinical practice is not clearly visible.

Recent trends in public mental health and in the organization of mental health service systems – at least in several European countries – could be judged as clearly contradictory to some of the core formulations in the Conventions quoted above. Examples include: the increasing numbers for days out of work and of early receipt of disability pensions due to mental disorders [39], the increasing social distance towards people with mental illness [40] and the tendency to socially exclude these individuals [41], the need for anti-stigma campaigns (see Chapter 2), the cross-national trend of reinstitutionalization as documented by increasing placements in homes and in institutions of forensic mental health care and rising rates of detained patients in psychiatric hospitals [22,42,43], and – as outlined later in this chapter – insufficient legal regulations for detainment and involuntary treatment in long-stay care units for people with mental and developmental disabilities, as well as for elderly persons with dementia or other disorders in care homes [44]. National and international recommendations for organizing or restructuring mental health care should emphasize the systematic identification of such trends and detailed measures to counteract these in order to protect and guarantee the human rights of the diverse subgroups of people with mental disabilities who are most vulnerable to human rights violations.

A high variation of legal regulations in the area of mental health laws might be seen as another source for concern in terms of patients' rights [45]. The lack of clear, internationally accepted standards for such regulations not only opens up opportunities for injustice and inequality in the field of mental health laws in general, but may also influence the important field of clinical practice as demonstrated by recent international research on involuntary hospitalization [46,47].

A standardized legal analysis of civil law issues associated with involuntary hospitalization in psychiatric establishments [48], performed within the framework of the EUNOMIA project [46], revealed major differences amongst the 12 European countries studied. Variations appeared in regard to basic conditions as well as additional criteria for involuntary admission, time periods for making decisions, the association between involuntary placement and treatment, patients' rights to register complaints, roles of relatives, and safeguard procedures of these processes.

In a prospective clinical study in 11 European countries [49] – another part of the EUNOMIA project – 2326 consecutive patients admitted involuntarily to psychiatric hospital departments were interviewed within one week after admission; 1809 were followed-up after one month, and 1613 were interviewed three months later. The outcome criterion was whether the patient viewed the admission as appropriate. In the different countries, after one month, between 39% and 71% found the admission appropriate, and between 46% and 86% after three months. Female patients, those living alone, and those with a diagnosis of schizophrenia had more negative views. Adjusting for confounding factors, differences between countries were significant. Patients' views on the appropriateness of their involuntary admission showed significant differences between sites in different countries, even when adjusted for other predictor variables. The *post hoc* comparisons showed that not all differences between sites at different countries were statistically significant, but the more substantial ones were. For example, the patients' views in England are significantly less favourable than those in Bulgaria, Greece, Spain, the Czech Republic, Italy, Germany and Slovakia, whilst patients' views in Slovakia are significantly more positive than in all sites other than those in the Czech Republic, Italy and Germany. Can the identified differences in patients' views of involuntary admission be linked to characteristics of the given legislation? There is no straightforward answer. The legislation in all countries is complex and has many features which are of potential importance. One possible criterion to classify the national regulations is the extent to which they protect the rights and interests of the patients concerned. Seven criteria that vary between countries and may be seen as relevant for the protection of the interests of the patients are as follows (note: the first option in each question is seen as more protective of the interest of the patients): (i) Is involuntary admission possible only when patients pose a risk to themselves and/or others, or also to avoid a more general threat to the patients' health? (ii) Can the admission be initiated only by authorities and medical doctors or also by other stakeholders? (iii) Does involuntary admission require the decision of a court or not? (iv) Is the period of time for which the hospital can decide to keep patients involuntarily on the wards without a formal decision for involuntary treatment shorter or longer than 24 hours? (v) Is legal support guaranteed or not? (vi) With respect to appeal procedures to independent bodies, are there binding time periods for a response, and are people and/or institutions other than the patient authorized to appeal, or not? (vii) Is the decision for involuntary treatment measures separate from the decision for involuntary admission or not? Although the answers to the questions are not always clear-cut, the authors of the study [49] established the number of criteria for each country. The resulting ranking has similarities with the order of outcomes in the multivariate analysis of this study (with the most protective legislation and most positive patient views in Slovakia and Germany, and the least protective legislation and most negative views in England), but the criteria still leave many of the differences in patients' views unexplained. Another possible factor accounting for differences could be clinical practice (the behaviour of professionals towards involuntary patients and the methods employed to support and treat them) which is likely to vary across Europe and impact on outcomes.

Measurement of the protection of human rights in the field of mental health care is an area in which empirical research has just begun, and thus data in this sensitive field is lacking. Having such measurement instruments available and used in clinical practice would enable setting-specific places and subgroups of people with mental disabilities bearing high(er) risks of human rights violations to be identified. Further, such information would stimulate the political and public debate on the need for specific improvements in health care guided by the aim to protect human rights. The following brief report on a recently completed European mental health services research project [50] illustrates the current state of a methodology being developed for reliably assessing and reviewing living situations, care and treatment practices in psychiatric and social care institutions, with a particular focus on human rights and the protection of the dignity of residents. The initial stages of development of the toolkit within this study (acronym: DEMoBinc) comprised a literature review of aspects of institutional care associated with service users' recovery and an international Delphi exercise investigating key stakeholders' views of the 'critical success factors' involved in promoting service users' recovery in these settings. The systematic review of the literature published internationally relating to quality of institutional care for people with longer-term mental health problems [51] identified eight domains that were key to service users' recovery: living conditions; interventions for schizophrenia; physical health; restraint and seclusion; staff training and support; therapeutic relationship; autonomy and service user involvement; and clinical governance. Because so few papers on the issue of human rights were found, the research group was not surprised that the protection of human rights could not be identified as a domain of its own. The international Delphi study involving 4 separate expert groups (service users, mental health professionals, caregivers, and advocates) in 10 European countries identified 11 broad domains of care important to recovery [52]: social policy and human rights, social inclusion, self-management and autonomy, therapeutic interventions, governance, staffing, staff attitudes, institutional environment, post-discharge care, caregivers, and physical health care. Developed empirically in these two stages, with an additional review of care standards in each of the 10 countries participating, human rights have finally achieved the rank of a domain on their own in the Quality Indicator for Rehabilitative Care (QuIRC) toolkit that has since been completed. Further, the instrument contains individual items which assess the potential degree of victimization or degrading treatment of individual patient groups.

The following examples from Europe underscore the current challenges and lack of prominence of institutions or bodies addressing the issues of patients' rights.

Article 1 of the European Convention for the Prevention of Torture and Inhuman or Degrading Treatment or Punishment [34], defines the mandate of the European Committee for the Prevention of Torture and Inhuman or Degrading Treatment or Punishment (CPT): 'The Committee shall, by means of visits, examine the treatment of persons deprived of their liberty with a view to strengthening, if necessary, the protection of such persons from torture and from inhuman or degrading treatment or punishment.' The CPT's members are independent and impartial experts from a variety of backgrounds. They are, for example, lawyers, medical doctors and specialists in prison or police matters. They are elected for a four-year term by the Committee of Ministers, the Council of Europe's decision-making body, and can be re-elected twice. One member is elected in respect of each Contracting State. The

CPT visits places of detention (e.g. prisons and juvenile detention centres, police stations, holding centres for immigration detainees and psychiatric hospitals), to see how persons deprived of their liberty are treated and, if necessary, to recommend improvements to States. Visits are carried out by delegations, usually of two or more CPT members, accompanied by members of the committee's secretariat and, if necessary, by experts and interpreters. The member elected in respect of the country being visited does not join the delegation. CPT delegations visit Contracting States periodically, but may organize additional 'ad hoc' visits if necessary. The Committee must notify the State concerned but need not specify the period between notification and the actual visit, which, in exceptional circumstances, may be carried out immediately after notification. Governments' objections to the time or place of a visit can only be justified on grounds of national defence, public safety, serious disorder, the medical condition of a person or that an urgent interrogation relating to a serious crime is in progress. In such cases the State must immediately take steps to enable the Committee to visit as soon as possible. Under the Convention, CPT delegations have unlimited access to places of detention and the right to move inside such places without restriction. They interview persons deprived of their liberty in private, and communicate freely with anyone who can provide information. The recommendations which the CPT may formulate, on the basis of facts found during the visit, are included in a report which is sent to the State concerned. This report is the starting point for an ongoing dialogue with the State concerned. The CPT has two guiding principles – cooperation and confidentiality. Cooperation with the national authority is at the heart of the Convention, since the aim is to protect persons deprived of their liberty rather than to condemn States for abuses. The Committee therefore meets in camera and its reports are strictly confidential. Nevertheless, if a country fails to cooperate or refuses to improve the situation in the light of the Committee's recommendations, the CPT may decide to make a public statement. Of course, the State itself may request publication of the Committee's report, together with its comments. In addition, the CPT draws up a general report on its activities every year, which is made public. To date, the Convention has been ratified by the 47 member States of the Council of Europe. Over its years of activity in the field, the CPT has developed standards relating to the treatment of persons deprived of their liberty. These standards, for example on health care services in prisons and on involuntary placement in psychiatric establishments, have been published in the brochure *The CPT Standards* ([53], see also www.cpt.coe.int). It may be because of the CPT's guiding principles, cooperation and confidentiality, that neither the detailed visit reports (282 visits as of February 2010), which include highly relevant recommendations for the improvement of services or clinical behaviour, nor the CPT Standards, which are of equal importance, have gained the high public attention or visibility they would deserve. Even in the field of psychiatry they have received little attention.

The European Court of Human Rights (ECHR), based in Strasbourg, is an international court set up in 1959. It rules on individual or State applications alleging violations of the civil and political rights set out in the European Convention on Human Rights. A recent review of the ECHR case law concerning psychiatric commitment revealed that of the almost 118 000 decisions taken by the ECHR in a 50-year period, only 108 dealt with situations concerning psychiatric commitment [54]. The most worrying conclusion was that the possibility of an individual having access to ECHR depends on the degree of democracy in his or her country and on the access to legal assistance through nongovernmental organizations or individual intervening parties.

Further results from the EUNOMIA project in 12 European countries on involuntary hospitalizations [46] illustrate the lack of clear standards for implementing the instruments or institutions responsible for clinical governance (or safeguard procedures of these processes) and that the impact of their reports on clinical practice is not apparent.

The most common authority responsible for checking and monitoring involuntary hospitalizations is a qualified Judge or a judicial Court, identified in 10 out of the 12 countries assessed [55]. In several countries other authorities play a more relevant role, however. A Public Attorney or Public Prosecutor might act as an intermediate agent between the applying family and the Judge, or assume supervising functions during the hospital stay on behalf of the Judge. Examples of this can be seen in Bulgaria, Czech Republic, Greece and Spain. In a few countries such as Bulgaria and Lithuania the health authorities themselves have taken some responsibility for this task. Paradigmatic is the case of Israel, where health professionals appointed as public officers exercise the full safeguarding and monitoring authority, though the Public Attorney might appeal the decision of the Psychiatric District Committee [56]. The institution of the ombudsman is mentioned in legislation in the Czech Republic, Greece and Sweden as a safeguarding or supervising agency, but country-specific legal reports [45] show that the practical impact does not seem to be highly significant in relation to people with mental illness admitted to the hospital against their will.

The complex, lengthy and bureaucratic procedural safeguards have been identified several times as the main explanation for the situation that emergency legal procedures (instead of the regular ones) have become the primary (and not the exceptional) method used for involuntary admissions. The Greek legal framework exemplifies this bureaucratic complexity. In that country, the Judge, the Public Attorney, and the Ombudsman, depending on the stage of the procedure, share the responsibility of supervision [57].

The general impression from these 12 European countries studied is that activities of supervising authorities are largely performed as formal routine [45]. Supervision includes checking that paperwork is completed correctly and signed, but does not stimulate or demand practical changes. Despite the complexity of the regulations, or perhaps because of them, a face-to-face interview between the person with mental illness and the supervising authority is exceptional. Changes to the patient's legal status dictated by an authority and not previously suggested by the health professionals are extremely rare. Although appeal proceedings of the patients are foreseen by most of the laws, they rarely occur.

Most of the regulations do not examine other coercive measures which might affect the patient while staying in the hospital. It seems that once the patient is placed in the hospital, the law delegates responsibility to the health professionals, and assumes that these professionals will always act in the best interest of the patient.

Another recommendation derived from this analysis would be that supervising authorities should not be established only irregularly or periodically. On the contrary, permanent and continuous mechanisms should be available to provide patients and their families the opportunity to have face-to-face interviews with both the health professionals and the supervising authorities in an effort to guarantee the correct application of legal regulations pertaining to coercive (treatment) measures. This is not only in the patients' interests. Health care providers also need to be legally protected and considered in the legislation so that they are supported by authorities supervising the correct application of legal principles.

## 8.3   Do new approaches in the field of mental health care endanger patients' rights?

Outpatient commitment (i.e. a treatment order, authorized by mental health legislation, which requires patients to comply with psychiatric treatment outside hospital) and laws on mental health care reporting serve as examples that might endanger patients' rights because – to the knowledge of the author – initiatives in these two fields recently stimulated controversial debates. One side of the discussion focuses on clear advantages for patients such as decreasing frequency of hospitalizations and significantly shorter hospital stays resulting from outpatient commitment, and an improvement of planning needs-specific community mental health services and thus better accessibility of such services as effects of regular public mental health reporting. The opposing side of the discussion emphasizes major disadvantages for patients including restrictions of personal freedom when living in the community and harm to their therapeutic relationships or an infringement of their data protection rights. Further, the heterogeneity of legal regulations on outpatient commitment and mental health care reporting across nations, the associated controversy and the lack of scientific evidence can all endanger patients' rights.

An analysis of mental health legislation in 12 European countries [45,48,58] revealed that outpatient commitment laws can be subdivided into 3 parts. Four countries (Czech Republic, Lithuania, Slovak Republic and Spain) have provided the legal framework for ordering outpatient commitment (for up to five years in a medical centre or a specialist social health care institution as in Spain) in their criminal legislation only, but not in their civil laws. Four countries (Germany, Greece, Poland and Sweden) provide no legal basis for involuntary outpatient commitment whatsoever. Sweden, however, reports that de facto, for example, depot injections are carried out in outpatient settings when legally involuntarily admitted patients are on long-term leaves granted by the relevant civil laws. Four countries (Bulgaria, England, Israel and Italy) have included options for outpatient commitment in their civil legislation, but three of them have added restrictions indicating special modes of treatment, clinical situations, and procedural aspects. In England, the Mental Health Act of 1995 defines the rarely used option of aftercare under supervision, which refers to residence and institutions but not to medication. In Italy, the local health authority can issue the proposal for involuntary admission *not* under hospitalization, but this is used only for emergency treatment measures that can be performed at day hospitals or at home. Finally, Israel defines outpatient commitment as an alternative to hospitalization for periods of six months each, with hospitalization as the automatic consequence in the case of a failure to comply.

These variations in legal regulations reflect a general uncertainty about this issue, and highlight the legal concerns in several (European) countries to legitimize this treatment option [58]. They also emphasize the need for high quality research on these issues, taking country-specific legal regulations into account. This should improve the national knowledge bases on a specific option of providing mental health care for the vulnerable subgroup of 'revolving door' patients with severe, mostly psychotic mental disorders, relapse profiles with a high risk of violent behaviour, a history of frequent involuntary hospitalizations, lack of insight, and poor medication compliance and adherence to treatment appointments in the community [59–63]; but, such research should also enhance the international evidence base on this sensitive issue.

A recent review article that assessed RCT and non-RCT evidence for the effect of compulsory community treatment summarized the international research perspective [61]. A meta-analysis of RCTs showed no statistical differences in 12-month admission rates between subjects on involuntary outpatient treatment and controls; time to admission was equivocal; patients receiving the intervention were less likely to have long-term hospitalizations when hospital stays were longer than 10 days; and no clear differences in treatment adherence emerged. In light of the limited evidence of positive effects of involuntary outpatient treatment as a less restrictive alternative to admission, a wide range of outcomes needs to be evaluated if this type of legislation is introduced. The lack of empirical European data showing the effects of this strategy, especially on violent patients, compounds the legal concerns mentioned above. The United Kingdom, having recently implemented a randomized controlled trial on the effects of community treatment orders [64], will be the first European country generating scientific evidence pertaining to the legal and clinical questions of whether or not it is justified to exclude or implement a care approach which might restrict patients' rights when being treated in the community.

Research from Finland on suicide provides the most convincing recent evidence for the importance of the availability of nationwide, or at least regional, comprehensive data on (in this case, adult) mental health service units and thus for a standardized reporting system including all of these services [65]. This study showed that well-developed community mental health services have a greater association with lower suicide rates than services orientated towards inpatient treatment provision. These data are consistent with the idea that population mental health can be improved by multifaceted, community-based, specialized mental health services. For mental health care planning, such results could stimulate the shift from inpatient treatment provision to community care where such reorganization towards community-based care has been less successful, thus increasing the potential for suicide prevention and strengthening patients' rights to the highest attainable standard of health.

The systems needed for providing regular mental health reporting must balance their range of information against relevant data protection issues [66]. In order to achieve this, the anonymized and standardized data set [5,66,67] recording the individual patients in all services of one area or country must be reduced to a minimum of variables which must not only respect relevant data protection laws, but must also be agreed on by all stakeholders, including the staff in these (mostly small) service units. Further, and particularly in fragmented care systems, the tasks of the independent institution designated to analyse and report on the data periodically, and the ways in which data are transferred to this institution, must be clearly defined. At best, all these definitions could be made in separate laws on mental health care reporting or in special sections of mental health laws on mental health care reporting. This would not only guarantee that institutions responsible for data protection are involved in the process of working out such laws, but would also clarify the responsibilities of service providers and assure patients that their rights concerning their personal data are respected.

## 8.4   Can promising initiatives for improving patients' rights be identified?

Revisions of national mental health laws, the elaboration of best practice guidelines for the use of coercive measures, and the formulation of psychiatric advance directives serve as promising examples of current initiatives for improving patients' rights, illustrated by the following analysis. The examples were chosen because they address different levels of responsibility for the practice of mental health care which may have significant impact on this field: the legal framework, the framework of professional behaviour, and the therapeutic relationship of the individual patient and his carers.

There is potential for improvement in this field, via revisions of national mental health laws to avoid issues not consistent with the protection of patients' rights. Szmukler and Dawson address this at a general level in this volume by proposing to 'fuse' incapacity and mental health legislation (Chapter 7). Other suggestions refer to specific issues such as the process of involuntary hospitalization, for which an international analysis has recently identified major cross-national differences of legal regulations important for clinical practice [48]. Without any intention to disregard long-standing and well-founded national legal and clinical traditions, specific issues with the potential or even need for cross-national harmonization appeared. In the opinion of the author, the following issues deserve special attention when revisions of (national) mental health laws address the process of involuntary hospitalization:

• The legal basis for treatment decisions (including the treatment setting) and the decision process itself must be simplified to the greatest extent possible.
• The powers of decision have to be clearly subdivided and assigned to different professional roles; standards of professional competency for these roles need to be defined.
• Time periods for the judicial decisions and performance of judicial authorities should be standardized across nations.
• Laws should be adapted with consideration for the clinical reality of high rates of emergency involuntary hospital admissions.
• During each stage of the judicial proceedings mandating involuntary hospitalization and coercive treatment measures, the patient should have the right to a legal representative.
• Regulations regarding the appeals process have to be as simple and transparent as possible.

Currently, no solid evidence base addresses whether and in which way such changes in the legal definitions would influence the practice of involuntary admission and stay in psychiatric hospitals [47], and if these would increase the acceptance of such coercive interventions by the patients, or if they would then evaluate their rights as better respected.

The development of best practice guidelines (Chapter 4; [68,69]) addressing the use of coercive measures is still a rather new movement. In particular, methodology in this field of various national and international activities, mostly driven by national associations of psychiatrists, is heterogeneous. Thus, existing documents cover a range from recommendations for best practice up to the most advanced guidelines according to the standard defined, for example, by the Association of Scientific Medical Societies (in Germany) or comparable national or international bodies.

Respect for patients' rights is further complicated because only recommendations on pharmacological treatment and prevention of aggressive and/or agitated behaviour are based on the highest possible level of evidence. In contrast, a lack of empirical studies available for critical appraisal in the guideline development process means that many recommendations on relevant issues of clinical behaviour in this field are given only at the lowest evidence level of good clinical practice rather than being deduced from empirical findings established at a high level of scientific evidence. This includes, for example, the protection of patients' rights, gender issues, pharmacological treatment of agitated patients with an intoxication syndrome, the treatment of ethnic minorities, aspects of the therapeutic relationship and the ward atmosphere, architecture and structural or organizational aspects of the institution, practical or technical details of the way in which individual coercive measures like mechanical restraint or seclusion are used, the evaluation of the measure afterwards and how to involve the patient in this procedure, and the aftercare for professionals who use coercive measures.

The largely unsolved issue of cross-national harmonization is also problematic. This is of special importance here because major differences at the national level in respecting patients' rights would suggest differences in terms of human rights requirements. Using local expert groups, the EUNOMIA research group aimed to establish recommendations for improving the clinical practice in the field of individual coercive measures in 12 European countries (the London site, with the established UK Code of Clinical Practice [70] was excluded) [46,71,72]. Several centres (Dresden, Prague, Naples, Wroclaw, Michalovce, Granada, Örebro) established regional expert groups of 10 to 15 individuals representing all parties potentially involved in the administration of coercive treatment measures (e.g. psychiatrists and nurses, municipal and police officers, members of patients' and relatives' organizations). These expert groups ran semi-structured discussions or focus groups to develop unanimous agreement on national suggestions. Some other centres (Sofia, Thessaloniki, Tel Aviv) implemented a written survey of selected national representatives of all parties involved in these treatment measures; the results were combined with information from personal interviews to create the final products. Within a second phase of the work, all centres in which local expert groups were established asked different national professional organizations (e.g. psychiatrists, lawyers or judges, patients and relatives, ministries) for comments on their suggestions. These comments were collected using structured or unstructured questionnaires, or discussions in specific thematic workshops; the expert groups modified the text of the local suggestions based on the comments received. All national suggestions were translated into English, and collected by the centre coordinating EUNOMIA in Dresden. This centre performed a qualitative analysis of the content to produce common suggestions. Two researchers from the Dresden centre extracted the information independently from the national suggestions and crosschecked their category assignments afterwards. For further analyses, 'summary tables' were developed. Subsequently, three researchers from the Dresden centre integrated the information into a proposal valid for all participating centres in each category. After completing the summary, the tables were sent to each centre to review the validity, comprehensiveness and completeness of each summary with regard to the situation in the respective countries. In the final step, researchers from the coordinating centre revised the summaries incorporating the feedback from the other centres. This process omitted all information which differed across the centres. Thus, the EUNOMIA research team developed a final version of the suggestions for best clinical practice in the use of involuntary hospital admission valid for the 11 project centres.

Published results from this research address the issues of mechanical restraint [71] and involuntary admission to a psychiatric hospital [72]. The following examples on these two specific issues demonstrate what was able to be achieved – and not achieved – by such an approach: (i) *Care of other patients and visitors when mechanical restraint must be administered at the ward* [71]. It is recommended that only essential personnel with specific tasks should be present when administering mechanical restraint. There shall be no spectators without tasks in the restraint. To avoid unnecessary trauma, other patients should be directed to their rooms. Furthermore, visitors are requested to go to secluded common parts of the ward, for instance the dayroom. Additional personnel should be appointed to care for the other patients; that is, being close to them and being available to notice reactions like fear and anger. Caring for other patients also includes calming them and briefly explaining events without violating patient confidentiality. The patient being mechanically restrained should have contact with other patients if this is according to his or her wishes, and if this is not too stressful for his or her health status or for the health status of the other patients. (ii) *Behaviour of judges in the process of involuntary admission to a psychiatric hospital* [72] . The judge, before formulating any decision about the patient's admission, must collect information from the patient her-/himself, relatives and community mental health professionals, enquiring about the patient's actual clinical situation directly from the ward psychiatrist. In cases where orders that led to an involuntary hospitalization were not carried out within 48 hours, the circumstances under which the orders were issued should be re-examined. If national legislation stipulates that a hearing is required (e.g. in the Czech Republic, Lithuania, Slovakia, Spain and Germany), this should take place in a comfortable and safe room, possibly located within the ward. During the hearing, the judge should involve the ward psychiatrist in order to integrate the available information with clinical details. The judge's decision should be made only after all persons participating in the involuntary admission procedure have been heard.

To date, many open questions remain concerning the content of such guidelines or recommendations and their implementation into clinical practice. As documented above, in particular when a broader consensus is sought, recommendations seem to be rather generalized and not adequately specific. Further, effects of implementing such guidelines or recommendations on complex situations into clinical practice are unknown. Thus, the potential of such documents to improve patients' rights remains unclear.

Psychiatric advance directives are legal documents that allow a patient to consent to or refuse future mental health treatment in the event of an incapacitating psychiatric crisis. Advance instructions or appointing of a surrogate decision-maker can be documented. The general intention behind this instrument is to support patients' self-determination at times when they are particularly vulnerable to loss of autonomy, to help them ensure that their preferences are known and respected, and to minimize unwanted and involuntary treatment. Empirical research showed a high potential demand from users for such documents but low completion rates, which could be increased by facilitation sessions [73]. Further, such research demonstrated that these directives may be an effective tool for reducing coercive interventions around incapacitating mental health crises [74]. Problems identified with implementing such documents much more widely into the practice of mental health care include the time-consuming and emotionally painful process for the patient of establishing such a document [21], the legal status of such documents that has yet to be defined well from an international perspective, and the indication by a significant number of psychiatrists that they would override a valid, competently executed psychiatric advance directive that refused hospitalization and medication [75].

Thus, further comprehensive activities are needed to ensure the legality of such documents, to generate acceptance amongst psychiatrists, and to support patients directly in establishing their advance directives in order to make these more influential for the common practice of mental health care. Such achievements would provide a solid basis for assessing the potential of such directives for improving patients' rights. At the moment, it is too early to make a valid statement on this issue.

## 8.5    Is autonomy still the supreme principle guiding recent socio-legal developments with regard to mental health care?

The current social climate in the Western (European) societies, at least, seems to be characterized by contradictory trends in the ways people with mental illness are seen and treated as members of society. The most important dichotomies might be expressed by the following key terms: high societal burden associated with increased indirect health care costs vs. decreasing budgets for direct mental health care costs; the reality of social exclusion as indicated by such examples as an increase in people with mental illness who are homeless or by their separation from the first working market vs. health policy goals focusing on social inclusion; and high thresholds for accessibility to specialized mental health services vs. initiatives to increase the public knowledge about mental disorders and threats to mental health ([2,6,39–41]; Chapter 2).

Such contradictory trends also seem to be represented in recent socio-legal developments. The right of the individual patient to choose a personal financial budget for health care of chronic mental illness (as defined in the German socio-legal system) [76] and the leverage from the social welfare system (see Chapter 3) are taken as examples demonstrating that autonomy for people with mental illness cannot be taken for granted in the current social climate.

Based on the general idea of empowering people with mental illness, of strengthening their competence to select health care providers who meet their individualized needs, thus increasing their influence and active participation in treatment, the German socio-legal system [76] introduced the opportunity for chronically (mentally) ill or disabled persons to choose a so-called personal (financial) budget for health care. This budget would subdivide money amongst the health care providers that patients selected for treatment or care according to their needs. This opportunity to respect the autonomy and decisional capacity of these individuals met the reality of a highly fragmented community health care system, however [5,6]. Fragmentation refers to financial carriers of health and social care elements, to (public or a range of private) providers of mental health services within the same catchment area, to the conceptualization of individual services themselves (e.g. supported housing), and to therapeutic relationships in a system in which no clear clinical case management systems are established [6]. Thus, the opportunity provided was not implemented in practice to the degree expected by policy-makers [77]. In fact, it increased the risk of dependency of people with chronic mental illness on agencies or care-givers legally appointed to guide these individuals through the complex bureaucracy required to receive such a personalized budget for mental health care.

The concept of leverage from the social welfare system, as outlined by John Monahan in this book (Chapter 3), and especially its (legal) conceptualization in terms of 'contract' instead of 'coercion' [78] are – to the knowledge of the author – not discussed in Western European countries with the same high visibility (supported by research activities) as in the US. This does not mean, however, that this kind of (hidden) leverage does not play a significant role in other socio-legal systems. In the spectrum of mental disorders, this seems to affect individuals with substance abuse disorders most frequently, as is also the case with leverage from the judicial system. In Germany, for example, a job agency or pension fund agency can ask applicants with substance abuse disorders who have been long-term unemployed to accept long-term treatment in specialized rehabilitation units before they are granted a disability benefit [79]. If the applicants refuse, their financial assistance while unemployed could be reduced or a decision on their disability benefit could be denied. On an international level, a recent review of socially sanctioned coercion mechanisms for addiction treatment presented substantial findings that such mechanisms, available for decades, such as licensure sanctions and employee assistance programs, while often perceived negatively are effective in initiating recovery and achieving positive clinical outcomes [80]. In contrast, social security disability benefits seem to be an area where an opportunity for 'constructive' coercion was missed in the treatment of substance abuse disorders. The authors call for implementing socially sanctioned mechanisms of coercion, although this may be seen as a paradigm shift in mental health treatment. This shift would involve an acceptance of the involuntary aspects of addiction as well as concern about the impact of addiction on society, but may need to occur because of the increased understanding of the impact of addiction on brain functioning with subsequent compromise of volitional controls. The authors conclude that the likelihood of this position attracting broader professional and societal support remains to be seen.

These examples, even if not representative, raise significant concern that societies pay lip service to protect the autonomy of people with mental illness, but significantly challenge this guiding principle for organizing mental health care in practice.

## 8.6   Are there legal areas that need clearer definitions in order to respect patients' rights?

The patient's freedom to choose a psychiatric hospital for inpatient care, and involuntary placement and treatment in long-stay care homes serve as two examples – chosen from the German perspective of the author – to analyse this question.

In Germany, hospital-based mental health care, as well as more and more services in the community, is organized following the principle of sectorization; that is, patients living in a geographical catchment area must be admitted to the psychiatric hospital (or receive care in community services) responsible for that catchment area [5,6]. This principle of providing community-orientated mental health care is written in the Mental Health Acts of the German Länder [81], which also define that the freedom to choose treatment should be respected. These Acts fail to define clearly which of these two principles of care is primary, however. In clinical practice, and in particular when hospitals are overcrowded as is the reality for under-financed community-orientated mental health services [6], this leads to an individual's freedom to choose treatment being restricted or overwhelmed by a principle representing a population-based approach to care. In contrast to community-orientated service provision which could be evaluated as positive for the individual patient also, freedom to choose treatment could be seen as the higher legally-protected right for the individual person because it respects her/his autonomy and decision-making capacity, and is in line with person-centred concepts such as empowerment and recovery [20]. Because of the importance of both of these principles, a legal, ethical and health policy discussion is needed to clarify which principle takes precedence over the other. Otherwise, chance and the clinical and economic reality of empty hospital beds become the deciding factors for the clinicians in individual clinical situations.

None of the German civil or public administrative laws covering mental health matters [45,81] contain specific regulations for involuntary placement in (long-stay) care homes. Because of a fragmented mental health care reporting system, national data on the frequency of such placements are not available. However, it is evident that clearly defined subgroups of chronically mentally ill patients (those with addictive disorders with multiple mental and/or physical disorders associated with drug abuse, chronic schizophrenic disorders, older persons with dementia) and developmentally disabled persons (with highly disturbed behaviour) are vulnerable populations for such placements. Estimations of the general frequency amount to 20 000 persons [82], and further increase can be expected. Therefore, the establishment of clear regulations for many issues around this topic is urgently needed [44]. The following is a selection of those concerns evaluated as being of outstanding importance:

- The relevant authorities for the inspection of homes must clearly decide if the conditions of an institution are adequate for performing involuntary placements; further, the authority must assign the task of performing involuntary placements to the individual institution, and regularly assess the quality of the performance of such placements.
- Laws must include regulations to guarantee that each person placed involuntarily receives a care plan comprising adequate care and treatment measures for meeting

his or her needs based on an individual assessment and aiming to socially reintegrate the person, and that this plan is updated on a regular basis.

- Concerning the implementation of the involuntary placement itself, the following issues must be clearly regulated: that the individual person or her/his legal guardian are informed of the rights and obligations during the placement and of the contents of the care plan; that the individual person or her/his legal guardian have the right to freely choose treating physicians; that the right of the individual to freely practice his or her religion is strictly respected.

- The following issues concerning the roles and obligations of the staff in such homes must be clearly regulated: who is authorized to order and perform any other coercive measures and especially those requiring the use of physical force; who is authorized to physically examine patients against their will and the way in which those examinations should be performed; who can decide to restrict the right to see visitors and the right to freely use telecommunication and to receive and send mail.

- Concerning any decisions on changes in the involuntary placement measure itself, the following issues must be clearly defined: the prerequisites modifying the placement, and the assignment of the responsibility for such decisions to certain staff members; the preconditions for sending persons on leave, for defining behavioural restrictions when persons are on leave, and for revising such decisions as well as the assignment of the responsibility for such decisions to certain staff members.

It is self-evident, in the opinion of the author, that the examples presented above of the patient's freedom to choose a psychiatric hospital for inpatient care and involuntary placement and treatment in long-stay care homes clearly demonstrate that legal areas that urgently need clearer definitions in order to respect patients' rights indeed exist! Because such areas may vary across countries, the obligation falls on each national mental health care system to implement review procedures which will enable it to systematically identify these sensitive and critical issues.

## 8.7 Conclusions

The field of psychiatry in its current status should be deeply concerned that the human rights of mental health patients – in their complexity and comprehensiveness that clearly exceeds the issue of coercive treatments – are, at least, not addressed and respected fully, and at worst, might even be severely endangered. Arguments underpinning this statement are as follows: current international health policy recommendations for organizing mental health care are not as clearly orientated to respect these rights comprehensively as they could or should be. Further, legal regulations in the area of mental health vary widely. Research on if and how the protection of human rights can be measured in the field of mental health care is still a work in progress. Institutions or bodies concerned with the issue of the respect of these rights are not well known, have a low-key profile, or can be not easily accessed by patients. These issues add to the concern that authorities responsible for clinical governance are not following a clear standard, and that the impact of their reports on clinical practice is not clearly visible.

Another source of concern is that patients' rights may be further endangered by new initiatives in the field of mental health care. For example, the legal basis for outpatient commitment is characterized by a variety of national regulations that reflects an uncertainty about dealing with this issue in general. Further, high-quality research on this issue, taking country-specific legal regulations into account, is needed. This should generate the scientific evidence required to address the legal, ethical and clinical decision of whether excluding or implementing an option of clinical treatment which might restrict the rights of a vulnerable subgroup of patients when being treated in the community is ever justified. Because of the sensitivity of data protection issues, separate laws on mental health care reporting or special sections of mental health laws on mental health care reporting could make the implementation of national or regional initiatives in this field easier, an important factor in organizing the best standard of health care. Building a solid legal basis would not only guarantee that institutions responsible for data protection are involved in the process of developing such laws, but would also assure patients that their rights concerning their personal health data are respected.

Adding to the scepticism outlined so far, the potential of recent initiatives intended to improve the rights of patients to influence the reality of mental health care provision in this direction is currently not as clear as desired. Revising national mental health laws which avoid issues currently identified as critical for patients' rights presents potential for improvement in this field. However and again, no solid evidence base is currently available about if and in which way such changes would influence clinical practice, and whether patients would then see their rights better respected. Recently established best practice recommendations or guidelines for the use of coercive measures seem to be rather generalized and not specific enough. Further, effects of implementing such documents into clinical practice remain unknown. In order to make psychiatric advance directives more influential for the routine practice of mental health care, further comprehensive activities are needed to ensure the legality of such documents, to generate acceptance amongst psychiatrists, and to directly support patients in establishing their directives.

Examples of recent socio-legal developments, even if not representative, significantly increase the concern already outlined because they demonstrate that societies pay lip service to protect the autonomy of people with mental illness, but in reality challenge this guiding principle for organizing mental health care.

Finally, legal areas indeed remain that urgently need clearer definitions in order to respect patients' rights as outlined. Examples include involuntary placement and treatment of patients with chronic mental illnesses (those with addictive disorders with multiple mental and/or physical disorders associated with drug abuse, chronic schizophrenic disorders, older persons with dementia), and people with mental and developmental disabilities (with highly disturbed behaviour) in (long-stay) care homes. Because such areas may vary across countries, each national mental health care system could be obligated to implement review procedures to systematically identify such sensitive and critical issues.

Thus in closing, the author considers that the compatibility of mental health care and patients' rights seems to be more of an extremely important general aim for health politics and the field of psychiatry than a reality at present!

## Acknowledgement

The multi-site research project *European Evaluation of Coercion in Psychiatry and Harmonization of Best Clinical Practice* (acronym: EUNOMIA) was funded by the European Commission (Quality of Life and Management of Living Resources Programme, contract no. QLG4-CT-2002-01036). The author gratefully acknowledges the assistance in text editing from Charlene Reiss.

## References

1. Thornicroft, G. and Szmukler, G. (eds) (2001) *Textbook of Community Psychiatry*, Oxford University Press, Oxford.
2. Becker, T., Bauer, M., Rutz, W. and Aktion Psychisch Kranke (2001) Psychiatric reform in Europe. *Acta Psychiatrica Scandinavia*, **104** (Supplement 410), 7–109.
3. Catty, J., Burns, T., Comas, A. and Poole Z. (2007) Day centres for severe mental illness. *Cochrane Database of Systematic Reviews* 1 (Art. No.: CD001710). doi: 10.1002/14651858. CD001710.pub2
4. Chilvers, R., Macdonald, G. and Hayes, A. (2006) Supported housing for people with severe mental disorders. *Cochrane Database of Systematic Reviews* 4 (Art. No.: CD000453). doi: 10.1002/14651858.CD000453.pub2
5. Salize, H.J., Rössler, W. and Becker, T. (2007) Mental health care in germany. *European Archives of Psychiatry and Clinical Neuroscience*, **257**, 92–103.
6. Eikelmann, B., Becker, T., Rössler, W. and Kallert, T.W. (2011) Versorgungsstrukturen in der Psychiatrie, in *Psychiatrie und Psychotherapie, 4. Auflage*, Volume 1 (eds H.J. Möller, G. Laux and H.P. Kapfhammer), Springer Verlag, Berlin, pp. 1143–1175.
7. Kallert, T.W. (2005) Is mental health services research in need of randomised controlled trials? (in German). *Psychiatrische Praxis*, **32**, 375–377.
8. Kallert, T.W., Priebe, S., McCabe, R. *et al.* (2007) Are day hospitals effective for acutely ill psychiatric patients? A multi-center European randomized controlled trial. *Journal of Clinical Psychiatry*, **68**, 278–287.

9. Marshall, M., Gray, A., Lockwood, A. and Green, R. (1998) Case management for people with severe mental disorders. *Cochrane Database of Systematic Reviews* 2 (Art. No.: CD000050). doi: 10.1002/14651858.CD000050

10. Marshall, M. and Lockwood, A. (1998) Assertive community treatment for people with severe mental disorders. *Cochrane Database of Systematic Reviews* 2 (Art. No.: CD001089). doi: 10.1002/14651858.CD001089

11. Burns, T., Catty, J., Dash, M. *et al.* (2007) Use of intensive case management to reduce time in hospital in people with severe mental illness: systematic review and meta-regression. *British Medical Journal*, **335**, 336.

12. King, R. (2006) Intensive case management: a critical re-appraisal of the scientific evidence for effectiveness. *Administration and Policy in Mental Health and Mental Health Services Research*, **33**, 529–535.

13. Johnson, S., Nolan, F., Pilling, S. *et al.* (2005) Randomised controlled trial of acute mental health care by a crisis resolution team: the north Islington crisis study. *British Medical Journal*, **331**, 599.

14. McCrone, P., Johnson, S., Nolan, F. *et al.* (2009) Economic evaluation of a crisis resolution service: a randomised controlled trial. *Epidemiologia e Psichiatria Sociale*, **18**, 54–58.

15. National Institute for Health and Clinical Excellence (2009) *Schizophrenia. Core Interventions in the Treatment and Management of Schizophrenia in Adults in Primary and Secondary Care*. NICE Clinical Guideline 82, NICE, London. Available at www.nice.org.uk (accessed 30 November 2010).

16. Burns, T., Catty, J., Becker, T. *et al.* (2007) The effectiveness of supported employment for people with severe mental illness: a randomised controlled trial. *Lancet*, **370**, 1146–1152.

17. National Institute For Health and Clinical Excellence (2006) *The Management of Bipolar Disorder in Adults, Children and Adolescents, in Primary and Secondary Care*. NICE Clinical Guideline 38, The British Psychological Society, Leicester and The Royal College of Psychiatrists, London. Available at www.nice.org.uk (accessed 30 November 2010).

18. Deutsche Gesellschaft für Psychiatrie, Psychotherapie und Nervenheilkunde (DGPPN) (2005) *Behandlungsleitlinie Psychosoziale Therapien*, Steinkopff Verlag, Darmstadt.

19. Mezzich, J.E., Berganza, C.E., von Cranach, M. *et al.* (2003) Essentials of the World Psychiatric Association's International Guidelines for Diagnostic Assessment (IGDA). *British Journal of Psychiatry*, **182** (Supplement 45), 373–461.

20. Amering, M. and Schmolke, M. (2009) Recovery in mental health, in *Reshaping Scientific and Clinical Responsibilities*, John Wiley & Sons, Ltd, Chichester, UK.

21. Henderson, C., Jackson, C., Slade, M. *et al.* (2010) How should we implement psychiatric advance directives? Views of consumers, caregivers, mental health providers and researchers. *Administration and Policy in Mental Health*. doi: 10.1007/s10488-010-0264-5

22. Priebe, S., Badesconyi, A., Fioritti, A. *et al.* (2005) Reinstitutionalisation in mental health care: comparison of data on service provision from six European countries. *British Medical Journal*, **330**, 123–126.

23. Gruskin, S., Mills, E.J. and Tarantola, D. (2007) History, principles, and practice of health and human rights. *Lancet*, **370**, 449–455.

24. Singh, J.A., Govender, M. and Mills, E.J. (2007) Do human rights matter to health? *Lancet*, **370**, 521–527.

25. Beyrer, C., Villar, J.C., Suwanvanichkij, V. *et al.* (2007) Neglected diseases, civil conflicts and the right to health. *Lancet*, **370**, 619–627.

26. Orbinski, J., Beyrer, C. and Singh, S. (2007) Violations of human rights: health practitioners as witnesses. *Lancet*, **370**, 689–704.

27. Dudley, M., Silove, D. and Gale, F. (eds) (in press) Mental Health and Human Rights, Oxford University Press, Oxford.

28. Kallert, T.W. (2010) Conventions of Human Rights – and their relevance for the field of psychiatry (in German). Die Psychiatrie, 2, 87–93.

29. Ishay, M.R. (2008) The History of Human Rights. From Ancient Times to the Globalization Era, University of California Press, Berkeley, CA.

30. Universal Declaration of Human Rights, Resolution 217 A (III) of the General Assembly of the United Nations (10 December 1948).

31. European Convention for the Protection of Human Rights and Fundamental Freedoms, Rome (4 November 1950).

32. International Covenant on Civil and Political Rights, Resolution 2200A (XXI) of the General Assembly of the United Nations (CCPR, 16 December 1966).

33. International Covenant on Economic, Social and Cultural Rights, Resolution 2200A (XXI) of the General Assembly of the United Nations (CESCR, 16 December 1966).

34. European Convention for the Prevention of Torture and Inhuman or Degrading Treatment or Punishment, Strasbourg (26 November 1987).

35. UN Convention Against Torture and Other Cruel, Inhuman or Degrading Punishment, Resolution 39/46 of the General Assembly of the United Nations (10 December 1984).

36. UN Convention on the Rights of Persons with Disabilities, Resolution A/RES/61/106 of the General Assembly of the United Nations (13 December 2006).

37. Hale, B. (2007) Justice and equality in mental health law: the European experience. International Journal of Law and Psychiatry, 30, 18–28.

38. Commission of the European Communities (2005) Green Paper: Improving the Mental Health of the Population. Towards a Strategy on Mental Health for the European Union. Brussels, 14 Oct, No. COM(2005)484 final.

39. Schneider, F. Zur Lage der Psychiatrie. Opening lecture, Kongress der Deutschen Gesellschaft für Psychiatrie, Psychotherapie und Nervenheilkunde 2009. Berlin, 25 November 2009. Available at www.dgppn.de (accessed 3 December 2010).

40. Angermeyer, M.C., Holzinger, A. and Matschinger, H. (2009) Mental health literacy and attitude towards people with mental illness: a trend analysis based on population surveys in the eastern part of Germany. European Psychiatry, 24, 225–232.

41. Eikelmann, B., Reker, T. and Richter, D. (2005) Social exclusion of the mentally ill – a critical review and outlook of community psychiatry at the beginning of the 21st century (in German). Fortschritte der Neurologie Psychiatrie, 73, 664–673.

42. Kallert, T.W. (2005) Legal involuntary admissions to general psychiatric hospitals in Germany: are the rates increasing? (in German). Die Psychiatrie, 2, 231–234.

43. Köhler, N. and Kallert, T.W. (2009) Forensic mental health hospitals in the new and old German Federal States: a comparison (in German). Forensische Psychiatrie, Psychologie, Kriminologie, 3, 56–66.

44. Böcker, F.M. (2008) Geschlossene Unterbringung im Heim: Rechtliche Aspekte, in 14. Bericht des Ausschusses für Angelegenheiten der psychiatrischen Krankenversorgung des Landes Sachsen-Anhalt, Landesverwaltungsamt Sachsen-Anhalt, Halle (Saale), Germany, pp. 37–48.

45. Kallert, T.W. and Torres-González, F. (eds) (2006) Legislation on Coercive Mental Health Care in Europe. Legal Documents and Comparative Assessment of Twelve European Countries, Peter Lang, Berlin.

46. Kallert, T.W., Glöckner, M., Onchev, G. et al. (2005) The EUNOMIA project on coercion in psychiatry: study design and preliminary data. World Psychiatry, 4, 168–172.

47. Kallert, T.W., Glöckner, M. and Schützwohl, M. (2008) Involuntary vs. voluntary hospital admission – a systematic review on outcome diversity. *European Archives of Psychiatry and Clinical Neuroscience*, **258**, 195–209.

48. Kallert, T.W., Rymaszewska, J. and Torres-González, F. (2007) Differences of legal regulations concerning involuntary psychiatric hospitalization in twelve European countries: implications for clinical practice. *International Journal of Forensic Mental Health*, **6**, 197–207.

49. Priebe, S., Katsakou, C., Glöckner, M. *et al.* (2010) Patients' views of involuntary hospital admission in psychiatry after one and three months: a prospective study in eleven European countries. *British Journal of Psychiatry*, **196**, 179–185.

50. Killaspy, H., King, M., Wright, C. *et al.* (2009) Study protocol for the development of a European measure of best practice for people with long term mental illness in institutional care (DEMoBinc). *BMC Psychiatry*, **9**, 36.

51. Taylor, T.L., Killaspy, H., Wright, C. *et al.* (2009) A systematic review of the international published literature relating to quality of institutional care for people with longer term mental health problems. *BMC Psychiatry*, **9**, 55.

52. Turton, P., Wright, C., White, S. *et al.*; the DEMoBinc group (2010) Promoting recovery in long-term mental health institutional care: an international Delphi study of stakeholder views. *Psychiatric Services*, **61**, 293–299.

53. European Committee for the Prevention of Torture and Inhuman or Degrading Treatment or Punishment (CPT) (2009) The CPT Standards. "Substantive" Sections of the CPT's General Reports. CPT/Inf/E (2002) 1 – Rev. Council of Europe, Strasbourg.

54. Niveau, G. and Materi, J. (2007) Psychiatric commitment: over 50 years of case law from the European Court of Human Rights. *European Psychiatry*, **22**, 59–67.

55. Conrady, J. and Roeder, T. (2006) The legal point of view: comparing differences of legal regulations related to involuntary admission and hospital stays in twelve European countries, in *Legislation on Coercive Mental Health Care in Europe. Legal Documents and Comparative Assessment of Twelve European Countries* (eds T.W. Kallert and F. Torres-González), Peter Lang, Berlin, pp. 349–374.

56. Musallam, M. (2006) Legal report – Israel, in *Legislation on Coercive Mental Health Care in Europe. Legal Documents and Comparative Assessment of Twelve European Countries* (eds T.W. Kallert and F. Torres-González), Peter Lang, Berlin, pp. 161–177.

57. Triantaphyllou, G. (2006) Legal report – Greece, in *Legislation on Coercive Mental Health Care in Europe. Legal Documents and Comparative Assessment of Twelve European Countries* (eds T.W. Kallert and F. Torres-González), Peter Lang, Berlin, pp. 139–159.

58. Hegendörfer, G. (2007) Compulsory outpatient treatment and mental health care: aspects of the legal discussion from the European and Israeli perspective (in German). *Psychiatrische Praxis*, **34** (Supplement 2), S227–S232.

59. Swartz, M., Swanson, J., Kim, M. and Petrila, J. (2006) Use of outpatient commitment or related civil court treatment orders in five U.S. communities. *Psychiatric Services*, **57**, 343–349.

60. Freedman, R., Ross, R., Michels, R. *et al.* (2007) Psychiatrists, mental illness, and violence. *American Journal of Psychiatry*, **164**, 1315–1317.

61. Kisely, S., Campbell, L.A., Scott, A. *et al.* (2007) Randomized and non-randomized evidence for the effect of compulsory community and involuntary out-patient treatment on health service use: systematic review and meta-analysis. *Psychological Medicine*, **37**, 3–14.

62. Dawson, J. and Mullen, R. (2008) Insight and use of community treatment orders. *Journal of Mental Health*, **17**, 269–280.

63. Swartz, M. and Swanson, J. (2008) Outpatient commitment: when it improves patient outcomes. *Current Psychiatry*, **7**, 25–35.
64. Burns, T., Rugasa, J., Dawson, J. *et al.* (2010) Oxford community treatment order evaluation trial (OCTET): a single outcome randomized controlled trial of compulsory outpatient treatment in psychosis. *Lancet*, in press.
65. Pirkola, S., Sund, S., Sailas, E. and Wahlbeck, K. (2009) Community mental-health services and suicide rate in Finland: a nationwide small-area analysis. *Lancet*, **373**, 147–153.
66. Schützwohl, M. and Kallert, T.W. (2009) Routinedaten im komplementären Bereich, in *Routinedaten in der Psychiatrie. Sektorenübergreifende Versorgungsforschung und Qualitätssicherung* (eds W. Gaebel, H. Spiessl and T. Becker), Steinkopff, Heidelberg, pp. 38–44.
67. Glover, G. (2007) Adult mental health care in England. *European Archives of Psychiatry and Clinical Neuroscience*, **257**, 71–82.
68. National Institute for Health and Clinical Excellence (2005) *Violence: The Short-Term Management of Disturbed/Violent Behaviour in Psychiatric In-patient Settings and Emergency Departments*, NICE Clinical Guideline 25, Royal College of Nursing, London. Available at http://guidance.nice.org.uk/CG25/NICEGuidance/pdf/English (accessed 22 November 2010).
69. Deutsche Gesellschaft für Psychiatrie, Psychotherapie und Nervenheilkunde (2009) *S2-Leitlinie Therapeutische Maßnahmen bei aggressivem Verhalten in Psychiatrie und Psychotherapie*, Steinkopff Verlag, Heidelberg.
70. Department of Health and Welsh Office (1999) *Government Guidance. Code of Practice Mental Health Act 1983*, The Stationary Office, London, UK.
71. Kallert, T.W., Jurjanz, L., Schnall, K. *et al.* (2007) Eine Empfehlung zur Durchführungspraxis von Fixierungen im Rahmen der stationären psychiatrischen Akutbehandlung. Ein Beitrag zur Harmonisierung bester klinischer Praxis in Europa (in German). *Psychiatrische Praxis*, **34** (Supplement 2), S233–S240.
72. Fiorillo, A., de Rosa, C., del Vecchio, V. *et al.* (2010) How to improve clinical practice on involuntary hospital admissions of psychiatric patients: suggestions from the EUNOMIA study. *European Psychiatry*. doi: 10.1016/j.eurpsy.2010.01.013
73. Swanson, J.W., Swartz, M.S., Elbogen, E.B. *et al.* (2006) Facilitated psychiatric advance directives: a randomized trial of an intervention to foster advance treatment planning among persons with severe mental illness. *American Journal of Psychiatry*, **163**, 1943–1951.
74. Swanson, J.W., Swartz, M.S., Elbogen, E.B. *et al.* (2008) Psychiatric advance directives and reduction of coercive crisis interventions. *Journal of Mental Health*, **17**, 255–267.
75. Swanson, J.W., van McCrary, S., Swartz, M.S. *et al.* (2007) Overriding psychiatric advance directives: factors associated with psychiatrists' decisions to preempt patients' advance refusal of hospitalization and medication. *Law and Human Behavior*, **31**, 77–90.
76. Sozialgesetzbuch (SGB) Neuntes Buch (IX) – Rehabilitation und Teilhabe behinderter Menschen, Artikel 1 des Gesetzes v. 19.6.2001, BGBl. I S. 1046 (19 June 2001).
77. Interessengemeinschaft Beratender zum Trägerübergreifenden Persönlichen Budget (January 2010) Stellungnahme der bundesweiten Interessengemeinschaft Beratender zum Trägerübergreifenden Persönlichen Budget.
78. Bonnie, R.J. and Monahan, J. (2005) From coercion to contract: reframing the debate on mandated community treatment for people with mental disorders. *Law and Human Behavior*, **29**, 485–503.
79. Retzlaff, R., Hildebrandt, M., Bechmann, M. and Ueberschär, I. (2009) Rehabilitation effizient und rentabel: Neue Zugangswege zur Entwöhnungsbehandlung. *Sucht aktuell*, **11**, 43–51.

80. Nace, E.P., Birkmayer, F., Sullivan, M.A. *et al.* (2007) Socially sanctioned coercion mechanisms for addiction treatment. *American Journal on Addictions*, **16**, 15–23.
81. Weig, W. and Cording, C. (eds) (2003) *Zwischen Zwang und Fürsorge. Die Psychiatriegesetze der deutschen Länder*, Deutscher Wissenschaftsverlag, Baden-Baden.
82. Salize, H.J., Spengler, A. and Dressing, H. (2007) Involuntary hospital admissions of mentally ill patients – how specific are differences among the German Federal States? (in German). *Psychiatrische Praxis*, **34** (Supplement 2), S196–S202.

# Section 3

## Ethical aspects of coercive treatment

# 9 Cross-cultural perspectives on coercive treatment in psychiatry

## Ahmed Okasha and Tarek Okasha

*Ain Shams University, Institute of Psychiatry, Faculty of Medicine, Cairo, Egypt*

## 9.1 Introduction

The use of coercive measures (seclusion, physical and chemical restraint) in the treatment of psychiatric patients is very common in psychiatric hospitalization. There is a remarkable lack of experimental studies concerning the use of these measures. From the legal viewpoint, ambiguity still exists in the regulation of the application of these measures [1]. The World Psychiatric Association ethical code, the Madrid Declaration, stated that when the patient is incapacitated and/or unable to exercise proper judgement because of a mental disorder, or gravely disabled or incompetent, the psychiatrist should consult with the family and, if appropriate, seek legal counselling, to safeguard human dignity and the legal rights of the patient. No treatment should be provided against the patient's will, unless withholding treatment would endanger the life of the patient and/or those around her/him. Treatment must always be in the best interest of the patient. Admitting a patient involuntarily does not

*Coercive Treatment in Psychiatry: Clinical, Legal and Ethical Aspects*, First Edition.
Edited by Thomas W. Kallert, Juan E. Mezzich and John Monahan.
© 2011 John Wiley & Sons, Ltd. Published 2011 by John Wiley & Sons, Ltd.

mean automatically to implement involuntary treatment. Many patients may accept treatment voluntarily following involuntary admission.

The necessity of applying coercive measures in certain circumstances singularly distinguishes psychiatry from most other medical disciplines. Due to the massive impact upon the liberty and freedom of the persons concerned, the application of coercive measures is regulated worldwide in a variety of mental health acts or other laws, which have to balance potentially contradictory intentions. The debate between human rights activists and psychiatrists regarding coercion in psychiatry is still controversial.

The attitude towards coercion varies in different cultures. It may be accepted in family-centred traditional societies where individual autonomy is sacrificed for the sake of family decisions, the opposite of Western cultures. Culture, religion and spirituality have an impact and influence on individual autonomy. In these traditional societies, informed consent is the family obligation, and involuntary admission is a family decision which should be respected, otherwise the individual faces marginalization from his or her society.

Against this background, the chapter will discuss the transcultural ethical aspects of implementing coercive management of psychiatric disorders, emphasizing the point that the human rights values of Western culture may disturb social conformity and religious adherence in some traditional societies and may be counterproductive for the social network of the patient in these societies.

## 9.2   Delivery of mental health care

The patient's rights to autonomy and to adequate treatment, even if the patient's competence to decide on this treatment is compromised, should be respected if public safety is not at issue. Depending on a variety of cultural or legal traditions, however, the frameworks for regulating these rights differ internationally to a considerable degree. As a consequence, practices of applying coercive measures also vary internationally.

An ongoing methodological challenge is to identify evidence for the relationship between coercive measures and the quality and effectiveness of mental health care. Methodologically sound studies and overall findings in this field are scarce, however, as demonstrated in recent literature reviews [2,3].

## 9.3   Selected studies in developing countries on involuntary hospitalization, seclusion and restraint

Unfortunately, no evidence at all is available from developing countries.

The most recent overviews on the state of human or mental health rights in Asian, African or Central American psychiatry date back to 2000, concluding that mental health care is not a high priority for many governments of socio-economically struggling developing countries. In these countries, access to mental health services of Western standards is scarce and restricted to a small minority of privileged citizens [4]. When the right of a mentally ill person to receive modern psychiatric care is not within the capacity of many developing countries, traditional treatments prevail. Most often these are applied against the will of the patients, include physical restraint, and can be considered as abusive or infringing on basic civil rights in Western contexts. However, coercive treatment is culturally accepted in these family-orientated societies [5]. Immigrants from non-Western countries also may experience more compulsory treatments. For example, a study from Norway reports that non-Western immigrants receive more involuntary treatment, although their referrals to psychiatric emergency departments are not more frequent than for the indigenous Norwegian population [6].

Egypt has about 6000 psychiatric beds for inpatients. In a population of 68 million, the number for involuntary admission in 2008 did not exceed 7.2% in state mental hospitals. In private hospitals, reaching 3000 beds in Egypt, involuntary admission did not exceed 7 patients, a phenomenon reflecting that family decision encroaching on individual autonomy is playing a pivotal role but accepted culturally and socially.

## 9.4  Coercive measures in child and adolescent psychiatry

Forcing a child into treatment initially is a legitimate role for parents or guardians and is validated by mental health professionals, who feel that this must be accepted as part of regular clinical work – especially in the case of school-age children, who only rarely can initiate requests for help. Further, the clinical use of power and persuasion has been addressed by a number of authors at both theoretical and pragmatic levels. Child psychiatrists deal with issues of coercion systematically and successfully in clinical practice. Although children often come into treatment against their will, sometimes because of physical pressures or threats and sometimes because of economic or emotional threats, they often can make use of a therapeutic relationship that is negotiated over time and gives careful attention to the child's identified needs and wishes. This experience leads one to recognize many seemingly overtly coercive treatment contexts which may be turned into effective treatment interventions. Exploration of the use of power and coercion as they relate to children, whether in normal development or in treatment, is helpful in the study of the psychopathology of adults who require limit setting, persuasion or coercion in their treatment, often quite possibly because their childhood developmental experience regarding issues of power was dysfunctional [7].

In traditional societies, the decision for involuntary or voluntary admission of children and adolescents is totally the responsibility of the family. Neither the judicial system nor the civil law has a role.

## 9.5    Attitudes towards coercion

In some traditional societies in Africa, South East Asia and the Middle East, the perception of mental illness varies between rural and urban areas. In rural areas it is still considered to be possession by evil spirits, magic, evil eye, or the wrath of ancestors, and to use coercive treatment and restraint to exorcise the evil eye spirit is socially acceptable and if not applied the society will consider the family as negligent.

## 9.6    Deprivation of liberty

In non-Western cultures, the acceptance by the patients of their family decision for involuntary placement may surprise Western practitioners. Patients are grateful to their family for pursuing the path to get rid of the evil eye or spirit or the wrath of the ancestors. Although we do not have any scientific studies of patient's perception in those cultures it is our impression that it does not leave any scar or anger or rejection as they returned to the path of virtue.

## 9.7    Transcultural aspects

Cultural variations of negative symptoms in the WHO International Classification of Diseases, ICD-10, for example avolition, anhedonia, indifference, blunting of affect in simple schizophrenia, schizotypal disorder, residual schizophrenia, cannabinoid use and chronic depression, can be considered desirable social traits in certain religious cults. Normal emotional expression in Anglo-Saxon culture may suggest a schizoid reduction of emotional response in a Mediterranean culture.

Religious and traditional families assess quality of life according to adherence to religious rituals, regardless of mental symptoms. Negative symptoms can be interpreted as deeper contemplation about God, and virtuous. And positive symptoms can be considered as gifted from God by the extraordinary perception of, for example, a special person. Religious interpretation of personality disorders challenges the concept of personality disorders in different cultures. This can be illustrated as follows: schizotypic as close to God, schizoid as a kind person, paranoid as careful, avoidant as following religious purity especially in mixing with the opposite sex, and obsessive-compulsive as meticulous in following religious rituals.

Traditional societies have high tolerance to negative symptoms that may have religious connotations such as piety and asceticism. Further, the peoples of traditional societies do not conceptualize such symptoms as belonging to the medical model. Positive symptoms associated with violence require an urgent intervention, according to their concept. Religious beliefs have a prominent influence on ethics, morals and deontological mistakes.

Okasha *et al.* [8], studying nine cultures, were impressed by the similarities rather than the differences amongst cultures: the denial of the self for the sake of others, the devotion of the individual for the promotion of the group, which characterize Indian, Chinese, Japanese, Latin-American and Arab cultures as well. Individual autonomy is observed in European and American cultures but is not empowering for traditional family-centred societies in Arabic, Sub-Sahara African, Indian and Japanese cultures. This difference may affect the use of involuntary admission, informed consent and religious psychotherapy, amongst other practices, in traditional versus Western societies.

Differences between the two types of societies are listed in Table 9.1. These differences are the mainstream norm and not an absolute description of a stereotyped behaviour. The table highlights that cultural diversity may influence the implementation of ethics in different societies. In traditional societies, the family is an extended one, decision-making is group- and family-orientated, and the Western attitude regarding individual autonomy does not exist. The concept of external control, dependence on God with regard to health and disease, and attribution of illness and recovery to God's will all maintain a healthy doctor–patient relationship, which makes trust, confidence and compliance characteristic in traditional societies.

**Table 9.1** Traditional versus Western societies: highlights of the main differences.

| Traditional society | Western society |
| --- | --- |
| Family and group orientated | Individual orientated |
| Extended family (not so geographical as before, but conceptual) | Nuclear family |
| Status determined by age and position in the family, care of elderly | Status achieved by own efforts |
| Relationship between kin obligatory | Determined by individual choice |
| Arranged marriages with an element of choice dependent on interfamilial relationship | Choice of marital partner, determined by interpersonal relationship |
| Extensive knowledge of distant relatives | Restricted to only close relatives |
| Decision-making dependent on the family | Autonomy of individual |
| Locus of control external | Locus of control internal |
| Respect and holiness of the decision of the physician | Doubt in doctor–patient relationship |
| Rare suing for malpractice | Common |
| Deference is God's will | Self determined |
| Doctor–patient relationship is still healthy | Mistrust |
| Individual can be replaced. The family should continue and the pride is in the family ties | Irreplaceable, self pride |

Arab culture includes traditional beliefs in devils, jinn, the evil eye and so on (delusional cultural beliefs). The family structure is characterized by affiliated behaviour at the expense of differentiating behaviour. Also, rearing is orientated towards accommodation, conformity, cooperation, affection and interdependence, as opposed to individuation, intellectualization, independence and compartmentalization. The extended family helps in managing intergenerational conflicts. Young individuals vacillate between two worlds, one following the values of Western societies and the other following the values and beliefs of traditional societies.

What if the decision-making process is not an individual one? In Arab and some other traditional cultures, issues of illness are dealt with as a family matter. Whether a patient is hospitalized, for example, or subject to electroconvulsive therapy or discharged from the hospital, is dependent not on what the patient wants him- or herself but on the estimation, need, or wish of the extended family. Patients may wish at times not to be burdened with the extra load of making decisions that may determine the patterns of the rest of their lives. The concept of shared responsibility is central in Arab and other traditional cultures, and most people in the Arab world would not like to be responsible for the outcomes of decisions made on their own.

The decision-making style in traditional cultures might be best described as family centred. The moral, social and psychological support for which extended families in developing countries are so well known is the result of collectivity of decision-making; that is, decision-making by consensus. An individual decision that differs from the collective decision leaves the decision-maker to bear the responsibility of the outcome alone and may deprive him or her of familial support. On the other hand, when a collective decision is acted on, negative consequences of the decision are not the patient's fault alone and he or she does not have to bear the guilt of making a wrong decision.

One illustrative example of the issue of consent and decision-making is hospital admission. In the United States, 73% of patients in psychiatric facilities are voluntarily admitted, whereas in Egypt, the rate is 90% [3,9]. In reality, the distinction between voluntary and involuntary admission is not as clear as is stated in law. Patients are often pressured into agreeing to voluntary admission. If voluntary admission were always strictly voluntary, the rate of involuntary admission would likely increase. The family plays a strong role in the rate of voluntary admission. In those cultures, respect for and compliance with family decisions is more important than autonomy of the individual, especially if responsibility for the outpatient rests with the family because there are no community social support systems. It is the responsibility of the family to learn the patient's diagnosis and prognosis and to make the difficult decisions needed. Studies in Italy, Greece, Spain and Egypt showed that a patient's learning of his or her diagnosis of cancer is not viewed as empowering. Rather, this knowledge is seen as isolating and burdensome to the patient, who is suffering too much and is too ignorant about his or her condition to be able to make meaningful choices. Knowledge of a diagnosis harms the patient by causing him or her to lose hope [8].

## 9.8  Conclusions

Preserving human rights at the expense of violating conformity, opposing traditions and deviating from religious norms is considered unethical in some traditional societies. Transcultural aspects of implementing ethics of coercion should be considered.

Involuntary admission and coercive treatment is viewed in some societies, where family decision adherence is valued more than individual autonomy, as a socially accepted value, and is revered by the patients to get rid of the vicious nature of their mental illness and to return to the path of truth and virtue.

## References

1. Mayoral, F. and Torres, F. (2005) Use of coercive measures in psychiatry. *Actas Españolas de Psiquiatria*, **33**, 331–338.
2. Katsakou, C. and Priebe, S. (2006) Outcomes of involuntary hospital admission – a review. *Acta Psychiatrica Scandinavica*, **114**, 232–241.
3. Kallert, T.W., Glöckner, M. and Schützwohl, M. (2008) Involuntary vs. voluntary hospital admission. A systematic literature review on outcome diversity. *European Archives of Psychiatry and Clinical Neuroscience*, **258**, 195–209.
4. Levav, I. and Gonzalea Uzcategui, R. (2000) Rights of persons with mental illness in Central America. *Acta Psychiatrica Scandinavica*, **101**, 83–86.
5. Alem, A. (2000) Human rights and psychiatric care in Africa with particular reference to the Ethiopian situation. *Acta Psychiatrica Scandinavica*, **101** (Supplement 399), 93–96.
6. Berg, J.E. and Johnson, E. (2004) Are immigrants admitted to emergency psychiatric departments more often than ethnic Norwegians? *Tidsskrift for den Norske Laegeforening*, **124**, 634–636.
7. Group for Advancement of Psychiatry (1994) *Forced into Treatment. The Role of Coercion in Clinical Practice*. Formulated by the Committee on Government Policy. Report no. 137. American Psychiatric Publishing, Inc., Arlington, VA, pp. 1–133.
8. Okasha, A., Arboleda-Flórez, J. and Sartorius, N. (2000) *Ethics, Culture and Psychiatry: International Perspective*, American Psychiatric Press, Washington, DC.
9. Okasha, A. and Okasha, T. (eds) (2009) *Contemporary Psychiatry* (in Arabic), 15th edn, The Anglo-Egyptian Bookshop, Cairo, pp. 42–71.

# 10 Historical injustice in psychiatry with examples from Nazi Germany and others – ethical lessons for the modern professional

## Rael Strous

*Tel Aviv University, Beer Yaakov Mental Health Center, Sackler Faculty of Medicine, Tel Aviv, Israel*

Psychiatry is a fine profession. It is characterized by the study of human behaviour and mental processes. Its mandated 'social contract' with the community is to describe, understand, predict and modify behaviour, particularly in cases of mental illness. Most importantly, treating psychiatrists are committed to assisting the individual in need and alleviating emotional pain. As such, they have privileged access to the human psyche and behaviour. This privilege demands responsibility and the primary duty to care for the mental health of their patients. This is what lies at the heart of the profession. To act otherwise would constitute abdication of professional responsibility [1].

Along with this tremendous responsibility, comes tremendous power. It would be expected that instances of abuse of this power are rare given the important calling and expected inherent sensitivity that many in the field inherently posses and express in

*Coercive Treatment in Psychiatry: Clinical, Legal and Ethical Aspects*, First Edition.
Edited by Thomas W. Kallert, Juan E. Mezzich and John Monahan.
© 2011 John Wiley & Sons, Ltd. Published 2011 by John Wiley & Sons, Ltd.

their professional dealings with patients. However, as with all human traits, when there is power it may be used by many in an inappropriate manner. This unfortunately may be the case in clinical and research psychiatry as well. While instances of inappropriate care and unethical professional behaviour are relatively rare, history does provide us with some important examples of crossing the boundaries of ethical health care in individuals with mental illness. This may occur with the individual behind the closed doors of the treatment room, as well as larger scale inappropriate behaviour which some may even consider as genocide.

Much of this unethical behaviour emanates from both subtle and prominent boundary violations. Just as it is important to learn the 'nuts and bolts' of psychopharmacology, psychotherapy and cultural sensitivity in the field of psychiatry, it is just as important to learn basic concepts of ethical practice and how these concepts apply to the day to day practice of psychiatry as well as more complex ethical dilemmas which crop up from time to time. However, learning the concepts alone is not enough. Most medical schools and professional organizations at least pay lip service to the study of these concepts as well as to the publications of ethical guidelines which may vary from medical subspecialty to subspecialty depending on the nuances of the field. However, studying the concepts and distributing ethical codes either by subspecialty or by national medical societies is insufficient. In 1931 the German medical society developed a code of medical ethics which at the time was considered one of the most advanced, if not the most advanced, in the world. Some maintain that in some areas it is even more comprehensive than the Helsinki code of ethical research conduct that exists today. However, all know how much effect this code had and what the German Nazi doctors did despite this code of medical ethics being in existence and which was expected to be well known and rehearsed by doctors at the time. Thus while many believe that ethics training in medical school and residency training ameliorates the risk that such practice will ever be repeated, this is not necessarily the case. Rather, ethics training without a focus on clinical and research psychiatric practice with examples from history would be fundamentally lacking. The reason for this is that many psychiatrists in history have believed that they were doing the right thing from a moral and scientific standpoint. While, often, following analysis of the situations it is easy to state that these psychiatrists were inherently 'evil', this is not necessarily the case. Often their gross misbehaviour and unethical conduct emanated from a belief they were doing the best in the interests of science and for the good of mankind, irrespective of the methodology including often profound coercion and disregard for human value and patient rights. Several examples may provide illustration of how ethics training and policy without a focus on history becomes futile.

Perhaps the most commonly quoted approach to medical ethics is consideration of the four cardinal ethical concepts. These values that commonly apply to medical ethics discussions are respectively: autonomy, beneficence, non-maleficence and justice. Two additional concepts in medical ethics are commonly invoked in conjunction with these four cardinal values. These are the principles of dignity and honesty. As a model to explain the concept of medical ethics and their importance, a brief explanation of the concepts will be given as well as examples from history where these concepts have been ignored or violated. Providing vivid examples from history of unethical practice increases the chance that lessons may be learned and that the concepts will be applied in a more appropriate manner.

## 10.1  Autonomy

Some would argue that, more than any other principle, the concept of autonomy lies at the heart of good ethical practice in medicine. In essence, autonomy may be defined as the right of a patient to decide their own treatment. This includes the right to accept or refuse any management or treatment plan offered to them. This respect for a patient's self determination allows the individual to make decisions about their own lives and does not leave all medical decision-making in the hands of the 'all-powerful physician'.

In the past it was often traditional for the approach to the patient being of a paternalistic nature as opposed to respecting patient autonomy in treatment decision-making. Many have attributed this to cultural factors, and which continues today in many parts of the world in medical practice. However others would argue that this is not a cultural phenomenon but rather an error in attitude by physicians which may over time have become cultural/traditional in certain societies. While in many cases a paternalistic approach, ignoring patient autonomy, does not lead to any serious problems for the patient, arguably the worst ever period in medical history regarding this subject occurred not so long ago. Around 70 years ago transpired, beyond any doubt, one of the most shocking episodes in the history of psychiatry with respect to denial of patient autonomy.

### 10.1.1  Example with historical context

During the Nazi era (1933–1945), psychiatrists, more than any other medical subspecialty, played a critical role in Nazi policy and their extermination regime. Their involvement encompassed many varied aspects of the killing including selection, identification and classification of mentally ill individuals sent for murder; culminating in the supervision and coordination of their killing. Psychiatrists carefully chose the psychiatric institutions and victims for 'euthanasia', and they were instrumental in optimizing the bureaucratic system in the implementation of the killing. Finally they selected and counselled the killers [2]. All this was carried out by means of a highly organized and efficient extermination process. Their involvement was rooted in many psychiatrists' belief in and support of the eugenics movement. Their views were reflected in the perceived needs of German society at the time, which were influenced by crisis in the economy and Hitler's meteoric climb to power, and all the nationalism and totalitarianism that it bred. One of the earliest and most prominent German psychiatrists in the early twentieth century to write about the mentally ill was the well-known German psychiatrist and professor of psychiatry at the University of Freiburg, Alfred Hoche. He co-published a book with Rudolf Binding (professor of law) entitled *The Permission to Destroy Unworthy Life* [3]. In this popular work, often referred to by prominent Nazi leaders, he stated that the 'principle of allowable killing should be extended to the incurably sick. . . the right to live must be earned and justified, not dogmatically assumed.' He wrote that those who are not capable of human feeling ('ballast lives' and 'empty husks') fill psychiatric institutions and have no sense of the value of life – therefore theirs is a life not worth living and their destruction is not only acceptable but also humane. A symbiotic relationship developed between the racial hygiene intentions of the psychiatrists to 'rid' the world of mental illness and disability and the Nazi's views of racial cleanliness (reviewed in [4]).

While precise numbers of psychiatrists involved in the atrocities to their patients are not available, it has been estimated that there were around 700–800 psychiatrists in Germany in 1933. Very few were known to have protested at the crimes against psychiatric patients. Thus the percentage of those involved is therefore believed to have been considerable. It is clear that psychiatrists played a prominent, if not critical, role in two principal categories of medical coercion and crimes against humanity: sterilization and euthanasia [5,6].

## Sterilization

Psychiatrists were central to the drawing up of policy plans and carrying out the compulsory sterilization of hundreds of thousands of individuals for whom it was considered undesirable to reproduce. One of the most prominent members of the team which designed the legislation for the compulsory sterilization of 'undesirables' in Germany was the distinguished psychiatry professor, Professor Ernst Ruedin [7]. He was well published and internationally acclaimed. He also functioned as the director of the Munich Psychiatric Institute and chairman of the Association of German Neurologists and Psychiatrists. Many today still consider him to be the 'father of psychiatric genealogy'. His writings remain well read. In 1933, he was selected by the Nazi regime to head the Society for Racial Hygiene. Ruedin made a statement calling for compulsory sterilization of 'ballast lives' (*ballastexistenzen*). He prided himself on being an author of the official manual instituting the law of compulsory sterilization for eugenic purposes. This legislation was passed into law on July 14, 1933 and was based on the thoughts and direction of eugenics scientists who called for compulsory sterilization of individuals mostly suffering from psychiatric and/or hereditary disorders. Many of the psychiatrists who participated actively were acting according to what they considered to be the genuine interests of society. Patients with psychiatric illness which required sterilization included schizophrenia, cyclothymia and mental retardation. Numbers in the entire sterilization programme have been estimated to range between 300 000 and 400 000. Most of the sterilizations took place in the years before the war (1934–1937) and required enormous effort by physicians. Based on the patient population to be sterilized, psychiatrists served a particularly important role in this programme (reviewed in [2,4,5]).

## Euthanasia

The second and most egregious stage of the psychiatrists' involvement in the Nazi racial hygiene project was the euthanasia project. This programme involved the German civilian population (both Jewish and non-Jewish) and began around the beginning of the war and continued through its early years, albeit in varying fashion and method of killing. The process was called the T4 programme, based on the address of its central coordinating office, No. 4 Tiergartenstrasse, situated in the centre of Berlin. There were two stages. The first began in 1939 and continued until its official closure in 1941, when the gassing phase of the operation was officially stopped. In this initial phase, where patients were gassed in specialized rooms for the purpose, 70 273 individuals with various forms of mental illness were forcibly murdered in the name of racial hygiene and medicine. In addition to adults with psychiatric illness, many of the murdered included children with psychiatric disorders. Their lives and subsequent deaths were explained by physicians as being similar to aggressive steps needing to be taken at times in order to preserve life – such as removal of a gangrenous appendix. After the official cessation of the euthanasia programme in 1941, the programme continued in an unofficial manner, termed 'wild euthanasia' with an estimated further 130 000 patients starved, poisoned, neglected and shot to death in German psychiatric hospitals in the years 1942–1945 [8]. With the cessation of the initial period of euthanasia, the killing resumed in the east,where larger scale genocidal operations by means of gassing took place primarily targeting Jews at camps including Treblinka, Belzec, Auschwitz, Sobibor and Majdanek. One psychiatrist, albeit with minimal training, Dr Irmfried Eberl, had served as the head of two (Brandenburg, Bernburg) of the six psychiatry hospitals (the others being Grafeneck, Hartheim, Sonnenstein and Hadamar) where gassing took place. With his extensive experience in gassing of the mentally ill, he was appointed to set up and run the Treblinka death camp [9]. Thus psychiatric institutions formed a bridge between euthanasia and the larger scale annihilation of Jews and others such as homosexuals and Gypsies in the process of racial purification and murder of 'undesirables'. This later became known as the Holocaust.

The killing of psychiatric patients amongst others was given legitimacy by the medical profession and psychiatrists who facilitated the programme. Their power was immense, only matched by the extent of the abuse of this power that transpired. The extent of extermination of psychiatry patients was considered to be so potentially successful that many psychiatrists were concerned for the future of the field and that the euthanasia programme would inevitably result in psychiatrists having no patients to treat [8].

Psychiatrists involved were not peripheral members of the profession. Many were very senior with international reputations as leaders in their field [2]. They included the director of the Gorden Psychiatry Hospital, Professor Hans Heinze; Dr Werner Heyde, head of Hitler's euthanasia project and full professor of psychiatry at Wurzburg; Professor Paul Nitsche of the Sonnenstein State Hospital who perfected the process of intravenous dosing for medical killing; Dr Hermann Pfannmuller, director of the prominent Children's Institution Eglfing-Haar who openly prided himself on the gradual starvation of 'undesirable children', as he described it, 'the most simple method'. Professor Max de Crinis, Psychiatry Chair at Charite Hospital, Berlin, mentioned above, was a further well-known psychiatrist who reportedly provided Hitler with the wording of his euthanasia letter where he gave permission to medical personnel to kill their patients (they were never ordered) (reviewed in [2,4,8]).

Several psychiatrists even managed to continue with prominent research during the war years, making use of prisoners, alive and dead, for their research development. Two psychiatrists in particular included Drs Julius Hallervorden and Dr Hugo Spatz. They were instrumental in describing for the first time the medical disorder whose eponym bares their name (Hallervorden–Spatz disease – a neurodegenerative disorder of basal ganglia characterized by extrapyramidal symptoms, mental deterioration, dementia and retinal degeneration). They were reportedly sent 697 brains of euthanized mentally ill individuals [5,8].

Apart from the psychiatrists themselves, psychiatric institutions with very few exclusions agreed to report lists of those hospitalized for over five years, the criminal mentally ill, and those who were not employable. Some of the goals of the morbid 'success' of the programme (200 000 dead) could never have been achieved without the cooperation of outpatient and private psychiatrists who appeared to readily submit lists of patients to the authorities in Berlin. Thus these patients' *autonomy* was irreversibly removed. Only a few psychiatrists refused to submit to social and political pressures and to unilaterally remove patient autonomy to the extent that it was. They include, most notably, the doctors Karl Bonheoffer, Martin Hohl Hans Creutzfeldt and Gottfried Ewald [2,8].

In some cases, what lay at the heart of these psychiatrists' involvement in the atrocities was often a genuine desire to serve society and science. Maintaining that they were 'just evil' minimizes the learning experience and desensitizes us to the breaches in ethical practice to an extent unknown in history. The psychiatrists erred in dramatic fashion by removing all respect for autonomy in patient care and management. Many maintained that patients were suffering and that as a result they were lives not worth living. They neglected to speak to patients inquiring as to what they want. The prominent and critical issues of autonomy in medical practice cannot be ignored. The practice of German Nazi psychiatry provides a most vivid picture of where they went wrong.

## 10.2  Beneficence

Beneficence may be defined as the need for the physician to always act in the best interests of the patient. While there are often competing interests, when a physician sits at his desk across from the patient or stands next to the bed of those in his care, what should interest him or her is the greatest good he or she can extend to the patient. Thus, for example, the personal interests of the family or the physician and even the health system should take second place in the physician acting for the good of the patient. Competing interests may also be financial for the institution, such as administering cheaper or the cheapest medications available but that may be less appropriate. Other competing factors may include publicity for the institution or physician, or research needs. While these interests may come to benefit the patient in the long run, though not always, the question is, does it benefit the patient now and has the patient been informed of these competing interests.

### 10.2.1  Example with historical context

The psychiatrist, Henry A. Cotton strongly held the belief of many physicians in the 1920s that the basis for all serious mental illness lay in infection, the source of which is not always clear. He was a student and avid admirer of Dr Adolf Meyer from the Johns Hopkins School of Medicine and arguably one of the most prominent and well-known psychiatrists of his day. Adolf Meyer held that infectious aetiology led to all mental illness and was the biological source of mental disorder. Thus if one could locate the source of this infection and eradicate it, mental illness could be cured for that individual. This belief came out from the knowledge that individuals who were delirious as a result of fever from infection would be psychotic and confused, however this would resolve on the fever and infection abating [10].

With the assistance and support of his mentor, Adolf Meyer, he became medical director of Trenton State Hospital at the relatively young age of 30, and implemented his 'infectious aetiology theory' in the treatment of patients, followed up by research. Genuinely interested in treating patients and relieving the burden of mental illness, he began his search for the source of this 'focal sepsis'. He implemented a treatment schedule by first removing the teeth of many patients in the hospital, considering that the source of infection lay there. If this failed, he went on to remove, often in random fashion, other sources of potential infection in the body. These included the tonsils, gall bladders, stomachs, spleens, cervixes, testicles and ovaries. In many treatment-resistant cases, shockingly he even removed the colons of patients. In an era before antibiotic medications this, not surprisingly, lead to significant mortality. It is estimated that at least 30% of his patients with colectomy died, and this figure may have even been closer to 45%. Dr Phyllis Greenacre, a student of Dr Adolf Meyer, was sent to provide an independent professional review of Dr Cotton's work. In light of her findings, the report of which was never officially published, she expressed great reservation regarding Cotton's research and clinical practice [10]. However, the outside community did not catch on to the problematic nature of his treatment and research and, in June 1922, the *New York Times* stated in a review of Cotton's work

> At the State Hospital at Trenton, N.J., under the brilliant leadership of the medical director, Dr. Henry A. Cotton, there is on foot the most searching, aggressive, and profound scientific investigation that has yet been made of the whole field of mental and nervous disorders... there is hope, high hope... for the future.

Cotton officially retired in October 1930 but continued an active involvement in the hospital. He died in 1933 and was eulogized as a very respectable and honourable physician with far-reaching contributions to the field of medicine. Despite a public hearing and investigation into his close-to-murderous practices, he was never brought to justice, and his surgical management techniques continued unabated while he was at the helm of this hospital [10].

Besides the dubious scientific value of his work and research (no control or double-blind conditions), no care was taken that informed consent was respected – with sceptical patients often being forced into the surgical operating room. In the face of Dr Cotton's rampant academic ambitions to serve his selfish research aspirations and to prove his own and his mentor's view of the source of psychotic illness, he paid no attention to the age-old medical dictum '*primun non nocere*' (first do no harm) and most importantly to always act in the best interest of the patient (beneficence).

## 10.3 Non-maleficence

Non-maleficence refers to the age-old dictum in medicine mentioned above, 'first, do no harm' (*primum non nocere*). The concept derives from the fact that, in certain circumstances and situations, it may be preferable for the physician not to intervene when his or her intervention may lead to more harm than good. Thus the doctor is always reminded that any intervention has risks and unwanted consequences. These need to be weighed up before any active intervention is undertaken.

### 10.3.1   Example with historical context

An intriguing example of this concept has occurred in the not so distant past. Alvin Bernard Ford was found guilty of murder in 1974 and was subsequently sentenced to death. At the time of arrest and conviction he was completely sane with no concerns as to his mental competence. However, beginning around 1982, he began showing evidence of mental illness. These signs deteriorated into obvious paranoid symptomatology with the belief that he was at the centre of a conspiracy involving the Ku Klux Klan encouraging him to commit suicide. His psychotic symptomatology, both paranoid and grandiose, extended to his jailers and fellow inmates. He was examined by several psychiatrists who concurred that he was suffering from psychosis. They all believed that Ford should be designated incompetent. A death order however was still signed by the Governor. Eventually, following appeal, the case was presented to the US Supreme Court, where it was decided that the State may not carry out the death penalty on an individual who is declared to be non-competent. The ethical dilemma lies in whether a psychiatrist should agree to assist in such a case, if called upon to treat the individual in order to return him to a state of competence. A state of competence is required prior to the death penalty so that he understands the reason why he is being sentenced to death. Thus the psychiatrist would be treating the individual in order to permit the state to execute him/her [11,12]. While the psychiatrist will be treating the patient, this treatment will lead to the patient's death. Similarly to the prohibition of physicians' involvement in executions, such involvement would violate similar medical ethics. Thus while treatment would return some level of sanity to the patient, if the treatment would lead to greater harm, it would violate the principle of non-maleficence and 'first do no harm' and thus be considered unethical. Others, albeit in the minority, would argue, however, that treating the individual would return some element of 'rational autonomy' which would enable the individual on death row to confront the results of his misdeeds with dignity, as well as open up the option of true repentance [12].

Following this interesting ethical dilemma resulting from several cases wherein psychiatrists did administer treatment, the General Assembly of the World Psychiatric Association (WPA), at its World Congress in Athens in October 1989, declared 'that the psychiatrist shall serve the best interests of the patient and treat every patient with the solicitude and respect due to the dignity of all human beings.' Therefore 'the psychiatrist must refuse to cooperate if some third party demands actions contrary to ethical principles.' Conscious that psychiatrists may be called on to participate in actions connected to executions, the WPA declared that the participation of psychiatrists in any such action would be 'a violation of professional ethics.' This is due to the fact that physicians are healers, not executioners. For obvious reasons it would be unethical for a physician to involve himself or herself in a procedure/treatment/management schedule that has as its principal purpose the death of an individual [13].

## 10.4  Justice

Justice refers to the concepts of fairness and equality in psychiatric practice. It has several applications in medical ethics including the fair distribution of health resources as well as situations concerning who gets which treatment. It may also be argued that the concept of 'justice' refers to the fair and just application of psychiatric knowledge, diagnosis and management to individuals who may or may not be suffering from mental illness.

An unwritten 'social contract' exists between psychiatrists and the community. This agreement allows psychiatrists to describe, understand, predict and modify behaviour, particularly in cases of mental illness. Above all, practitioners are committed to helping the individual and alleviating emotional pain. The field of psychiatry thus is an academic discipline, a profession and a science, with psychiatrists being granted special and privileged access to the human psyche and behaviour. While there is agreement to this role more or less across the board, the privilege is associated with responsibilities and the crucial duty to care for the mental health of their patients. To ignore this key consideration in placing the patient first, over and above any other consideration, would constitute abdication of professional responsibility and would herald the slippery slope to psychiatric coercion. History is replete with examples of exploitation of psychiatry in order to advance political ideology or to suppress political opposition. This would be considered a profound boundary violation and directly and profoundly negate the objectives of the field [1].

### 10.4.1  Example with historical context

There have been many cases in distant and recent history where psychiatrists have been inappropriately called upon to assist in the 'solving' of problems of society. Based on the inherent power in the field and potential to control and modify behaviour, various totalitarian regimes have attempted, and in many cases have succeeded, to exploit psychiatrists in order to carry out their aims of coercion and behavioural control. Examples of such misuse include in the areas of political discourse and activism, including interrogation and evaluation to the extreme of torture and cooperation with executions as described above. By participating and acquiescing to such involvement in political process and governmental coercion, psychiatrists compromise their standards of professionalism and ethical conduct.

Several key illustrations exist of this practice in recent history. One prominent case in point is the cooperation of many psychiatrists in the use of psychiatric repression as a tool of the government to punish political dissidents. In this manner, many individuals who were open opponents to the political system and oppressive activities of the Soviet Union were targeted for psychiatric confinement [14]. This practice surfaced in the early 1970s, resulting in condemnation of the psychiatrists involved. This was followed by the resignation of the Soviet Union psychiatry organization from the World Psychiatric Association several years later. Only in 1989, following perestroika and glasnost did the full picture begin to emerge. It became clear that psychiatric coercion was in full force during the prior years, whereby many individuals without any evidence of mental illness who had conveyed their opposition to state practices on theoretical and ethical grounds were deemed to be mentally unstable and committed involuntarily to psychiatric institutions, even to the extent of being treated with antipsychotic medication. Treatments also included insulin coma and physical restraints. These 'patients' were not allowed any legal representation or recourse to any form of appeal. Many of these political admissions received the diagnosis of 'sluggish schizophrenia' with the ambiguity and subjectivity of psychiatric diagnosis and classification being exploited for the benefits of state repression. This 'hyperdiagnosis' of psychiatric disorder, not uncommon in other parts of the world, led to much improper labelling of patients and subsequent hospitalization [14]. While the case of psychiatrists in the ex-Soviet Union is presented as one particular example, it is not unique, and involvement of psychiatrists in governmental repression has been alleged in other countries including Argentina, South Africa, Serbia and China [14,15].

While the above four examples of psychiatric coercion from history represent clear instances of the abuse of the inherent power of psychiatry and abdication of the key ethical principles in the medical profession (autonomy, beneficence, non-maleficence and justice), they all also indicate a clear violation of two other key concepts often mentioned along with these four principles. These are the principles of dignity and honesty, so fundamental to ethical practice of medicine in general and psychiatry in particular.

## 10.5 Abuse of power

Arguably, the central theme that runs throughout these four principal examples of ethical breeches of conduct in the history of psychiatry lies in 'abuse of power'. These cases provide evidence of what transpires when the authority and control of psychiatric practice goes unchecked. Coercion using the forces and qualities of psychiatry is extremely perverse, since it inculcates the exploitation and repression of the 'weakest' of the population – often those with no voice. Doctors who allow themselves to participate in such actions as demonstrated by the above examples breach fundamental aspects of norms of behaviour and psychiatric ethics. Often this abuse of psychiatry is subtle, such as the issue of hyperdiagnosis and introduction of so-called 'cultural ambiguities' in diagnosis and management [14]. However, in most cases this is not the case and coercion is readily recognizable to all. As with the Nazi German psychiatrists, probably the case with the most blatant disregard for patient autonomy leading to extermination of patients, medicine and psychiatry may become the underlying source of the momentum which drives the application of coercion to the population, thus giving some respectability to the practice.

It should be stated that while there have been several instances of gross violations of ethical behaviour by psychiatrists in history, most of clinical psychiatry practiced by members of the profession is carried out in an ethical, professional and dedicated manner. The violations when present are so damaging to the field in general and patients in particular that it becomes important to place some emphasis on these practices in order to prevent any recurrence. This is most crucial for teaching purposes when students and residents of the profession are required to learn about ethical and professional practice. Simply teaching the concepts is insufficient. Trainees should know where psychiatrists have transgressed in the past and how they have wandered from the path of the straight and narrow regarding ethical practice of the profession and paternalistic lack of respect for patient needs. For example, with respect to the practice of psychiatry during the Nazi era, student trainees need to know that several crucial errors led to their misconduct. These include allowing philosophical constructs to define clinical practice, focusing exclusively on prevention of mental illness, allowing political considerations to influence practice, and falsely believing that good science and good ethics always coexist [16]. Most importantly they need to know that it is often the 'average psychiatrist' who participates in these unethical behaviours. Attributing unethical behaviour to physicians and psychiatrists who are 'evil' simply misrepresents the truth. This realization is important to relay to trainees so that a constant awareness of the issues is maintained, and so that risk is minimized in order that coercion will not continue in any form or manner amongst practitioners of psychiatry.

While providing no guarantee, pertinent safeguards, including ethical codes and ongoing medical education, are required in order to minimize potential risks of unethical behaviour by members of the profession. This includes, for example, being aware of outside pressures influencing clinical care, be they political, economic or research related. While the risks are great, there is great benefit in averting such behaviour and transmitting the most important values of our field in patient care. These include those of empathy, dedication, resilience, self-sacrifice, honesty, respect, dignity, confidentiality, perseverance and devotion. Our sick deserve no less.

# References

1. Strous, R. (2007) Commentary: political activism: should psychologists and psychiatrists try to make a difference? *Israel Journal of Psychiatry and Related Science*, **44**, 12–17.
2. Lifton, R. (1986) *The Nazi Doctors: Medical Killing and the Psychology of Genocide*, Basic Books, New York.
3. Binding, K. and Hoche, A. (1920) *Die Freigabe der Vernichtung lebensunwerten Lebens: Ihr Mass und ihre Form*, F Meiner, Leipzig.
4. Strous, R.D. (2006) Hitler's psychiatrists: healers and researchers turned executioners and its relevance today. *Harvard Review of Psychiatry*, **14**, 30–37.
5. Proctor, R.N. (1988) *Racial Hygiene: Medicine Under the Nazis*, Harvard University Press, Cambridge, MA.
6. Kater, M. (1989) *Doctors under Hitler*, University of North Carolina Press, Chapel Hill, NC.
7. Gejman, P.V. (1997) Ernst Ruedin and Nazi euthanasia: another stain on his career. *American Journal of Medical Genetics*, **74**, 455–456.
8. Friedlander, H. (1995) *The Origins of Nazi Genocide: From Euthanasia to the Final Solution*, University of North Carolina Press, Chapel Hill, NC.
9. Strous, R.D. (2009) Dr. Irmfried Eberl (1910–1948): mass murdering MD. *Israel Medical Association Journal*, **11**, 216–218.
10. Scull, A. (2005) *Madhouse: A Tragic Tale of Megalomania and Modern Medicine*, Yale University Press, New Haven, CT.
11. Appelbaum, P. (1986) Treating death row prisoner – an ethical dilemma. Clinical Psychiatry News (August).
12. Kermani, E.J. and Drob, S.L. (1988) Psychiatry and the death penalty: dilemma for mental health professionals. *Psychiatric Quarterly*, **59**, 193–212.
13. Black, L.J. and Levine, M.A. (2008) Ethical prohibition against physician participation in capital punishment. *Mayo Clinic Proceedings*, **83**, 113–114.
14. Bonnie, R.J. (2002) Political abuse of psychiatry in the Soviet Union and in China: complexities and controversies. *The Journal of the American Academy of Psychiatry and the Law*, **30**, 136–144.
15. Hollander, N.C. (1992) Psychoanalysis and state terror in Argentina. *American Journal of Psychoanalysis*, **52**, 273–289.
16. Strous, R.D. (2007) Psychiatry during the Nazi era: ethical lessons for the modern professional. *Annals of General Psychiatry*, **27**, 8.

# 11 Paternalism in mental health – when boots are superior to Pushkin

## Tom Burns

*University of Oxford, Warneford Hospital, Oxford, UK*

## 11.1 Patient autonomy and the demise of paternalism

Paternalism and paternalistic are not neutral words. In psychiatry they are currently used to criticize or to indicate something to be avoided. Accused of being paternalistic, we are often frankly embarrassed. 'Protecting and promoting patient autonomy' is the dominant theme in current ethical and legal discourse in both general and mental health care. The concept of capacity, and its effective definition and assessment, has become a central determinant in this debate. This increase in interest in capacity arose from an international re-evaluation of the fundamental relationship between doctor and patient. There has been a shift in the developed world from a broadly paternalistic approach in medicine to a greater emphasis on the individual's own treatment decisions [1]. Psychiatry is not immune to this shift, and the American Psychiatric Association proposed a model stature based around a mental capacity test [2] as the legal and ethical basis for mental health legislation.

Protecting patient autonomy is not, however, generally proposed as absolute and has required careful consideration of how its limits can be defined. This is

*Coercive Treatment in Psychiatry: Clinical, Legal and Ethical Aspects*, First Edition.
Edited by Thomas W. Kallert, Juan E. Mezzich and John Monahan.
© 2011 John Wiley & Sons, Ltd. Published 2011 by John Wiley & Sons, Ltd.

particularly pressing in psychiatry, where imposing treatments against a patient's clearly expressed wishes is a common and recognized practice. Traditionally, mental health legislation has been based primarily on need – the need to protect an impaired individual from risk to themselves or others. Recently, proposals have been made to replace this approach with one based predominantly on capacity, arguing that to treat the mentally ill differently to other medical disorders is discriminatory and possibly stigmatizing [3–5].

## 11.2    Capacity and risk in mental health law

Capacity, long an important consideration in the assessment and management of dementia, is now the subject of increasing research interest in general psychiatric patients [6,7]. A systematic review of studies of mental capacity in psychiatric patients [8] identified 37 papers using 29 different measures of capacity and found that nearly a third of patients were judged to lack capacity. A semi-structured interview for assessing capacity, the MacArthur Competence Assessment Tool for Treatment (MacCAT-T) [9] has been used in several of these studies and shown to have good inter-rater reliability [6,8]. The existence of a well-respected assessment tool is both a measure of the level of interest in the subject but also a guarantor of further increases in that interest and research activity.

Modern mental health Acts have increasingly used the language of risk. Proposals to move towards a capacity-based mental health law invariably provide for some form of override if a capacitous or borderline capacitous patient is deemed to pose a risk to others [10,11]. This risk criterion usually also includes significant risk to the self. How strictly risk to self is interpreted varies markedly between different national and health care contexts. In its strictest interpretation, it can be taken to require an imminent threat of physical harm (suicidal or reckless behaviour for instance). In the UK, however, risk to self in the recent (2007) amendment to the Mental Health Act is still interpreted very widely to include a deterioration in health because of failure to take appropriate treatment. Many UK clinicians strongly opposed this amended wording emphasizing risk. They were concerned that it would result in either a distortion of language to continue to admit at the older threshold, or that a higher risk threshold could leave seriously ill patients untreated.

This preoccupation with capacity reflects a need to delineate circumstances (and find an ethical justification) for when patient autonomy can be overridden. The centrality of capacity and patient autonomy in the Richardson proposals for the reform of the Mental Health Act in England and Wales [11] led to a bruising head-on collision and its rejection by a pragmatic government. Despite this, the current debate privileges patient autonomy almost exclusively. In their recently published proposal, Szmukler and colleagues [10] state '...protecting the autonomy of patients with capacity *is not the only important ethical principle*. . . another concerns the need to protect other people. . .' In its most logical expression, this view labels any mental health legislation as discriminatory and unnecessary, insisting that capacitous individuals should be subject to normal legal processes [5]. Thomas Szasz [12] even went further and argued for patients' equal rights to be punished for their crimes and to refuse treatment whatever their mental state. All in all, paternalism seems anachronistic, embarrassing and dismissed in mental health care.

## 11.3   Paternalism's continued existence

There may, however, be a more widespread and legitimate acceptance of paternalism than this current discourse suggests. Paternalism and beneficence are alive and well in mental health practice. Independent of the clinical setting, the language used or the legal system espoused, clinicians (psychiatrists, psychiatric nurses and psychiatric social workers) regularly override autonomy when they consider it in the patient's best interest. The language of psychiatry from its inception has stressed the alienation of the ill patient from their normal self, and recovery was described as their being 'restored to reason'. Paternalistic decisions are usually based on an assumption that the professional can, in an assessment, form a judgement of what that person would want where they 'their normal self'. Being absolutely clear that this judgement reflects the patient's best interests and their 'normal self' wishes and not what the practitioner thinks is best for them based on his or her own values is, of course, a difficult and murky area. It is not, however, a completely impossible distinction and most of us make it regularly in our interactions, both professional and private. A paternalistic approach would need to be alive to this possibility and guard against it.

## 11.4   Paternalism's philosophical legitimacy

The idea that people can have different wishes and desires at different times and in different states and that some form of precedence can be established between them is recognized by philosophers. Indeed the philosopher Harry Frankfurt considers it the defining quality of being a person. He outlines the concept of first- and second-order desires [13] and argues that *the* defining characteristic of a human being is their capacity for 'second-order desires'.

All animals can want things, but only human beings can 'want to want'. For example, any creature can experience a desire to eat or a desire not to eat, but only a human (what Frankfurt calls rather precisely 'a being with personhood') can experience a desire to not desire to eat. This is a second-order desire. There may be times when our more fundamental long-term wishes are overwhelmed by temporary ones. Frankfurt uses the example of the alcoholic who, while he wants to drink, wants not to want to drink. Such a view of humans forms the possible justification for denying, or frankly contradicting, their expressed wishes. In mental illness we may believe that the illness is overwhelming and obscuring the patient's fundamental (second-order) desires. In compulsory treatment we thus act against their first-order desires (e.g. flight from delusional persecution) to protect their second-order desire (to remain well and stay with their family).

## 11.5  Conflicting moral principles

John Stuart Mill's *On Liberty* [14] has established the primacy of individual rights in Western thinking. It is not, however, the only moral framework available to us. Isaiah Berlin argued that there are often several moral principles relevant to a decision and that they may at times conflict. Liberté, égalité, and fraternité do not always point in the same direction. The Nobel Laureate Amartya Sen [15] has been particularly concerned with how one can arrive at meaningful moral judgements about competing claims for individual freedoms. How can justice be achieved and identity respected in vastly different settings and with competing claims?

Sen is part of a wider movement that rejects the traditional search for a single, articulated theory for a just society, based on certain principles from which ethical guidance is then derived. This approach has been most clearly summarized in the work of the moral and political philosopher John Rawls [16], whose concept of a 'social contract' is based on the principle that fairness is justice. Sen argues for a 'social choice' approach to justice and ethical decisions. While we may not all agree on the exact configuration of the just society, Sen insists that most of us can readily agree on the presence of manifest injustice. He argues the need for empirical work to identify what he calls 'circumscribed congruence' to include those competing moral forces that we can agree are relevant to make a just decision in a specific situation. There is not a single, consistent dominant moral principle that will always guide us.

Psychiatric ethical debates seem immune to this later, more person-centred and complex philosophical framework and remain focused on an either-or, two-dimensional approach. Either it is autonomy or paternalism, and we appear to assume that everyone else (lawyers, economists, philosophers, politicians) has jettisoned paternalism. It is just us left struggling with this otherwise extinct and anachronistic concept. However, this is not so. There is an extensive literature on acceptable forms of paternalism in modern societies within several disciplines that warrant closer consideration by psychiatry.

## 11.6  Political theory

John Stuart Mill did not consider that liberty was an end in itself. He valued it as a basis for social progress, 'utility in the largest sense, grounded on the permanent interests of *man as a progressive being.*' [14, p.53] Isaiah Berlin's famous inaugural lecture *Two Concepts of Liberty* [17] proposed a negative and a positive liberty. He argued that Mill had restricted himself to the negative form – that which defines the area within which others may not tell you what to do. The boundary of this area is, however,

> . . .a matter of argument, indeed of haggling. Men are largely interdependent, and no man's activity is so completely private as never to obstruct the lives of others in any way.

Berlin argues that the exercise of freedoms (and indeed their existence) is *not* independent of the condition of individuals. The freedom to starve is simply not a freedom. Positive liberty depends on being able to exert your freedoms, and his illustration is particularly relevant to mental health:

> . . .to offer political rights, or safeguards against intervention by the State, to men who are half naked, illiterate, underfed and diseased is to mock their condition; . . . First things come first – there are times when boots are superior to Pushkin

In Berlin's thesis, liberty is equivalent to 'patient autonomy' in mental health considerations. He argues that it is more than simply the absence of frustration or coercion. In a moral society it may occasionally be necessary to make decisions for someone in order to promote their true liberty. There can be interventions against someone's will which may increase their liberty; an obvious example is universal education. Berlin was intensely sensitive to the potential misrepresentation of this position by totalitarian regimes. He distinguished it strongly from the sophistry that such temporary coercion is 'not coercion' because it serves the interests of the individual's 'true self'. It *is* coercion and any moral justification proposed for it must recognize this.

Like Anatole France ('The law, in its majestic equality, forbids the rich as well as the poor to sleep under bridges, to beg in the streets, and to steal bread') [18], he highlights how a narrow configuration of liberty can be used to protect the consciences of the wealthy and powerful in their exploitation and neglect of the vulnerable and powerless. The practice of some low-tax states in permitting homelessness and neglect of the severely mentally ill, on ostensibly libertarian grounds, has been pithily characterized as 'the freedom to die with their rights on' [19].

## 11.7   Economic theory

'Soft (or Liberal) Paternalism' has been proposed by economists as one sensible response to the complex challenges of evolved systems. Chicago economists Sunstein and Thaler argue that 'libertarian paternalism is not an oxymoron' [20].

Soft paternalism is the introduction of economic regulations for individuals' best interests even when we can be sure that, asked directly if they wanted those regulations, they would be highly likely to decline. Common examples are comparing opt-in to opt-out arrangements in pension schemes, such as the recent US legislation 401(k), which requires an opt-out, spurred on by the spectre of increasing old-age poverty in an ageing population. Success is measured in the difference between the rates of how many people remain enrolled through inertia than would actively choose to do so. The 401(k) legislation doubled the number of savers. The authors' justification for supporting this approach is:

> Often people's preferences are ill-formed, and their choices will inevitably be influenced by default rules, framing effects and starting points. In these circumstances a form of paternalism cannot be avoided.

They aim to 'unsettle the Libertarian dogma that people generally make decisions in their best interests', pointing out that this implies 'complete information, unlimited cognitive abilities and no lack of will-power'. In their recent internationally influential book, *Nudge: Improving Decisions about Health, Wealth and Happiness* [21], they describe this liberal paternalism as 'choice architecture' and their discipline as 'behavioural economics'. Thaler and Sunstein argue that it is disingenuous to ignore the ubiquitous pressures that people are subject to simply because they are undeclared. Much of this economic social engineering is so familiar to us that we hardly notice it. The current debate about opt-in or opt-out for organ donation [22,23] (where 90% of the UK population support organ donation and only 23% have registered their wish to donate) contrasts sharply with the ready acceptance of taxes for universal health care and schooling.

Considering the even starker problems of extreme poverty in sub-Saharan Africa, the economist Jeffrey Sachs calls for increased economic paternalism:

> We should embrace market economics, but also recognise that free market economics are passé. We need an active role for the state to help the poorest break out of their poverty trap [24].

## 11.8   The feminist critique of autonomy and paternalism

Feminism might be anticipated to be paternalism's strongest critic. By championing women's autonomy and individual rights, they have challenged and eroded their traditional exploitation and suppression in patriarchal societies. However the picture is not monochrome.

Both philosophy and sociology contain pointed feminist critiques of individualism, particularly as it is used in the defence of an impersonal code of justice and individual rights. Feminist social scientists such as Ann Oakley [25] have even argued that the dominance of quantitative over qualitative research reflects a masculine world view; a world view which excessively emphasizes independence (i.e. counting the numbers) over interdependence (i.e. acknowledging the relationships).

The 'ethics of care' movement, drawing on the work of the psychologist Carol Gilligan [26], questions the neutrality and impartiality of traditional ethical frameworks and stresses the centrality of close relationships. It emphasizes the positive moral value of being *partial* toward those individuals with whom we have special and valuable relationships. There is a moral basis for responding to such persons as particular individuals with characteristics that demand a quite specific response that we do not extend to others.

> ... men tend to embrace an ethic of rights using quasi-legal terminology and impartial principles... women tend to affirm an ethic of care that centers on responsiveness in an interconnected network of needs, care, and prevention of harm. *Taking care of others is the core notion.*

> ... many human relationships involve persons who are vulnerable, dependent, ill, and frail... [and] the desirable moral response is *attached attentiveness to needs, not detached respect for rights* [27].

This view understands moral behaviour as built up from close personal experience and increasingly extended to a wider group. It is predicated on behaviour leading to the elaboration of ethical guidelines, rather than vice versa where theoretically constructed guidelines prescribe behaviour (as in classical deontology). Sachs [24] observed that it was those countries that already devoted high tax revenues for generous welfare states which went on to donate most in international aid. He concluded that it was familiarity with, and commitment to, supporting welfare locally that primes the individual, or state, to extend it internationally.

With women's unique relationship with newborn and dependent children, it should come as no surprise that they recognize the centrality of interdependence and build their thinking upon it. The Psychoanalyst Donald Winnicot caught the essence with his declaration '*there is no such thing as a new-born baby*' [28]. Mother and newborn is the fundamental unit. In this most intense human relationship interdependency is not an optional extra; it is the very prerequisite for survival.

In post-institutional psychiatry, women's opinions matter, and they probably should matter more than men's. It is overwhelmingly women who do the caring for the severely mentally ill [29]. They shoulder the responsibility and have the experience, so they may be more realistic about the moral challenges. The human rights agenda is an important one but it is only one of several.

## 11.9   Not dead and gone

Paternalism undoubtedly plays a decreasing role in our increasingly egalitarian and well-educated societies. It can easily slip over into authoritarianism and it remains contested in several areas of moral discourse. However it is a day-to-day reality in our provision of humane mental health care, and moral reasoning which ignores it is incomplete. We need to examine its place in managing the ethical dilemmas we constantly face, and not delude ourselves that it is either dead and gone, or that it is irrelevant.

## Acknowledgements

My thanks to John Dawson, Professor of Law at Otago University, New Zealand, for his most helpful comments and guidance on an earlier draft of this article.

## References

1. Schneider, C. (1999) *The Practice of Autonomy*, Oxford University Press, New York.
2. Stromberg, C. and Stone, A. (1983) Statute: a model state law on civil commitment of the mentally ill. *Harvard Journal on Legislation*, **20**, 275–396.
3. Richardson, G. (2007) Balancing autonomy and risk: a failure of nerve in England and Wales? *International Journal of Law and Psychiatry*, **30**, 71–80.
4. Dawson, J. and Szmukler, G. (2006) Fusion of mental health and incapacity legislation. *British Journal of Psychiatry*, **188**, 504–509.
5. Szmukler, G. and Holloway, F. (1998) Mental health legislation is now a harmful anachronism. *Psychiatric Bulletin*, **22**, 662–655.
6. Cairns, R., Maddock, C., Buchanan, A. *et al.* (2005) Reliability of mental capacity assessments in psychiatric in-patients. *British Journal of Psychiatry*, **187**, 372–378.
7. Appelbaum, P.S. (2007) Assessment of patient's competence to consent to treatment. *New England Journal of Medicine*, **357**, 1834–1840.
8. Okai, D., Owen, G., McGuire, H. *et al.* (2007) Mental capacity in psychiatric patients. Systematic review. *British Journal of Psychiatry*, **191**, 291–297.
9. Grisso, T., Appelbaum, P.S. and Hill-Fotouhi, C. (1997) The MacCAT-T: a clinical tool to assess patients' capacities to make treatment decisions. *Psychiatric Services*, **48**, 1415–1419.
10. Szmukler, G., Daw, R. and Dawson, J. (2010) A model law fusing incapacity and mental health legislation. *Journal of Mental Health Law, Special Issue*, **20**, 11–22, and 101–126.
11. Department of Health (1999) *Report of the Expert Committee: Review of the Mental Health Act 1983*, Department of Health, London.

12. Szasz, T.S. (1972) *The Myth of Mental Illness: Foundations of a Theory of Personal Conduct*, Paladin, London.
13. Frankfurt, H.G. (1971) Freedom of the will and the concept of a person. *The Journal of Philosophy*, **LXVII**, 5–20.
14. Mill, J.S. (1859) *On Liberty*, Parker, London.
15. Sen, A. (2006) What do we want from a theory of justice? *The Journal of Philosophy*, **CII**, 215–238.
16. Rawls, J. (1971) *A Theory of Justice*, Harvard University Press, Cambridge, MA.
17. Berlin, I. (1958) *Two Concepts of Liberty*, Clarendon Press, Oxford, UK.
18. France, A. (1894) *The Red Lily*, Paris.
19. Treffert, D.A. (1973) Dying with their rights on. *American Journal of Psychiatry*, **130**, 1041.
20. Thaler, R.H. and Sunstein, C. (2003) Libertarian paternalism is not an oxymoron. *University of Chicago Law Review*, **70**, 1159–1202.
21. Thaler, R.H. and Sunstein, C. (2008) *Nudge: Improving Decisions About Health, Wealth and Happiness*, Yale University Press, New Haven, CT.
22. English, V. (2007) Is presumed consent the answer to organ shortages? Yes. *British Medical Journal*, **334**, 1088.
23. Wright, L. (2007) Is presumed consent the answer to organ shortages? No. *British Medical Journal*, **334**, 1089.
24. Sachs, J.D. (2005) *The End of Poverty: Economic Possibilities for Our Time*, Penguin, London.
25. Oakley, A. (1998) Gender, methodology and people's ways of knowing: some problems with feminism and the paradigm debate in social science. *Sociology*, **32**, 707–731.
26. Gilligan, C. (1982) *In a Different Voice*, Harvard University Press, Cambridge, MA.
27. Beauchamp, T.L. and Childress, J.F. (2001) *Principles of Biomedical Ethics*, 5th edn, Oxford University Press, New York.
28. Winnicott, D.W. (1964) *Further Thoughts on Babies as Persons. The Child, the Family, and the Outside World*, Penguin, London.
29. Harvey, K., Burns, T., Sedgwick, P. *et al.* (2001) Relatives of patients with severe psychotic disorders: factors that influence contact frequency. Report from the UK700 trial. *British Journal of Psychiatry*, **178**, 248–254.

# Section 4

## Users' views on coercive treatment

# 12 The moral imperative for dialogue with organizations of survivors of coerced psychiatric human rights violations

**David W. Oaks**

*MindFreedom International, Eugene, OR, USA*

## 12.1 Overview – coerced psychiatric procedures lead to an insurmountable power imbalance

I personally experienced coerced psychiatric procedures in a variety of ways over a three-year period as a young adult. Because of what I perceived as my unjust and harmful mental health care, I felt passionately motivated to become a community organizer in the field of human rights in mental health. In my opinion, the coerced psychiatric procedures I was subjected to were significant violations of my human rights that profoundly traumatize me to this day.

*Coercive Treatment in Psychiatry: Clinical, Legal and Ethical Aspects*, First Edition.
Edited by Thomas W. Kallert, Juan E. Mezzich and John Monahan.
© 2011 John Wiley & Sons, Ltd. Published 2011 by John Wiley & Sons, Ltd.

As a grassroots activist in the field of mental health advocacy for the past 35 years, I have heard moving stories from hundreds of other individuals who identify themselves as survivors of coerced psychiatric human rights violations, often far more traumatic than mine. I feel privileged, humbled and thankful to call many of these psychiatric survivors my lifetime friends and colleagues. Because of my unique career, I have had a front seat watching the beautiful resilience of the human spirit overcome not only their original mental and emotional crises, but also the insidiously complex trauma that occurs when one feels betrayed by those who are charged and licensed by our society to provide care, healing and protection.

Too often, individuals, who for the first time hear about our little-known social change movement led by survivors of psychiatric abuse, claim that the kinds of violations that I and other leaders suffered decades ago were remnants of a dark age and no longer occur. As the director for the past 25 years of an international non-governmental organization (NGO) that works for the human rights of people in the mental health system, MindFreedom International, I can testify that nearly every day our office receives new, moving, poignant, personal reports of abuse in the contemporary psychiatric care system, usually related to some type of coercion. The types of abuse I hear about have continued unabated throughout all these years, to the present time. My subjective perception is that this psychiatric coercion is increasing, and in fact appears to be expanding rapidly into poor and developing countries.

I discuss coercion in psychiatric care here neither as an academic with an advanced degree, nor as a licensed mental health professional with clinical experience, because I am neither. Instead, I question coercion in the mental health field as a psychiatric survivor activist who has devoted his adult life to promoting human rights as the very foundation of mental and emotional well being. I will briefly review what I have learned from my vocation, and discuss what I categorize as three general types of psychiatric coercion:

## 1. Force: physically imposed mental health care over the expressed wishes of the subject

For example, some individuals diagnosed with psychiatric disorders are now under court order to take prescribed psychiatric pharmaceuticals over and against their expressed wishes, even though they are living peacefully and legally outside of an institution, in a community setting in their own home. In many instances, if such an individual refuses to take a prescribed psychiatric drug, then he or she can be immediately institutionalized. Known by a variety of terms such as 'involuntary outpatient commitment' or 'compulsory community treatment', this approach is an example of the expansion of coerced psychiatric treatment from the back wards of locked psychiatric institutions, to the front porch of our own homes in our own neighbourhoods. This spread of what often amounts to coerced psychiatric drugging in our communities has become widespread in North America, Europe and Australasia [1].

2. **Fraud: misinformation by licensed mental health professionals in order to alter the behaviour of mental health clients**

   For example, as we will see, back in the 1970s I was told by my psychiatrist that I would absolutely need to take prescribed psychiatric pharmaceuticals for the rest of my life because, he alleged, I had a scientifically proven, genetically caused, chemical imbalance. While I respect others who make the personal health care decision to take prescribed psychiatric medications, apparently my psychiatrist was misinformed. I have been off of all psychiatric medications since 1977.

3. **Fear: the terrifying belief by an individual seeking mental health care that he or she has no alternative available, other than a very narrow range of choices, typically limited to a conventional medical model**

   For example, many individuals, contacting our office to complain about their mental health care, report that they are not offered psychotherapy or other non-drug psychosocial approaches at all; instead, they are often prescribed a perplexing and frequently changing combination of many psychiatric medications. A wide array of non-drug alternatives is being utilized by other individuals who are diagnosed with severe mental and emotional problems to reach recovery, but these options are often not readily offered or available to the general public. One of the more promising fields is the use of peer support to augment or replace other types of psychiatric care [2].

In order to explore the psychosocial and ethical impact of these three forms of psychiatric coercion, I believe that open, mediated dialogue between mental health professional organizations and organizations representing those who have experienced psychiatric human rights violations is a moral imperative. I argue that a number of psychiatric survivor organizations have attempted such dialogue, but so far these invitations have not been enthusiastically reciprocated. While we must never give up, I conclude that we must learn from other successful social change movements in history who have represented extremely marginalized and disempowered populations, such as the US civil rights movement led by African Americans. We must consider the necessity of moving into an era of international nonviolent direct action, including peaceful cultural and civil disobedience protests.

## 12.2    On the sharp end of the needle – my recruitment to human rights activism

My personal introduction, to what I feel can be an astounding power imbalance between psychiatrist and client, arrived when I was a college student experiencing overwhelming mental and emotional problems. I had grown up in a working class neighbourhood on the south side of Chicago in a household with loving parents, and I won several scholarships to attend Harvard. Unfortunately, five times during my sophomore, junior and senior years I entered into severe mental and emotional crises, and ended up inside of psychiatric institutions. During my stays on these psychiatric units, I would often feel pressured by staff to take powerful psychiatric pills, and I often tried to refuse. More than once, staff brought me to an empty solitary confinement room, held me down on a bare mattress, pulled down my pants, injected me in my buttocks, and then left me there alone for a few hours to a few days.

The subjective experience of being forcibly injected with psychotropic drugs and left isolated has created one of my longest-standing recurring nightmares. There I was, a confused and frightened young person. I felt at the time that I needed respite, advice, support and comfort. Instead, the impact of the coerced psychiatric drug felt like a wrecking ball to the cathedral of my mind, a mind which was indeed troubled, but which I valued nonetheless. While on coerced neuroleptic psychiatric medication, also known as antipsychotics, the more I tried to focus and think, the more difficult I found the task. I developed a number of physical side effects to the medications that some might consider trivial, but that I found upsetting, such as muscle contortions in my neck and blurry vision. All in all, I felt humiliated, disrespected and defiant. I certainly did not feel a high level of trust with my mental health providers that might have been more conducive to a therapeutic relationship.

I was exposed to a variety of coercive acts while in psychiatric institutions. For instance, upon admission my basic rights were immediately taken a way, and then slowly given back as privileges for behaviour that was considered appropriate. My every movement was monitored and controlled. Any seemingly peaceful rebellion by me – such as questioning staff – could be misinterpreted as violent, and result in another forced drugging. For example, once, when I complained to staff about something on the ward, a staff member condescendingly gave me a cookie in a paternalistic gesture. I took the cookie and crumbled it in my hand. Immediately guards were summoned for another forced drug injection, even though I quickly and compliantly dropped every crumb of the cookie into the garbage can. My frantic gesture of cleanliness was futile, because the machinery of another forced psychiatric drugging had already been triggered.

The impact of these experiences alienated me far more from our society than anything I had experienced before or after. I remember with special clarity one particular moment when I was standing in my solitary confinement room after another forced psychiatric drug injection. I was looking out of the cell window, which was covered by an impenetrable steel mesh. I symbolically pounded the mesh a few times with my fist, slowly and methodically, doing no damage to either the mesh or my fist. But I vowed that when I got out I would seek to change how the mental health system treated people. I now refer to that solitary confinement room on the ground floor of Bowditch Hall at McLean Hospital in Belmont, Massachusetts, as my recruitment room to become a community organizer of mental health consumers and psychiatric survivors.

In my senior year, I am grateful that Harvard's social service agency, Phillips Brooks House (PBH), placed me as an intern in one of the early psychiatric survivor activist organizations in Cambridge, Massachusetts. Inspired by the ferment of the times, these groups began springing up in the USA, Europe and Canada in the early 1970s. The moment I entered the little store front where this group of psychiatric survivors met, I discovered I was not alone. Finding courage through mutual support, we exchanged our personal stories, and learned that others were seeking to significantly change the mental health system. This is where I met Judi Chamberlin, who was preparing to publish what would become an influential book, *On Our Own*, which proposed to transform the mental health system by creating peer-run alternatives [3]. Judi would become an internationally influential advocate for mental health consumers and psychiatric survivors. She was later to write about what brought her into this work:

> Being a patient was the most devastating experience of my life. At a time when I was already fragile and vulnerable, being labeled and treated only confirmed to me I was worthless. It was clear my thoughts, feelings, and opinions counted for little. I was presumed not to be able to take care of myself or to make decisions in my own best interest, and to need mental health professionals running my life for me. For this total disregard of my wishes and feelings, I was expected to be appreciative and grateful. In fact, anything less was taken as a further symptom of my illness, as one more indication I truly needed more of the same. [4]

The fifth and final time I was institutionalized, I was able to contact this grassroots group and ask for advocacy and moral support. Thankfully, my family, which had at first been compliant with suggestions by mental health professionals, had become more sceptical. As recounted in the book, *A Way Out of Madness: Dealing with Your Family After You've Been Diagnosed with a Psychiatric Disorder* [5], my family began to question the wisdom of the aggressive mental health care I was experiencing. Even today, I find the fact that my family took steps to protect my human rights decades ago as personally healing. As I prepared to assert my rights and leave my last psychiatric institutionalization, the mental health authorities apparently contacted my family to enquire about the possibility of seeking a court order to prevent me from leaving McLean Hospital. My mother famously replied on behalf of my family, 'If our David wants to try freedom we support him.'

After this final institutionalization, I wrote my senior paper at Harvard about my experience of volunteering with Judi and others. I explored how people, who have been hurt in such a deep way, appeared to feel compelled to innovate unique, empowering styles of organizing their group, in an attempt to prevent authoritarianism which might retraumatize them. Somehow, despite all of my problems and institutionalizations, I managed to graduate with honours from Harvard in 1977.

During the decades since I have noted that the scientific literature in psychiatry frequently hypothesizes about a possible chemical imbalance as being at the root of many serious mental and emotional problems. As we will see, strong scientific evidence for such a chemical imbalance apparently remains illusive to research scientists. However, as a community organizer I can offer my personal observation that a vast power imbalance exists between the psychiatric profession and their customers. When there is such a disparity in power, I have often found a silencing effect that can mute or distort the voice of the individual who finds him- or herself so shunned and discounted.

The enormity of the emotional harm caused by coercion in mental health care can be emotionally devastating, and even physically deadly. In an attempt to maintain the memory of those whose lives have been shortened due to mental health abuse, many of us call ourselves, as I do, 'psychiatric survivors'. I have listened to stories of individuals who have received the overt brutality of repeated electroshock (also known as electroconvulsive therapy or ECT), against their passionately expressed wishes. I have heard stories of being held in restraints for hours, or even days. I have several friends who personally experienced the now-abandoned insulin coma therapy, describing the pain of the forced experience as torture [6]. It is impossible to rank all the types of psychiatric coercion by the harm that is caused. A common denominator is that psychiatric survivors say that the unjust deprivation of liberty itself is always harmful.

One of the leaders I met when I first became active as a community organizer was Ted Chabasinski, a well-respected leader in the social change movement led by psychiatric survivors, who would later become an attorney working as a mental health advocate. As a child in the 1940s, Ted was subjected to well-documented and unfathomable abuse in a programme in New York State that was experimenting with the administration of ECT on children as young as three [7]. Ted was only six years old when he received his own experimental involuntary electroshock [8].

Ted recalled the memories in an interview he provided to MindFreedom International. He remembered thinking as a child, 'I won't go to the shock treatment, I won't!' Ted said it took three attendants to hold him:

> I wanted to die but I really didn't know what death was. I knew that it was something terrible. Maybe I'll be so tired after the next shock treatment I won't get up, I won't ever get up, and I'll be dead. But I always got up. Something in me beyond my wishes made me put myself together again.

Even as such a young, frightened child, Ted tried to find ways to somehow maintain his identity. Said Ted,

> I memorized my name, I taught myself to say my name. 'Teddy, Teddy, I'm Teddy. . . I'm here, I'm here, in this room, in this hospital. And my mommy's gone. . .' I would cry and realize how dizzy I was. The world was spinning around, and coming back to it hurt too much. I want to go down, I want to go where the shock treatment is sending me, I want to stop fighting and die. . . and something made me live, and to go on living I had to remember never to let anyone near me again.

Ted recounts that he spent his seventh, eighth and ninth birthdays locked in solitary confinement at Rockland State Hospital.

> I had learned the best way to endure this was to sleep as much as possible, and sleeping was all I could do anyway. . . Sometimes there was nothing in the room, nothing at all, and I would lie on the mattress and cry. I would try to fall asleep, but I couldn't sleep 24 hours a day, and I couldn't stand the dreams. I would curl into a ball, clutching my knees, and rock back and forth on the mattress, trying to comfort myself. And I cried and cried, hoping someone would come. 'I'll be good,' I said.

Psychiatric survivor Janet Foner, one of the founders of the support coalition united through MindFreedom International, listed some of the more distressing aspects of her institutionalization:

> The worst parts of being in an institution were: Being locked in seclusion twice. Being on drugs and not being able to stay awake, be aware, or move much. Gaining 30 pounds. Being made to stay there in confinement so long. Boredom. Not getting to go outside much. I wasn't allowed outside at all until a month had gone by. Not ever knowing when I would get out. Seeing most of the women on my ward come back from electroshock. Hearing them scream while in seclusion or restraint. Terrified the whole time that I would get shock. [9]

In my community organizing work, I have also come across positive stories that give me hope, including the history of allies who may be risking their professional careers by calling for deep change in mental health care. These dissident mental health providers have taught me that there is an antidote to the silencing caused by the power imbalance in mental health care, and that is the power of civil dialogue. A friend of mine who was a psychiatrist, Loren Mosher (1933–2004), did much to show me during the last years of his life what an ally within the psychiatric profession could do to help psychiatric survivors [10].

As I learned more about Loren's past, I found out that at the same time I made my vows in solitary confinement in a psychiatric institution as a Harvard student to become an activist, Loren was one of the national leaders in the USA on mental health care, and held a position as Chief of the Center for Studies of Schizophrenia at the US National Institute of Mental Health [11]. We did not know each other at that time, but Loren was attempting to prevent the type of mental health system bullying I was experiencing.

Loren helped create 'Soteria House' which, from 1971 to 1983, provided evidence that promoting caring relationships with people in crisis in a non-coercive, non-medical environment can produce positive outcomes [12]. As courageous as creating an alternative centre was, Loren did far more. Like civil rights activists who inspired our social change movement, Loren stood with us psychiatric survivors and spoke out. He agreed that activism to protest oppression was necessary, and he often did this with wit and humour. In a now-famous letter, Loren publicly resigned from the American Psychiatric Association. He wrote in the first paragraph 'The major reason for this action is my belief that I am actually resigning from the American Psychopharmacological Association. Luckily, the organization's true identity requires no change in the acronym.' [13]

Trauma meted out by the mental health system may naturally lead to anger and distrust in some psychiatric survivors. To whom can we turn for help, when it is the healing profession itself that we feel has most wounded us? Unfortunately, far too often we take this anger out on each other, or on our allies. Loren drew the line at tolerating personal abuse or unethical behaviour from anyone, including psychiatric survivors. Loren also realized that taking public action side by side with us, as uncomfortable as that might be, was important for transforming the system, and for our personal recovery from abuse. Loren spoke to the media, to his fellow psychiatrists, to the World Psychiatric Association, to the public, to anyone about our human rights, and what he saw as the truth about the failures of mental health care today.

I keep the example of Loren Mosher in mind when I am getting to know a sympathetic provider in the mental health field. I try to determine if this professional has taken any public action, no matter how modest, to better and humanize that system. Many mental health practitioners privately tell me, to paraphrase, 'Within my office, in my practice, behind closed doors, I provide clients with voluntary, gentle care that respects self-determination. But I never speak out publicly.' I feel this is a missed opportunity. Psychiatric survivors need their provider to be more than what I call a 'closed-door ally'. To such providers I say, I cannot tell you what way of breaking the silence is most aligned with your personal principles and inspiration. However, I can say that to be a truly great ally like Loren Mosher one must be willing to protest openly in some way, and break the silence about the emergency of human rights violations inherent in coerced psychiatric care.

To psychiatric survivors I say, if you have rage over the trauma caused by mental health system abuse, I understand. I do, too. But remember that Martin Luther King, Jr said 'Human salvation lies in the hands of the creatively maladjusted.' [14] I am not perfect, but I try to find a safe place to express my unfocused anger with trusted peers who understand. However, when taking public action with one another, it is in our individual and collective best interests to creatively channel our passion into unity. In my over-three decades of experience, I've seen division amongst psychiatric survivors be one of the main preventable obstacles to the nonviolent revolution in mental health care that I feel is so desperately needed.

By coincidence, all of the personal stories I have cited so far are by present and former board members of MindFreedom International. On our board of directors, we have had survivors of coerced psychiatric abuse such as Chamberlin, Foner and Chabasinski; but we have also had mental health professionals such as Mosher. All have bravely spoken out in their own ways for a complete overhaul of our mental health care system.

Activists in other movements on behalf of extremely disempowered constituencies have discovered the power of combining resistance with civil dialogue with opponents. Mahatma K. Gandhi, for example, believed that finding reconciliation was necessary to build a sustainably peaceful society. One of Gandhi's most memorable traits was his interest in seeking to convert his opponents by engaging in dialogue [15]. As Gandhi himself put it, 'A nonviolent revolution is not a program for the seizure of power. It is a program for the transformation of relationships ending in a peaceful transfer of power.' [16] In fact, I feel this mutual respect is at the root of peer support, which has helped so many of us receiving mental health care find a path to sustained, full recovery following severe mental and emotional problems. The moral principle of mutual respect applies not only to peer support between people diagnosed with psychiatric disorders who are in mental health care; this principle applies to everyone, including those who have taken away our rights. While I seek to change the laws so that coerced psychiatric procedures are an illegal, criminal offence, punishable in severe instances with fair prison sentences, I do not wish inhumane retribution or revenge on anyone.

One of the most prominent national psychiatric survivor activists in the USA is Pat Risser, and he described the power of mutual support to me this way:

Every time I'd tell a psychiatrist or therapist that I was suicidal, I'd get locked up, forcibly drugged, secluded and restrained. I survived over 20 hospitalizations including one hellish stay at a State hospital. Nothing, and I repeat, *nothing* that the system did to me or for me worked. Everything they tried just seemed to make matters worse. The only thing that helped was being accepted as a 'real' person by my fellow patients. Eventually, I realized that I could receive that sort of support without going into a hospital [17].

Just as Pat found the beginning of his own recovery by being acknowledged as a 'real person', so I believe dialogue between representatives of psychiatric professional organizations and psychiatric survivor organizations may help each see that the other is a real person.

It is difficult to express how the intrusion of coerced psychiatric care can feel so shattering to our very being that we may keep silent about our stories of mental health abuse. Dialogue can at least help instruct and warn others about the true cost of such violent and counterproductive mental health coercion. Repeatedly, in preparing this chapter I have reflected back to times in history when other enormous power imbalances have been addressed in dialogue. I recall a famous dialogue I read about from ancient days, recounted by Thucydides in his *History of the Peloponnesian War* [18]. I am referring, of course, to the dialogue between representatives of the inhabitants of the small, vulnerable island nation of Melos, and Athenian negotiators who demanded that Melians immediately submit and become Athenian allies in the imperial contest with Sparta. Plaintively, the Melians suggested a way to peace near the end of the dialogue, saying, 'We invite you to allow us to be friends of yours and enemies to neither side, to make a treaty which shall be agreeable to both you and us, and so to leave our country.' The Melians predicted in the dialogue that if Athens continued to choose crushing brutality in dealing with small nations like Melos, then Athens would eventually lead itself to self-destruction. While the Athenians did indeed decimate the population of the Island of Melos, in the long run the Melian prediction came true, Athens fell, and the wisdom of Melos rings down through history.

So, too, the often-ignored call for dialogue by representatives of organizations of psychiatric survivors is about more than venting over the harm caused to our constituency by coerced psychiatric human rights violations. We are in fact making a call to psychiatric professionals to redeem their own humanity, and to save their own profession. Perhaps a more contemporary example of the power of such dialogue may be the way South Africa has attempted to heal from Apartheid by having Truth and Reconciliation Commissions [19]. Of course, Apartheid first had to be made illegal for any lasting healing to occur.

Another example of the purpose of dialogue may be the way survivors of abuse while children within the Catholic Church have organized to call for systemic change throughout that religion's hierarchy. Too often we hear from leaders of the mental health industry that human rights violations by psychiatric professionals are the result of a 'few bad apples'. But the stunning silence of psychiatric professional organizations failing to address these human rights issues, or to even agree to dialogue about them, threatens to doom the credibility and future of the entire psychiatric profession itself. Dialogue is for the benefit of both sides of a power imbalance, because the humanity of both sides is robbed by that imbalance. Though I'm not a psychologist, I know that reward is more powerful than punishment. Therefore, in subtle ways those on the dominant end of an unfair power imbalance may be more trapped in this toxic relationship than those who are oppressed.

In June 2007, several organizations representing mental health consumers and psychiatric survivors did unite to engage in a hopeful dialogue with the World Psychiatric Association (WPA). The European Network of (ex-)Users and Survivors of Psychiatry, World Network of Users and Survivors of Psychiatry, and Mind-Freedom International, issued a statement, 'Declaration of Dresden Against Coerced Psychiatric Treatment', with the intent of making clear a coordinated position on force and psychiatry at the World Psychiatric Association Conference, *Coercive Treatment in Psychiatry: A Comprehensive Review*, that was held in Dresden, Germany [20].

In part, this 'Declaration of Dresden Against Coerced Psychiatric Treatment' stated,

> Our organizations are in a unique position to speak on this issue because we have experienced forced psychiatry and know the damage it has done to our lives and those of our members, colleagues, and friends. . . We believe that people who have been coerced by psychiatry have a moral claim to making the definitive statement concerning such coercion. We stand united in calling for an end to all forced and coerced psychiatric procedures and for the development of alternatives to psychiatry.

The united statement emphasized the historic nature of a treaty adopted in January 2007 by the United Nations General Assembly, entitled *Convention on the Rights of Persons with Disabilities* [21]. MindFreedom International is an NGO with United Nations Consultative Roster Status, and therefore our delegation, mainly composed of people who had personally experienced coerced psychiatric care and headed by our board president Celia Brown, worked side by side with hundreds of disability advocates from all over the world inside UN headquarters in New York City to craft and pass this binding international treaty. The Declaration of Dresden refers to this treaty, stating:

> We all have a right to refuse psychiatric procedures, since this Convention recognizes the right to free and informed consent with no discrimination based on disability. Even

more important, the Convention guarantees to people with disabilities the right to make our own decisions (legal capacity) on an equal basis with others, and requires governments to provide access to non-coercive support in decision-making, for those who need such support.

The very specific human rights violation of involuntary electroshock was explicitly cited in the Declaration of Dresden, because opposition to this extreme practice unites many mental health organizations, including the World Health Organization [22]. From the Declaration:

> We note that the World Health Organization (WHO) has stated its opposition to all involuntary electroshock, which is also known as electro-convulsive therapy (ECT). Involuntary electroshock is increasing internationally, including in poor and developing countries where it is most likely to be used without anesthesia. In particular, we call for the abolition of involuntary ECT in every country.

The Dresden statement also discusses the interest of international health bodies in developing self-help approaches for people in emotional distress that are less discriminatory. The statement read,

> Organizations of people who have experienced psychiatric treatment have taken the lead in developing self-help programs that are based on equality and choice, rather than on coercion, and have been successful in helping people lead integrated lives in the community. We know that healing can only occur when people are respected as humans with free will and when there are alternatives beyond psychiatry which are based on ethical approaches, which see the whole person, and which support recovery, while force makes recovery impossible.

The Declaration of Dresden also singles out involuntary outpatient commitment, the practice discussed above in which court orders can require individuals who are living out in the community in their own homes to take prescribed psychiatric medication against their wishes. States the Declaration,

> We note that in many countries of the world, there is an increasing use of forced psychiatric procedures, including court ordered treatment which requires that people living in their own homes take psychiatric drugs against their will or lose their freedom. This practice is a violation of our human rights as set forth in the UN Convention.

Those of us who worked on the Declaration of Dresden realized that our vision of eliminating and replacing psychiatric coercion is many years away, but we felt compelled to at least state our dream. We ended the statement by saying,

We invite all supporters of human rights to join and support us in demanding a world free of forced and coerced psychiatric procedures, and we call for adequate funding and support for voluntary self-help services and for alternatives to psychiatry which respect our humanity and dignity.

In the Dresden event, I personally felt hope that there may be more extensive and ongoing dialogue between representatives of mental health professional organizations, and psychiatric survivor organizations. We held informal meetings and a news conference with leaders from psychiatric professional organizations. The only discordant note was that apparently some representatives of pharmaceutical exhibits had objected to our style of grassroots activism in the conference. For whatever reason, as of this writing, I unfortunately must report that our offers for mediated dialogue following Dresden have generally not been accepted.

As a community organizer, it helps me to understand how a Declaration of Dresden can apply to real human beings in real circumstances. In my own workshop in Dresden, I suggested that, to assist in communicating with the public, it would be helpful to describe human rights violations involving coerced mental health care as falling generally into three categories: Force, Fraud and Fear. I'll provide here a few examples of each.

## 12.3 Forced psychiatric procedures over our expressed wishes

A contemporary example of forced psychiatry has taught all of us at Mind-Freedom International valuable lessons. I was in the MindFreedom office in October 2008 when we were phoned by an individual, Ray Sandford of Minnesota, who claimed that he was receiving ongoing, involuntary, outpatient electroshock procedures against his expressed wishes, on a weekly basis. We immediately investigated, because I had never heard of involuntary outpatient commitment being used for coerced electroshock of an individual living out in the community.

I contacted Ray's mental health workers and his mother, and read his court records. I found that there was no secret about it. Ray lived in a small group home in the Minneapolis area. Each Wednesday morning he was awoken early and escorted several miles to a nearby hospital where he received electroconvulsive therapy, and sent home until the next week. He had become determined to stop his regular, coerced outpatient electroshocks. However, while I considered Ray's abuse to be unconstitutional, all the proper Minnesota court orders gave the mental health authorities the legal power to give Ray this coerced electroshock each and every week [23].

It was a moving experience to speak to Ray on the phone before several of these involuntary electroshocks over his expressed wishes. He somehow managed to stay calm on the phone, and expressed in a reasoned but poignant way why he didn't want to have another coerced electroshock. He complained about memory problems he attributed to the procedures. He also objected to other aspects of the procedure, including being forced to undergo anaesthesia. Mainly, he reasonably found forced electroshock to be 'scary'.

We model MindFreedom International's work on the much more famous human rights organization, Amnesty International, so we quickly fashioned a human rights alert to distribute internationally to tens of thousands of concerned people, many of whom began responding immediately by contacting the Governor of Minnesota, and by forwarding the alert to others. We expected that as soon as the matter was brought to light, Ray's forced electroshocks would end. However, even though alert after alert went out, and outraged citizens would contact more and more mental health authorities and elected officials, Ray's involuntary electroshock continued. After further investigation we found a network of more than 30 agencies and services that received public funding and were mandated to help Ray, including protecting his rights. While a few agencies were assisting Ray in his efforts to end his electroshock, many of these 30 agencies were not supporting his efforts to win his human rights at all. Some agencies were in fact passionately fighting in court to continue Ray's forced electroshocks [24]. In a public relations disaster for the mental health system, one of Ray's forced electroshocks – which would turn out to be his last – was on 15 April 2009, which is USA tax day. While I do not have a scientific survey, my impression is that taxpayers generally do not appreciate their scarce resources being used to take a fellow citizen from his home over his objections for regular forced electroshocks.

We redoubled our efforts. Several of us, including myself, flew to Minnesota for peaceful protests. Ray received more attention, including national publicity [25]. Once we convinced members of the public, we quickly were able to outnumber the network of agencies surrounding Ray. We helped Ray to replace his attorney, psychiatrist and guardian. Finally, the forced electroshock ended and his rights were enforced. It is important to note that, throughout his campaign, Ray was not a mute or incoherent individual who was receiving electroshock. Ray was consistently outspoken and clear about why he did not want to receive involuntary electroshock, and he was consulted throughout on the campaign.

We had been told that Ray could not survive without his weekly involuntary electroshock. However, as I write this, it's been over one year since Ray's last electroshock. He calls me at the office about once or twice a week to check in, and I consider him a friend. I remind Ray that every day that he does well, every day that he thrives, he disproves the claim that he absolutely had to have coerced electroshock to survive.

We learned from Ray's victory. We learned that human rights violations like this were systemic, and so would require a systemic and organized nonviolent direct response mobilizing hundreds or even thousands of individuals and groups. Once more, we also found that once the public was informed with convincing evidence of such an outrageous violation as forced outpatient electroshock, we received astounding levels of support. I have found the vast majority of the public – both conservative and liberal – express revulsion and disgust about the continued existence of involuntary electroshock over the expressed wishes of the subject. The fact that such a violation can continue to this day internationally, including throughout the USA, shows that mental health system endorsement of principles, such as human rights, empowerment, peer support and advocacy, may not be entirely convincing to psychiatric survivors.

I feel that all involuntary psychiatric procedures can lessen an individual's level of dignity and self-determination, which are necessary resources for long-term sustained recovery. All involuntary psychiatric procedures undermine an individual's trust with their provider and the community, and this trust ought to be a cornerstone in rebuilding the relationships we all need for mental and emotional well being. All involuntary psychiatric procedures can feel unjust, because an individual is losing their liberty due to a psychiatric diagnosis, rather than because of violating a law created by duly elected representatives that is fairly applied to everyone equally.

However, especially troublesome is the intersection between involuntary psychiatric treatment, and particular procedures which – by their very nature – are intrusive and potentially irreversible. In other words, forced counselling may be humiliating, but one can choose to ignore the mental health counsellor. For example, if a judge offers a convicted drunk driver an educational programme as part of creative sentencing, this is part of due process, and is not coerced psychiatric care. However, procedures such as electroshock, psychiatric drugging and psychosurgery cannot be ignored, and therefore are especially problematic, even when administered to an individual who has been deprived of their liberty because of violating a criminal law. In other words, coerced electroshock, psychiatric drugging and psychosurgery are always wrong, even for individuals in the criminal justice system, because they are inherently cruel and unusual punishment.

Our social change movement is not alone in expressing opposition to all involuntary psychiatric procedures. We have especially found support amongst those working for the human rights of people with disabilities. The US National Council on Disability (NCD) is an independent federal agency empowered by law to provide policy recommendations to the President and Congress on issues involving disability. As one of the highest authorities associated with the US federal government addressing disability matters, the NCD produced a special report in 2000 about coercion in the mental health system, holding a unique public hearing and gathering evidence from psychiatric survivors. The report is entitled *From Privileges to Rights: People Labeled with Psychiatric Disabilities Speak for Themselves* [26].

In the Executive Summary, the NCD describes the process used to create this groundbreaking report:

> NCD heard testimony graphically describing how people with psychiatric disabilities have been beaten, shocked, isolated, incarcerated, restricted, raped, deprived of food and bathroom privileges, and physically and psychologically abused in institutions and in their communities. The testimony pointed to the inescapable fact that people with psychiatric disabilities are systematically and routinely deprived of their rights, and treated as less than full citizens or full human beings.

NCD produced 10 'core recommendations'. The first recommendation provides a hopeful vision on the subject of coercion and psychiatry:

> Laws that allow the use of involuntary treatments such as forced drugging and inpatient and outpatient commitment should be viewed as inherently suspect, because they are incompatible with the principle of self-determination. Public policy needs to move in the direction of a totally voluntary community-based mental health system that safeguards human dignity and respects individual autonomy.

The NCD report also spelled out their reasons for this courageous stand:

> Involuntary treatment is extremely rare outside the psychiatric system, allowable only in such cases as unconsciousness or the inability to communicate. People with psychiatric disabilities, on the other hand, even when they vigorously protest treatments they do not want, are routinely subjected to them anyway, on the justification that they 'lack insight' or are unable to recognize their need for treatment because of their 'mental illness.' In practice, 'lack of insight' becomes disagreement with the treating professional, and people who disagree are labeled 'noncompliant' or 'uncooperative with treatment.'

NCD showed great sensitivity and empathy about why we often do not hear from survivors of psychiatric abuse in our society:

> After years of contact with a system that routinely does not recognize their preferences or desires, many people with psychiatric disabilities become resigned to their fate and cease to protest openly. Although this is described in the psychiatric literature as 'compliance,' it is actually learned helplessness (also known as 'internalized oppression') that is incompatible with hope and with the possibility of recovery.

NCD said that, according to their public hearing, involuntary psychiatric interventions often harm people emotionally, which is the direct opposite of the goal of mental health care:

> The overwhelming amount of testimony concerned the harmfulness of involuntary interventions on people's sense of dignity and self-worth, and, further, contended that such interventions were seldom helpful in assisting people either with their immediate problems or with their long-range ability to improve their lives. NCD heard numerous eloquent pleas for services that were responsive and respectful, and which allowed recipients the same rights and freedoms other citizens take for granted.

The unique nature of trauma from involuntary psychiatric procedures means that it is difficult to elicit public statements from those who have experienced it. In other words, to whom does one turn for help, when one has reason not to trust the helpers? This conundrum can silence those who need to speak out about the coercion they have experienced.

From the NCD report,

> It is important to keep in mind that the hearing was one of the rare opportunities for people labeled with psychiatric disabilities themselves to be the major voice in a government-sponsored inquiry into mental health issues. It is common for mental health policy discussions never to mention words such as 'involuntariness' or 'force,' because these topics are seldom addressed except by people who have suffered because of them. In fact, there seems to be a tacit acceptance among policymakers and the media that people labeled with psychiatric disabilities 'need' to be forced 'for their own good,' and the question of whether such force belongs in a system of medical treatment rarely is systematically examined.

## 12.4   Fraud – coercion by misinformation

As in any complex field, there is ongoing, vigorous debate within the mental health profession about the scientific validity of many psychiatric practices and theories. In the case of coerced psychiatric procedures, this uncertainty and ambiguity becomes troublesome. A licensed mental health provider has been granted an enormous amount of authority by society. One could argue that in coerced psychiatric procedures, some of the most powerful individuals in our society have authority over some of the most disenfranchised, and discredited citizens. Because of this power imbalance, the veracity of claims by mental health professionals ought to be held to the highest scientific standards, because an error may destroy what many of us hold most precious: our liberty.

One of the most devastating experiences for me in my mental health care was misinformation. While being held down on a mattress and forcibly injected with a psychiatric drug was dramatic and degrading, the experience that almost broke my spirit was when, as I discussed above, a respected mental health professional provided to me disempowering disinformation about my psychological issues. I remember sitting down during my fifth psychiatric institutionalization with a Harvard psychiatrist in the recreation room of our ward. He looked me in the eye and told me he was certain that I had a genetically caused, incurable chemical imbalance, and therefore – just as a diabetic needs insulin – I would absolutely have to take powerful prescribed psychiatric medications such as neuroleptics for the rest of my life. Because of support from family, friends, advocacy groups and better mental health professionals, I was able to become sceptical of the claims of this psychiatrist. However, I well remember how close he came to convincing me to become a lifetime mental patient. I believe this psychiatrist was well meaning, but whether intentional or not, his misinformation amounted to fraud. His immense authority, combined with his unscientific message of hopelessness, was in fact a dangerous type of coercion.

I will give just a few examples of mental health controversies where I believe unscientific information may be misleading individuals in mental health care to make decisions different from those they would make if they were offered full and complete information.

## 1. Psychiatric diagnosis

One of the common legal requirements to justify a coerced psychiatric procedure is a psychiatric diagnosis. However, as a lay activist, I watch in amazement as leaders within the psychiatric industry cannot agree about the future of psychiatric diagnosis itself, as the American Psychiatric Association prepares the next edition of their highly influential *Diagnostic and Statistical Manual* (DSM), which influences psychiatric diagnosis internationally.

In a column entitled 'It's not too late to save "normal"', published in the *Los Angeles Times*, Allen Frances, MD, issues a clarion call of warning [27]. Dr Frances chaired the American Psychiatric Association (APA) task force that created the fourth edition of the *DSM* which was published in 1994. He wrote,

I learned from painful experience how small changes in the definition of mental disorders can create huge, unintended consequences. Our panel tried hard to be conservative and careful but inadvertently contributed to three false 'epidemics' – attention deficit disorder, autism and childhood bipolar disorder. Clearly, our net was cast too wide and captured many 'patients' who might have been far better off never entering the mental health system.

What is even more remarkable is the way Dr Frances directly challenges those working on the next version of the DSM. Referring to a draft that the APA posted online, Dr Frances said,

[it] is filled with suggestions that would multiply our mistakes and extend the reach of psychiatry dramatically deeper into the ever-shrinking domain of the normal. This wholesale medical imperialization of normality could potentially create tens of millions of innocent bystanders who would be mislabelled as having a mental disorder. The pharmaceutical industry would have a field day – despite the lack of solid evidence of any effective treatments for these newly proposed diagnoses.

I have to wonder, how accurate is a psychiatric diagnosis when there is such fierce struggle between those who have been the leaders for creating these diagnoses? No elected officials are involved in discussing, creating and voting upon the list of behaviours in the DSM, even though these diagnoses often have the force of law, and could mean the difference between freedom and liberty. 'We the people' have no direct representation in the decisions that create this powerful guideline for our behaviour.

## 2. Chemical imbalance

It is far beyond the scope of this chapter to explore, confirm, refute or even adequately explain some of the current theories in mental health care today. However, I have heard many statements over the years from leaders of various mental health organizations that major psychiatric disorders such as schizophrenia and bipolar are 'biologically based'.

Readers may find it relevant to know about a nonviolent direct action that I and a number of other MindFreedom International activists took together in 2003 on this topic: a hunger strike. Journalist Robert Whitaker has suggested that our hunger strike was a model in how individuals may question the current mental health system [28]. Our Fast for Freedom in Mental Health had a simple demand of the American Psychiatric Association: to produce evidence of this 'biological basis'.

We asked: 'Has science established, beyond a reasonable doubt, that so-called "major mental illnesses" are biological diseases of the brain?' We also asked: 'Does the government have compelling evidence to justify the way it singles out for its primary support this one theory of the origin of emotional distress and of pharmaceutical remedies for its relief?' [29].

For example, we requested evidence for a physical diagnostic exam – such as a scan or test of the brain, blood, urine, genes and so on – that can reliably distinguish individuals with these diagnoses (prior to treatment with psychiatric drugs), from individuals without these diagnoses. We refused to eat until we received a reply from the American Psychiatric Association and other psychiatric organizations, and the nonviolent conflict resulted in significant national media attention [30].

To its surprising credit, the American Psychiatric Association entered into a helpful and extensive back and forth written dialogue with our MindFreedom Scientific Panel. Several of us hunger strikers also met with the elected APA president. In the end, the APA did not claim to have any scientific evidence for a biological basis for psychiatric disorders. The concluding statement by the MindFreedom Scientific Panel on 15 December 2003 raised a final question that is especially applicable to this chapter:

The hunger strikers asked the APA for the 'evidence base' that justifies the biomedical model's stranglehold on the mental health system. The APA has not supplied any such evidence, which compels the scientific panel to ask one final question: on what basis does society justify the authority granted psychiatrists, as medical doctors, to force psycho-active drugs or electroconvulsive treatment upon unwilling individuals, or to incarcerate persons who may or may not have committed criminal acts? For, clearly, it is solely on the basis of trust in the claim that their professional acts and advice are founded on medical science that society grants psychiatrists such extraordinary authority.

## 3. Long-term effects of psychiatric medications
As I've explained, I personally came very close to believing that I needed to be kept, these past 34 years, on continuous neuroleptic psychiatric medications, also known as antipsychotics. Therefore, the long-term impact of this particular family of medications is especially relevant to my own life. In the last few years, mainstream science has used modern research, brain scans, animal studies and autopsies to study whether long-term neuroleptics may be inducing structural brain change, including to the brain's frontal lobes, which are linked to higher-level functions [31]. It is beyond this chapter's scope and my expertise to summarize and analyse these findings here. I will, however, quote from the abstract of just one recent study, which concluded:

Some evidence points towards the possibility that antipsychotic drugs reduce the volume of brain matter and increase ventricular or fluid volume. Antipsychotics may contribute to the genesis of some of the abnormalities usually attributed to schizophrenia. [32]

Attorney James Gottstein, who directs the public interest law firm PsychRights, is utilizing reviews of scientific studies about the impact of neuroleptics on the brain in his courtroom battles on behalf of clients who are attempting to prevent their involuntary psychiatric drugging [33]. In my work as a mental health advocate, I have never seen a written informed consent for neuroleptic psychiatric drugs which explains this finding, which is especially relevant to the controversy of coerced psychiatry. When a psychiatric procedure can be shown to induce significant changes to the structure of the brain, this means that enforcing the treatment raises special ethical issues similar to the older controversy of involuntary psychosurgery.

We frequently hear that coerced psychiatric procedures are justified because we lack insight into our condition, and that we don't understand the necessity of our treatment. However, I find that many patients, families, elected officials, the media and even many mental health professionals are often not adequately informed by the medical community about such urgent controversies as the impact of long-term neuroleptics on our brains. In fact, in my informal estimation, many psychiatric survivor activists are more informed about these scientific matters than some busy mental health professionals.

## 12.5   Fear – one choice is no choice

While force and fraud are more obvious ways to gain compliance without the true full informed consent of the individual, there is another category of coercion that I would consider to be the most common, which I sum up as *fear*, fear that one cannot find an alternative to the few mental health approaches that tend to be offered, which seem to mainly be medical model approaches such as psychiatric drugs.

MindFreedom International and I are pro-choice about personal health care decisions, and many of our members choose to take prescribed psychiatric drugs. Others like me do not. But we are united in speaking out about the immense power and domination of the psychiatric drug approach that seems to squeeze out other choices. We feel there are humane, effective, voluntary non-drug approaches that are often not readily made available to people who need that help. For example, the book *Alternatives Beyond Psychiatry*, co-edited by psychiatric survivor Peter Lehmann and psychiatrist Peter Stastny, brings together 61 authors from all over the world to examine more empowering and humane psychosocial options to help individuals seeking mental health care, other than coerced psychiatric procedures based on a primarily medical model [34]. When an individual in crisis is offered only one type of mental health care, this is a kind of Hobson's choice. That is, offering one choice is not really a choice.

In my hometown of Eugene, Oregon, the City of Eugene Human Rights Commission chose to address human rights in mental health as a priority issue for several years, and one result was the crafting of a resolution on the topic of choice in mental health as a human right. On 26 October 2009, the City Council of Eugene unanimously passed Resolution 4989, which states that the availability of more non-drug options in mental health care is the right of every citizen [35]. I conclude with the text of this unique resolution, below, because I find it to be a hopeful example of democracy beginning to get more hands-on and proactive about mental health care, rather than to defer that authority to a fairly small group of medical professionals. With a more empowered and informed public, perhaps we can address and end the immense power imbalance between those on the receiving end of coerced psychiatric procedures, and mental health providers.

RESOLUTION NO. 4989

A RESOLUTION AFFIRMING THE CITY'S COMMITMENT TO HUMAN RIGHTS AND MENTAL HEALTH CARE.

The City Council of the City of Eugene finds that:

A. The City Council of the City of Eugene recognizes that the diversity of our population is vital to our community's character, and that we have a long tradition of protecting and expanding human rights and civil liberties protections for all of our residents, including persons with all types of disabilities.
B. U.S. Courts have affirmed a number of rights for people diagnosed with mental disabilities. At the national level, the right to choose to live in the least restrictive environment that is reasonably available has been affirmed. At the state level, a number of courts have affirmed a person's right to refuse psychotropic medications, even when the state has a "compelling interest" in providing treatment, if less intrusive, effective treatment alternatives exist. These decisions are consistent with the principle that all people have the right to lives free of unnecessary restrictions and intrusions.
C. Many people determine that psychiatric medications are quite helpful for their mental and emotional conditions, and are grateful to have the opportunity to take them. Others find medications to be harmful to their health, unhelpful and/or excessively intrusive and problematic. When people seek treatment and are offered medication as the only treatment option, they may feel coerced into choosing that option. Many of the medications currently provided are typically associated with significant medical risk, are often experienced as subjectively harmful, and their long-term effectiveness remains controversial. Furthermore, there are widely researched psychosocial alternative treatments likely to be at least as effective for many, with fewer harmful effects.
D. Many mental health problems are caused by trauma and human rights violations, such as child abuse, war, racism, lack of housing and economic opportunities, domestic violence, and others. A key element in any kind of trauma is the denial of choice. When people who have been traumatized are denied choices in recovery, an effect may be retraumatization.
E. Serious psychiatric disorder is often thought of as inevitably a permanent condition requiring a lifetime of medication, however research shows that a substantial fraction of those with even the most serious diagnoses do fully recover, eventually not requiring treatment. Treatment choices, designed to foster rehabilitation and recovery, which include working, living, and participating in the life of the community, have been shown to increase such recovery.

NOW, THEREFORE, BE IT RESOLVED BY THE CITY COUNCIL OF THE CITY OF EUGENE, a Municipal Corporation of the State of Oregon, as follows:

Section 1. All mental health service providers within the City of Eugene are encouraged to incorporate self determination and consumer choice as much as possible, with accurate information provided to consumers and to families about those choices. Special emphasis should be placed on providing diverse alternatives in treatments, including non-drug alternatives, whenever possible.

Section 2. All mental health service providers within the City of Eugene are urged to offer a full range of choices designed to assist in complete recovery.

Section 3. This Resolution shall become effective immediately upon its adoption.

The foregoing Resolution adopted the 26 day of October, 2009.

## 12.6    Conclusion – offering dialogue and calling for demonstrations

Those of us who have allied ourselves with the less powerful side of the imbalance inherent in coerced psychiatric procedures need to learn from other social change movements throughout history who have turned to nonviolent direct resistance through creative civil disobedience. I realize that some in the psychiatric profession who say they support our concerns may oppose the idea of protest.

In his famous letter from the Birmingham Jail on 16 April 1963, Martin Luther, Jr, wrote this to those who cautioned him to slow down his protests:

> You deplore the demonstrations taking place in Birmingham. But your statement, I am sorry to say, fails to express a similar concern for the conditions that brought about the demonstrations. I am sure that none of you would want to rest content with the superficial kind of social analysis that deals merely with effects and does not grapple with underlying causes. It is unfortunate that demonstrations are taking place in Birmingham, but it is even more unfortunate that the city's white power structure left the Negro community with no alternative. [36]

## References

1. Kisely, S. and Campbell, L. (2007) Methodological issues in assessing the evidence for compulsory community treatment. *Current Psychiatry Reviews*, **3**, 51–56.
2. Clay, S., Schell, B. and Corrigan, P.W. (eds) (2005) *On Our Own, Together: Peer Programs for People with Mental Illness*, Vanderbilt University Press, Nashville, TN.
3. Chamberlin, J. (1978) *On Our Own: Patient Controlled Alternatives to the Mental Health System*, Hawthorn Books, New York.
4. Chamberlin, J. (1998) Confessions of a non-compliant patient. *Journal of Psychiatric Nursing*, **36**, 49–52.
5. Daniel Mackler, D. and Morrissey, M. (2010) *A Way Out of Madness: Dealing with Your Family After You've Been Diagnosed with a Psychiatric Disorder*, AuthorHouse, Bloomington, IN.
6. Bassman, R. (2007) *A Fight to Be: A Psychologist's Experience from Both Sides of the Locked Door*, Tantamount Press, Albany, NY.
7. Boodman, S.G. (1996) Shock Therapy ... It's Back. The Washington Post (24 September), p. 14.
8. Chabasinski, T. (2001) MindFreedom Personal Stories: Ted Chabasinski. www.mindfreedom.org/personal-stories/chabasisnskited (accessed 6 June 2010).
9. Foner, J. (2001) MindFreedom Personal Stories: Janet Foner. www.mindfreedom.org/personal-stories/fonerjanet (accessed 6 June 2010).
10. De Wyze, J. (2003) Still Crazy After All These Years. San Diego Weekly Reader (9 January). www.sandiegoreader.com/news/2003/jan/09/cover-still-crazy-after-all-these-years/ (accessed 4 December 2010).
11. Bernstein, A. (2004) Contrarian Psychiatrist Loren Mosher, 70. The Washington Post (20 July), p. B06.

12. Calton, T., Ferriter, M., Huband, N. and Spandler, H. (2008) A systematic review of the Soteria paradigm for the treatment of people diagnosed with schizophrenia. *Schizophrenia Bulletin*, **34**, 181–192.

13. Mosher, L. (1998) Letter of Resignation from the American Psychiatric Association: 4 December 1998. www.moshersoteria.com/articles/resignation-from-apa/ (accessed 3 December 2010).

14. King, M.L. (1963) *Strength to Love*, Augsburg Fortress Publishers, Minneapolis, p. 27.

15. Eichhorn, H.J. (2004) Theory and practice of Gandhian non-violence, in *Mahatma Gandhi: At the Close of Twentieth Century* (ed R. Kumar), Anmol Publications, New Delhi, p. 52.

16. Gandhi, M. and Merton, T. (eds) (2007) *Gandhi on Non-Violence*, New Directions, New York.

17. Risser, P. (2001) MindFreedom Personal Stories: Pat Risser. www.mindfreedom.org/personal-stories/risserpat (accessed 6 June 2010).

18. Smith, W. (1885) (transl.) *Thucydides, History of the Peloponnesian War*, Volume 2, Harper, New York, pp. 123–131.

19. Truth and Reconciliation Commission of South Africa (1999) *Truth and Reconciliation Commission of South Africa Report*, Palgrave Macmillan, London.

20. ENUSP, WNUSP, MFI and BPE (2007) Declaration of Dresden Against Coerced Psychiatric Treatment. Signatories Peter Lehmann and Judi Chamberlin; June 7. Available from www.enusp.org/dresden.htm (accessed 6 June 2010).

21. UN Convention on the Rights of Persons with Disabilities, Resolution A/RES/61/106 of the General Assembly of the United Nations (13 December 2006). Available at www.un.org/disabilities (accessed 6 June 2010).

22. World Health Organization (2005) *WHO Resource Book on Mental Health, Human Rights and Legislation*, WHO, Geneva, p. 64.

23. Snyders, M. (2009) Minnesota Mental Health Patient Ray Sandford Forced into Electro-Shock Therapy. Minneapolis City Pages (20 May), p. 1.

24. Karnowski, S., Associated Press (2009) Minn. Patient Wants Right to Refuse Electro-shocks. Star Tribune (10 May). www.startribune.com/lifestyle/health/44672722.html?elr= KArksUUUoDEy3LGDiO7aiU (accessed 4 December 2010).

25. MindFreedom International (2009) Ray Gateway: Campaign Ended Forced Outpatient Electroshock of Ray Sandford (22 Oct). http://mindfreedom.org/ray (accessed 6 June 2010).

26. National Council on Disability (2000) From Privileges to Rights: People Labeled with Psychiatric Disabilities Speak for Themselves. www.ncd.gov/newsroom/publications/2000/privileges.htm (accessed 6 June 2010).

27. Francis, A. (2010) It's Not Too Late To Save 'Normal'. Los Angeles Times (1 March). http://articles.latimes.com/2010/mar/01/opinion/la-oe-frances1-2010mar01 (accessed 4 December 2010).

28. Whitaker, R. (2010) *Anatomy of An Epidemic: Magic Bullets, Psychiatric Drugs and the Astonishing Rise of Mental Illness in America*, Crown Publishers, New York, pp. 331–334.

29. MindFreedom International (2003) MindFreedom Hunger Strike (16 August). www.mindfreedom.org/kb/act/2003/mf-hunger-strike (accessed 6 June 2010).

30. Edds, K. (2003) Raising Doubts About Drugs: Calif. Hunger Strike Challenges Use of Antidepressants. The Washington Post (30 August), p. A08.

31. MindFreedom International (2010) Brain Damage Caused by Neuroleptic Psychiatric Drugs. www.mindfreedom.org/kb/psychiatric-drugs/antipsychotics/neuroleptic-brain-damage (accessed 6 June 2010).

32. Gottstein, J. (2010) Psychrights: Neuroleptics. http://psychrights.org/research/Digest/NLPs/neuroleptics.htm (accessed 6 June 2010).

33. Moncrieff, J. and Leo, J. (2010) A systematic review of the effects of antipsychotic drugs on brain volume. *Psychological Medicine*, **20**, 1–14.

34. Lehmann, P. and Stastny, P. (eds) (2007) *Alternatives Beyond Psychiatry*, Lehmann Publishing, Berlin.

35. Oaks, D. (2009) Eugene Recognizes Mental Health Patients Have Rights, Too. The Register-Guard (10 December), p. A11.

36. King, M. (1963) Letter from Birmingham Jail: April 16, 1963. http://abacus.bates.edu/admin/offices/dos/mlk/letter.html (accessed 6 June 2010).

# 13 Resisting variables – service user/survivor perspectives on researching coercion

## Jasna Russo[1] and Jan Wallcraft[2,3]

[1]*Mental Disability Advocacy Centre, Budapest, Hungary*
[2]*University of Birmingham, Centre for Excellence in Interdisciplinary Mental Health, Birmingham, UK*
[3]*University of Hertfordshire, Centre for Mental Health Recovery, College Lane, Hatfield, Herts, UK*

Coercion in psychiatry and the fight against forced treatment are two of the main topics in the mental health service user/psychiatric survivor movement worldwide. At the same time, our own user-led or survivor-controlled research in this field is almost nonexistent. This chapter explores some of the structural obstacles to including service user/survivor perspectives in psychiatric research on coercion. Without aiming to provide a systematic or complete review, in the first part of the text we take a closer look at several psychiatric studies on coercion, and discuss their overall approaches and the methodologies applied. Our standpoints are informed by our own research practice, by our activism in the international movement of psychiatric survivors, and by our personal experiences of forced or coercive

*Coercive Treatment in Psychiatry: Clinical, Legal and Ethical Aspects*, First Edition.
Edited by Thomas W. Kallert, Juan E. Mezzich and John Monahan.
© 2011 John Wiley & Sons, Ltd. Published 2011 by John Wiley & Sons, Ltd.

treatment. This contribution aims to extend the debate on the ethics of coercion beyond the notions of 'treatment effectiveness' and 'perceived coercion' by raising questions about how coercive methods impact individual lives. The second part of the text will outline some of the principles and values that we consider essential for comprehensive and responsible research on coercion.

## 13.1    Limitations of psychiatric research on coercion

Legislation and policy are certainly not informed by research outcomes solely, but they do aspire to be evidence based. Human rights monitoring of different psychiatric settings, which has become a requirement under the UN Convention on the Rights of Persons with Disabilities [1] that 'expressly stipulates that civil society, in particular persons with disabilities and their representative organizations, shall be involved and participate fully in the monitoring process' (Article 33.3) [2]. In contrast to this requirement, scientific research on coercion is still dominated by the psychiatric approach and mostly undertaken by clinicians themselves. We think that the lack of independent research on coercion contributes to the outcomes of psychiatric studies being taken for '*the* evidence', reinforced by the medical authority behind them. One systematic review of 18 psychiatric research studies on coercion, for instance, reports that the percentage of patients who perceive their involuntary hospitalization as helpful can reach 81%, whereas the proportion of those who perceive no benefits or even feel harmed by the compulsory treatment can be as low as 6% [3].

We do not aim at any complete or systematic review of the up-to-date research on coercion, as such work would exceed the purpose of this chapter; however, we wanted to take a closer look at the nature of psychiatric research evidence, focusing on its inclusiveness of the perspectives, experiences and truths of persons subjected to forced treatment. We started with a small, non-systematic literature search of psychiatric studies on coercion both in institutional settings and in the community, mainly looking for those that we had already heard about. Our special interest was in some of the recent research on community treatment orders, because of its potential to inform current changes in legislation and debates around public safety and the extension of forced treatment from institutions into the community. We included peer-reviewed journal articles, about six quantitative [4–9] and about three qualitative research studies [10–12]; two systematic reviews [3,13]; and the online self-presentation of one randomized controlled trial currently being conducted in the UK [14]. The studies we included were conducted in the USA [4,7–9], the UK [6,12], New Zealand [5,10] and Sweden [11] in the course of the last 15 years. As researchers ourselves, we observed some major structural obstacles that stand in the way of service user/survivor knowledge of coercion entering these studies and forming their constitutional part. These refer to the language applied, to the understanding of what constitutes a 'sample', and to the research questions and methodologies applied. We consider these aspects of the research process to be decisive in shaping study outcomes, and think that their illumination must come before any debate about the findings of psychiatric investigations of coercion. We therefore focused primarily on the research process and tried to avoid discussion of the outcomes reported.

The perspective we take and the issues we raise are directly informed by both our background in user-led and survivor-controlled research and our experience in collaborative projects and participative methods. We also share the view that there is no such thing as a value-free investigation of social reality, and that transparency and attentiveness to the investigator's own standpoint are critical for the whole research process, starting from its design. Discussing the notion of 'evidence-based medicine', Alison Faulkner and Phil Thomas say:

> No matter how 'scientific' we aspire to be, clinical decisions always will involve value judgements and it is a serious mistake to pretend otherwise. [15]

Similarly, regardless of how 'objective' they aim to be, current studies on coercion in psychiatry are informed by the biomedical approach which directs their design and their outcomes. Systematic reviews of such studies from service user/survivor perspectives could be a way of moving towards informed and sound dialogue amongst different parties, in accordance with Mary O' Hagan's claim:

> The stakeholders who dominate this debate, such as mental health professionals, politicians and families tend to support and promote the legalised use of force. Their views are well known, well documented and well reflected in laws around the world that allow for compulsory intervention. But the views of users and survivors who want to see less or no force are relatively marginalised. As yet our views have not exerted any major influence on thinking, legislation or practice. This needs to change. [16]

Our attempt to briefly tackle some of the main limitations of psychiatric research on coercion in this chapter can certainly not replace such already overdue process.

## 13.2  Language

The terms which are used in psychiatric debates to describe persons subjected to coercive measures are 'patient' and 'service user' or 'consumer'. We find these terms both contradictory and inappropriate to the context of coercion: 'patient' implies the healing potential of coercion, while 'service user' or 'consumer' imply that coercive measures are one option amongst many mental health services on offer, which are to be freely chosen and used. Free choice is a false concept in psychiatric settings because of the very limited number of available alternatives to pharmacological treatment.

Choice is even less applicable to coercive methods since they are not chosen at all in the way the words 'user' or 'consumer' would suggest. The language of psychiatric studies on coercion represents one of the fundamental obstacles if the investigation of this topic is ever to open up to the perspectives of persons subjected to forced treatment. We wonder how a person can be considered a user (or consumer) of services which are imposed on them. How can restraint, seclusion and forced medication or electro-convulsive therapy (ECT) be understood as 'mental health services'?

In the context of researching coercion, we find the term 'patient' to some extent more appropriate and more honest, although being a patient is only one aspect of a person's identity, usually a temporary one. If the impact of coercion on a *person* is to be investigated, then persons must be perceived as more than treatment-responders, as Faulkner and Thomas suggest:

> Although EBM [*evidence-based medicine*] may be valuable in discriminating between the claims made by advocates of different treatments, patients are left feeling that their concerns are forgotten and that they are little more than a disease being treated. [15]

If research aims at inclusion and understanding of our perspectives, then the first step is to invite and welcome these perspectives instead of structurally excluding them with political terminology. This is, however, never simply a matter of the words applied, but rather of the concepts they stand for. What remains implicit in psychiatric research on coercion is the notion of research subjects. Either reduced to the role of passive patients or misleadingly reconstructed as 'service users' or 'consumers', the participants in research are perceived and treated as 'subjects'. This tradition remains implicit and persistent in psychiatric studies on coercion and stands in the way of acknowledging a *person* being subjected to forced treatment. This very fact pre-defines what is possible and restricts what is open to question and exploration in psychiatric research. If they are to enter an equitable dialogue, *persons* subjected to forced treatment must be seen as capable of reflecting upon their experiences and providing general judgements.

At present, the necessity of coercion seems to be taken for granted, and the main issues remaining to investigate concern the effectiveness of its different modalities. When the 'subject's' perspective appears on the research agenda, it remains reduced to a *perception of coercion*. The translation of the real coercion exerted and experienced into the reductive term 'perceived coercion' so common in psychiatric research [4–7] masks the actual incidence of coercion and its profound impact. As coercion is certainly not just a matter of perception, we fail to understand how such a construct can take a central role and guide investigations of coercion.

Psychiatric research has also so far failed to acknowledge the political organizing of people with psychiatric diagnoses and the fact that a large portion of participants in this movement define themselves as 'survivors of psychiatry'. The notion of a survivor is certainly not value-free; it is obviously disturbing as a working term because of its strong implication that psychiatric treatment is something to survive. But as the terms 'patient' and 'service user' (consumer) applied in psychiatric research on coercion are in no way neutral either, we plead for the acknowledgement and inclusion of uncomfortable survivor perspectives. We are convinced that these perspectives are directly relevant to research on coercion and that they should find their place in knowledge production, and constitute evidence.

## 13.3   Composition and perception of the 'sample'

Very often clinicians and other professional staff are the first ones to decide about their patients' capacity to take part in research on coercion. The process of obtaining participants' informed consent starts after the first selection has already taken place. This type of recruitment seems to be embedded in research studies in such an automatic and natural way that it is rarely even described. It is usually briefly mentioned, in some cases also providing information about the number of patients left out, but normally without any reflection on the possible impact this might have on creating a sample bias:

> Initially, personnel at the mental healthcare centres... were asked to select patients suitable for an interview. [11]

> The key workers (or case managers) of those patients were then approached, with an initial request to assess the patient's capacity to participate in the research, in consultation with their psychiatrist. [10]

> The exclusion criteria for participation in the study were... patient incompetence to participate as determined by the patient's "responsible clinician" and primary nurse... [5]

> Clinicians will identify patients and ask them if they will see the researchers. [14]

Just one amongst the nine reviewed studies provided a detailed 'recruitment and follow-up flowchart' [6]. Its focus was on involuntary hospital admissions, and although it just aimed to present the reasons for patients' nonparticipation or dropping out of the research, this rare chart, in our opinion, provides closer insight into the role of the professional staff in determining the study sample. Of all the reasons reported for the failure to contact patients, just one related explicitly to those patients' will – 'patient refusing to see anyone' (this reason related to 14 out of 136 patients whom the researchers failed to contact). The other five reasons included:

staff refused contact (too ill); staff refused contact (reason unspecified); staff refused to contact (too violent/dangerous/unpredictable); patient sedated; and patient sleeping [6].

Further on, we observed that psychiatric studies on coercion are limited to persons currently being subjected to forced treatment or who received it relatively recently. The usual follow-up period does not exceed one year [3]. This also refers to studies investigating compulsory treatment in the community. In the sample of one qualitative study which reports patients' generally positive attitudes to community treatment orders (CTOs), 52% of participants were still under the CTO at the time of the interview [10]. Despite such an outcome, the same study reports:

> Many service users who were still under the CTO at their interview wished to be discharged from the order, and the majority of those already discharged were pleased with their voluntary status. [10]

Given the fact that the possibility of forced treatment profoundly affects every person with a psychiatric diagnosis, we don't think that the investigation about its impact should be reserved only for those immediately affected. We consider this to be a serious restriction to comprehensive research on coercion, which is why we fully agree with the following remarks by survivor Peter Campbell:

> I do not intend to argue either for or against the use of legal compulsion in treatment. But the fact of its existence has repercussions for all service users, and these must be recognised.

> That an individual can be compelled to receive psychiatric treatment affects each in-patient regardless of whether his stay is formal or informal. It is hardly possible to be unaware that you are being cared for within a legal framework that allows for treatment against your will. [17]

The context in which psychiatric treatment happens, and its potential to turn into forced treatment, means that the legal definition of coercion is much narrower than the coercion actually exerted and experienced. In support of some of our statements, we will quote from a recent consultation exercise with service users/survivors across 15 European countries about their perspectives on human rights, which one of the authors was in charge of [18]:

> I see it less as a process of the legislation because coercion works on so many levels. Yes, there's the level of the legislation where you know people are sectioned against their will but then there's so many other little things you see in hospitals, you know people told – well unless you do this then this will happen and you know and that's not, that's not a legal process. [18]

Psychiatric patients don't have to be legally compelled in order to find themselves in situations of having no other choice but to adhere to treatment and to institutional or community psychiatric rules.

> And then I remember one, one thing that stuck into my mind that suddenly a male nurse comes to say to me that now – you have to take a shower that well, now if you don't take a shower, well, by that and that time, we will come all male nurses and wash you in the shower and I was totally terrified, that oh my God, what is this and first they fixed the deadline to eight o'clock and said now you must take a shower but then they made it quicker, I had to take a shower by six o'clock. [18]

Without seeking to equate forced treatment with voluntary treatment, what we want to emphasize is the coercive potential of psychiatric treatment itself. This is what restricts freedom of choice when undergoing psychiatric treatment to begin with; it is also what extends coercion far beyond what is captured by its legal definition. Inside a system based on the option of using force, the question of whether a person is legally coerced or not may become a side issue on an experiential level. Nevertheless, the patient's legal status as voluntary or involuntary remains what most psychiatric studies on coercion focus on; they don't investigate what exactly comprises the coercive treatment [4–7,9–11,14].

Some psychiatric research studies showed no significant differences in 'perceived coercion' between voluntarily and involuntarily admitted patients [19–21]. We also encountered recognition of the fact that 'coerced hospitalisation or treatment may occur in the absence of legal involuntary status.' [4] But further investigation of possible causes for such outcomes focused on demographic and clinical characteristics of patients [4,5] rather than any exploration of the treatment that they were actually experiencing.

In our opinion, an approach truly aiming to investigate coercion and understand its impact on both voluntary and involuntary patients – that is, the way it affects people's lives – requires a radically different perception of research participants. We are aware that the term 'perception' is reserved for patients only and never applied to clinicians and researchers because the only 'perceived' thing is coercion. No one mentions 'perceived treatment outcomes', 'perceived treatment need' or 'perceived psychiatric disorder'. We argue that even if never addressed, there is a *perception* of patients or research subjects inherent to psychiatric research which narrows its potential for ample investigation of coercion. To overcome this constraint, patients would need to be seen as capable of making reflections and judgements which reach beyond their individual and immediate situation, in the same way as all the other stakeholders. As long as we remain perceived as study subjects only, we will not be encouraged to reflect and will be forbidden to generalize, unlike everybody else involved. By the nature of our designated role, we will also not be invited to take part in dialogue, as no authentic dialogue can take place via psychometric scales. Hiday *et al.* report:

> In trying to understand causes of perceived coercion, negative pressures, and process fairness, our three dependent variables, we expected sociodemographic characteristics to be important because these characteristics place individuals in groups that experience legal and medical authority differently. Age, gender, racial, and socioeconomic groups vary in their norms and experiences which affect others' reactions to them and their own interpretations of the commitment process. [4]

This might be true (and proved true to a certain extent within this particular study), but we ask: how can such an investigation improve the understanding of the complex reality of coercion which does not take place only at a perceptual level or only as a correlate of sociodemographic characteristics?

Research on coercion needs to question, rethink and change researchers' perceptions of participants, as well as to move beyond attempts at approaching our lives as an interplay of dependent and independent variables.

Comprehensive research will also have to reach beyond persons being currently or recently subjected to forced treatment and their relatives or the professionals involved. Research on coercion needs to include the larger community of service users/survivors and build on their experiential knowledge, not just on their observable characteristics and the scores they produce on numeric scales. It also needs to radically redirect its focus from 'perceptions of coercion' towards an all-inclusive investigation of *actual* coercion capturing the range of modalities of its incidence.

## 13.4   Research questions and methodologies

The quantitative studies that we reviewed focused on measuring patients' perceptions of coercion and placing them in relation to their legal status [5], their socio-demographic and clinical characteristics [4], their adherence to treatment [7], their service evaluation [8] and factors associated with treatment outcomes [6,9,14]. Of the three qualitative studies that we included in this review, two aimed at understanding patients' experience of involuntary hospital admissions [11,12] and one explored patients', family members' and mental health professionals' views on community treatment orders [10].

In contrast with the detailed descriptions of the patients' socio-demographic and other characteristics, hardly any article provided even minimal information about the researchers' profiles and their background. Of the studies reviewed, the only exception to this rule was the one that reported and reflected on the collaborative nature of the investigation that included co-research with mental health service users [12]. One review of the 18 quantitative studies of involuntary hospital admissions states that 'most involuntary admitted patients show substantial clinical improvement over time.' [6] The fact that two-thirds of the studies used interviewers responsible for patients' treatment is mentioned when describing the methodological quality criteria for this review. However, the way this potentially influenced the outcomes goes entirely ignored.

We argue that the closeness of the research on coercion to the psychiatric treatment context reduces the ability of these studies to achieve a reliable and true picture of the topic under investigation. Some of the typical mechanisms applied include clinicians preselecting the sample, employing researchers who are part of the treatment team, conducting interviews and assessments at the same venues where persons receive psychiatric treatment, and recruiting participants who are still under forced treatment, or have been subjected to it very recently.

This problematic proximity between compulsory treatment and its psychiatric research is also reflected in the research questions guiding most of the studies. Too often we encountered quite an explicit and straightforward concern solely to identify factors that could predict patients' perception of coercion [4–9,14]. There also seemed to be a strong interest in making patients feel better about being subjected to forced treatment rather than searching for alternatives to it.

Improving the percentage of patients stating that the admission was justified might be a sensible aim for both policy and clinical practice. [6]

Approximately two-fifths of our sample reported little or no negative pressures and little or no process exclusion in their hospital admission. These findings suggest that involuntary admission to a mental hospital can permit patients to feel like they have voice and validation, and can avoid force even in the absence of choice. The challenge is to try to extend to all patients at the time of their admission a demonstration in word and action that they are persons with opinions, desires, rights, and dignity, and not just mental patients in an acute crisis. [4]

How to predict the way patients will feel about the coercive measures imposed on them seems to be a far more challenging question for modern psychiatric research than investigating possibilities for rethinking and replacing treatment based on force with something different.

Even those studies which attempt to explore the outcomes of compulsory treatment take a predominantly clinical perspective when defining those outcomes. The findings of these studies differ, showing that involuntary treatment may have negative, positive or no significantly different outcome in comparison with voluntary treatment, but what they have in common is the nature of the outcome measures applied. Besides measures like hospital re-admissions [6,9], arrest or homeless-ness [9], in six of the nine studies we reviewed, the attempt to understand the impact of coercion took place through asking patients to rate items on different scales or to assess a number of pre-formulated statements as 'true' or 'false'. Most of the articles we included do not describe the instruments that they applied in detail, but their technical and quantitative nature is clearly implied by their names: Perceived Coercion Scale, the Negative Pressure Scale and the Voice Scale [5]; true–false items of the MacArthur Interpersonal Relations Scale [4]; Client's Assessment of Treatment Scale, Global Assessment of Functioning, Brief Psychiatric Rating Scale [6]; Lehman Brief Quality of Life Interview [9]; subscales from the Therapeutic Limit Setting Measure, Modified Admission Experience Survey, Session Impacts Scale, the Working Alliance Inventory, Short Form [8]. Four of the six quantitative studies applied the MacArthur Perceived Coercion Scale [4,6,7,9]. This obviously popular and respected measure consists of the following five items which can only be assessed as either true or false and scored accordingly [4,7]:

- 'I felt free to do what I wanted about coming to the hospital';
- 'I chose to come into the hospital';
- 'It was my idea to come to the hospital';
- 'I had a lot of control over whether I went into the hospital'; and
- 'I had more influence than anyone else on whether I came into the hospital.'

Aside from noting that this measure is an oversimplified and therefore inappropriate tool to explore any aspect of coercion, we would like to raise two issues around its trustworthiness. Firstly, the answers on this scale relate only to the circumstances of hospital admission and hold no information about the person's perspectives on coercion from that moment onwards. Secondly, the scale ignores the fact that people may hold themselves ultimately responsible for most things in their lives; this does not mean they are unaware that force has been imposed over them.

Research on coercion obviously uses an approach similar to that of diagnostic tests and different instruments of psychiatric assessment. Psychiatric survivors, like Louise Pembroke, argue that this is a way of systematically depriving people of their experiences and the meanings these hold:

I have come to the conclusion that *people* are not studied by psychiatry and psychology, merely categorised and described. That their rigid frameworks serve only to fragment people, turning a break-up into a breakdown. In categorising the distress the distress itself is not acknowledged. The individuals' right to *own* the experience has been stolen. [22]

Research on coercion needs to become interactive and engage in a dialogue with different protagonists instead of celebrating one-way assessments. But this is hard, if not impossible, within a biomedical framework which perceives people as passive respondents to treatment and is traditionally based on observing and measuring them rather than engaging and attempting to understand and share their realities.

Coercion primarily takes place *between* people (and not as an isolated internal process) and so that is how and where we think it should be explored.

Qualitative methodological approaches in psychiatric research can certainly come closer to the complexity of persons' experiences, and we agree with Johansson and Lundman that 'using a narrative method increases the possibility to study coercion identified by the patient' [11]. Despite our critical stand on their method of recruiting the interviewees (through asking the personnel from mental health centres to 'select patients suitable for an interview'), we do appreciate the approach they take when trying to understand what coercion means for patients:

> A primary way of giving meaning into experience is to make stories of it. This is especially relevant when dealing with changes in life and trauma. [11]

This study, together with another qualitative one which was conducted in collaboration with mental health service users [12], we consider to be of the highest quality amongst the selection of nine which we reviewed for the purpose of this chapter.

But we want to stress that we consider neither service user involvement nor a qualitative approach as such to be guarantees of good quality research on coercion. When service users are employed just for data collection that takes place via quantitative clinical instruments alone, the experiential knowledge they bring will not have much influence on the whole process or enrich and reshape the research [23]. Similarly, the research topics and questions of qualitative studies can still be dictated by the same clinical/biomedical paradigm. In concluding their review of five qualitative studies on coercion, Katsakou and Priebe write:

> Although the perceived impact of involuntary treatment is fairly clearly described, differences between distinct patient groups are not examined. Future research should investigate such differences in order to inform relevant policy decisions for particular groups. [13]

Qualitative research can also remain driven by narrow attention to finding answers within the individuals or their 'particular groups' rather than broadening the focus to the larger treatment context in which coercive measures are applied. Despite the availability of participants' original quotes from qualitative research, some authors and reviewers feel free to draw conclusions which obviously reflect their own views rather than any evidence they encountered:

> Overall, people suffering from mental health problems are particularly sensitive against any intrusions into their autonomy and privacy. Coercive interventions are often viewed as an attack on their overall ability to self-regulate. [13]

We are not aware of any studies in which academic researchers, clinicians and others 'not suffering from mental health problems' were subjected to coercive measures for the sake of experiment and comparison. If we were to positively argue for randomized controlled trials, then these could be applied to test the statement above. We would hypothesise, though, that the 'others' would react much worse to 'intrusions' than service users/survivors because we have already been exposed to psychiatric force and might have learned some coping strategies. But we are not suggesting an experimental approach to research on coercion, and want instead to draw attention to the statement above as an example of the interpretative freedom exercised in 'scientific' reviews. The concluding part of this review illustrates what we have already observed to be the either explicitly suggested or frequently implied direction of modern psychiatric research on coercion:

> However, when patients feel that professionals genuinely care about them and offer them some degree of participation in their treatment, such interventions are viewed in a less negative light and do not have a negative impact on people's sense of self-value. Thus, it seems important to enhance people's perceived participation even when being treated involuntarily. [13]

As we don't share this conviction, in the second part of this chapter we will try to outline some alternative principles and values for research on coercion.

## 13.5 Towards comprehensive research on coercion

As we have already said, we are aware that research outcomes are just one of the factors that inform mental health legislation and policy, and presumably not the most important one. Nevertheless, taking into account that the premises of psychiatric studies as well as the way they are designed and conducted inhibit comprehensive research on coercion, we think that their further funding should be scrupulously reconsidered. If this broadly relevant topic is to be seriously investigated, the research will have to take a new direction: forced psychiatric treatment is a human rights issue, and there is no reason for further investments in strictly medical studies of it. The first step that needs to be taken is to let ethical, legal and social perspectives enter the arena of the investigation of forced treatment.

This has started to some extent through the work of bodies like the Committee for the Prevention of Torture [24] or the UN Special Rapporteur on Torture [25], but despite their considerable importance, short monitoring visits to places of detention cannot substitute for systematic explorations of coercive treatment, its incidence and its impact. Such visits are also not applicable to exploration of forced treatment outside of institutions.

Trying to envisage ample research on coercion, we agree with Mary O'Hagan that we should first of all encourage and listen to the perspectives of those people whose voices are stifled by forced treatment.

> In recent decades users and survivors have found their voices after centuries of virtual silence. You simply cannot engage in a fair and full debate on force with us, unless our voices lead the way. [16]

There is a growing body of available texts authored by people who identify themselves as mental health service users/psychiatric survivors. We consider these to be an invaluable source of guidance when developing questions of relevance for research on coercion. Referring to some of those texts, we will now let our voices lead the way by raising a few issues that we consider important when investigating coercion. As with our small-scale review of psychiatric studies on coercion, however, the following suggestions give only a snapshot of the work required to develop a comprehensive and socially responsible framework for research on coercion.

## 13.6   Importance of independent research

We are convinced that any sound research on coercion must take place completely independently from the provision of psychiatric treatment. As long as clinicians in charge of forced treatment are the same ones making decisions about the research, there will be no chance of a true and complete investigation. We have already criticized the method of recruiting study participants through clinical staff. We have also criticized the research on coercion being conducted by members of the treatment team, since it entirely ignores the power imbalance in the coercion situation, which we consider to be a matter of common sense.

> I had to learn not to express anger and frustration towards what felt like torture. I could not express my pain and anger to the people who were controlling every aspect of my life. [22]

Many written accounts by service users and survivors confirm that honesty cannot be expected in a coercive context and that a person needs to have sufficient distance not only physically but also in terms of time in order to freely report their experiences. We doubt that statements like the one below could have been obtained at the time when treatment was taking place.

> I signed the consent form because I hoped at the time that I would die under the anesthetic. This was the view that informed many of my future signatures on ECT and

over the next six years I received approximately 60, each justified by continually changing labels which ranged from psychotic depression to schizophrenia. [26]

Any research studies aiming at all-inclusive investigations of coercion will have to develop alternative ways of approaching potential participants, earning their trust and obtaining informed consent from them. Furthermore, the researcher should not be obliged to brief the clinician on the outcomes. There are parallels to attempts at investigating guardianship [27] while having to obtain guardians' consent to even talk to the persons in custody. Research ethics committees need to carefully consider such vicious circles and set different rules. Independent research on coercion must be demanded and allowed. The intimate link between the conduct of forced treatment and research about it will have to be broken in order for the topic under investigation to be brought out of the individual treatment context and become subjected to different perspectives.

## 13.7   Redirecting the research focus

Judgements of the 'effectiveness' of coercion, which remain the focus of most current research, should only come *after* a thorough explanation of coercive measures and how they take place. If something proves effective, this doesn't mean that it is good and acceptable. The fact that weapons are effective in fulfilling their goals does not mean that they should be recommended. Perhaps the goals themselves need to be brought into question. Even if there are people who anecdotally report that coercive measures have saved their lives, research should still be able to tackle the quality of those lives and continue raising questions about how things can be done in a better way. It is a matter of not assuming that because a practice is long established, this means it is necessary and right and unchallengeable. Many routine practices such as child labour, slavery, foot binding and forced marriages have been changed and even prohibited as new generations begin to see their inherent inhumanity.

In order to make complex judgments, everybody should be entitled to a detailed and comprehensive picture of what coercion looks like and what it consists of. Such topics are almost excluded from the current research on coercion. The fact that somebody is involuntarily committed or is under community treatment order does not say anything about the treatment they receive. One user-led study of experiences of hospital admissions confirms:

> . . . the coercion of being detained was not attributed to the legal process involved but rather to coercive events that service users were subject to as a consequence of detention. [28]

There is a lack of communicable knowledge of what ordinary psychiatric treatment imposed on a person looks and feels like.

What we are experiencing is a hierarchy of disempowerments that stretches from the psychiatrist's consulting room to the queue for bread and jam at bed time. It is interlinked and greater than the sum of its parts. In the end, it is sustained by our own suspicions that we are truly inferior. We come out of these isolating places and we are much too afraid to tell ordinary people what it was like. [29]

... the truth is that most of the interference with choice actually occurs in much more mundane, routine, noncrisis kinds of matters. Things like when we eat, when we're allowed to use the telephone, who we can associate with, and what we do with our time. And while these issues don't have the "glamour" of the high-risk situations we hear about, I really believe that that's where the most of us have felt the most intruded upon and where the lack of choice has really been a burden to us over the years. [30]

The definition of coercion needs to be enlarged to include all the single occurrences where people are denied a choice about basic things in their lives. Researching coercion should focus on its incidence and the methods used; it should be able to answer how, by whom and with what kind of justification coercive methods are applied.

From the already mentioned large consultation exercise with service users/survivors around 15 European countries [18], we learned that a person can be locked up for a week in solitary confinement (Belgium); that the nurse in charge of close observation does not speak to a patient at all (Finland); that patients who are not allowed to leave the ward have to wear pyjamas at all times in order to be easily distinguished from the others (Austria). We learned that there is often no access to a toilet in the isolation room and that the patient can be forcibly cleaned with the same mop with which the floor is cleaned (Greece). We would like to see research on coercion capable of examining and documenting such situations and providing complete and unbiased data. We expect the research on coercion to disclose all treatment methods, providing accurate information about their use, the decision-making processes behind them and their therapeutic justification.

As psychotropic medication is what constitutes psychiatric treatment, coercive measures are predominantly used in order to assist with administering drugs. The already mentioned user-led study of hospital admissions [28] confirms this.

There was a strong link between medication and coercion. All physical restraints reported were followed by forcible injection ... [28]

The European consultation exercise with service users/survivors [18] about their perspectives on human rights has also shown that refusing medication is not really an option in psychiatric treatment, both in hospitals and in the community.

I see it as a right for people to choose to not take medication as well as taking it and I don't feel that any country allows for that... We are all different and I totally respect everyone's right to take it or not take you know it's not a case of drugs are good or bad it's a personal choice but I don't feel we are allowed the right to not take it. It's very easy if you want it, you can have it by the shed load but if you don't want it – it is very difficult. [18]

You can refuse chemotherapy if you have cancer even if you are going to die but it can be made impossible to refuse medication [18]

Comprehensive research on coercion will therefore have to include independent, reliable and accessible information about the drugs administered, explaining both their main and side effects. The fact that current research pays no attention to such explanations completely leaves out the most crucial aspect of coerced treatment:

I guess for me the worst human rights violation is the forcing of physical treatments – drugs and ECT because for some people they can cause lasting damage whereas mechanical restraints are not as likely to cause lasting physical damage. [18]

Ron Bassman writes that:

The spirit-breaking component of forced drugging is reflective of the rationale used to justify past psychiatric treatments. A review of the history of psychiatry reveals that spirit-breaking was an important first step in treatment and a major justification for the psychic and physical torture of patients. [31]

Investigations of coercion need to move their focus away from *subjects'* perceptions and reactions, as these never take place in isolation. We would like to see research that reflects on the traits of clinical staff, their values and beliefs, while documenting the possibilities of monitoring their work.

Furthermore, the process of granting consent to treatment is well worth investigating in the psychiatric context, and studies should therefore never be limited to involuntary patients only. The fact that a person agreed to treatment does not guarantee that they have made a free and informed choice.

When I signed my consent form for ECT it was completely lacking in information. Nobody told me what the possible side effects would be, nobody told me that I might have memory loss. The information sheet didn't mention that, you know – so under what circumstances was I giving this consent? [18]

Studies of coercion should be designed to bring light to concrete practices, the entities in charge of them, and the whole interaction process. Before judging the outcomes, one should be able to explore and understand from multiple perspectives what constitutes the system of coercion and how this system operates.

While there is no space for a full discussion in this chapter, we believe that systematic investigations of the values, principles, practices and achievements of alternatives to coercive psychiatric treatment [32] should be called for as a necessary component in informed public debates about this issue.

## 13.8    Rethinking treatment outcomes

The outcome of coercive treatment cannot be quickly assessed from an outsider perspective. The impact of coercive treatment on people's biographies has to be tackled in terms of those biographies, as their owners are in the best position to report what happens in their lives. The notion of effectiveness of coercion as applied in psychiatric research remains just one amongst the variety of ways to think about treatment outcomes.

> Much of the research on outcomes involves time specific snapshots measuring recidivism and symptom reduction while ignoring the demonstrated non-linear path of recovery. Funding decisions that favour research to find ways to improve drug taking compliance limit the prospect for studies that reflect the richness and the complexity of the human condition. [31]

When service users/survivors talk about the impact of forced treatment, they seem to be thinking in terms of their whole lives. The first encounter with the psychiatric system usually marks a turning point in a person's biography [33], and forced treatment is often seen as incompatible with healing.

> And the truth is, you can't heal me without my cooperation, you cannot. There's no such thing as forced healing. [34]

> . . . people who have recovered are people who have made choices on their own. Choice is an integral part of the healing process. It's not just something that we can tack on to treatment when we feel it's convenient. If choice isn't available, then healing cannot occur. [30]

There seem to be historical disagreements around the question of whether 'healing' is at all amongst the intended goals of psychiatric interventions [35], including forced ones. Psychiatrist Peter Stastny distinguishes between medical practitioners respecting the Hippocratic Oath 'First do no harm' in contrast to those 'who practice social control under the guise of psychiatric treatment' [36].

The understanding of the scope of psychiatric intervention is closely connected to the question of who should define its outcomes and against which criteria. Many service users/survivors share demands such as those articulated by Lauren Tenney and Ron Bassman:

> Recovery is no longer the exception. Recovery is the expectation. [37]

> ... it is imperative that you see the individual and value that special individual by engaging in a collaborative search to find understanding, meaning, and connection in this person's unfolding life narrative. [38]

If psychiatric intervention is intended to help and heal, and if recovery and achieving a life worth living belong amongst its goals, then the outcomes of treatment need to be measured against the fulfilment of these goals. But such goals must also be articulated and revisited by persons themselves. The two treatment outcomes described below might have achieved a positive assessment if judged by any outside criteria.

> Introverted, dazed and abused by forced feeding and vast cocktails of tranquillisers, anti-depressants and sleeping pills, life had no meaning, no reality – no hope – even my dreams, all I had to live for, had been brutally shattered at my feet, I was imprisoned in a cage where no-one could reach me; even myself. [39]

> I did not manifest any of my internal distress, because I did not show any evidence of internal life at all. This is not the same as the absence of madness. Yet it was the gauge by which the success of treatment was measured. [40]

Even those outcomes which appear 'objective' and easy to define, such as 'employment' or 'maintaining work', give no information about their appropriateness for actual persons measured against their individual abilities and aspirations. We can't judge the realization and the fulfilment of somebody else's life without taking into account that person's unique criteria and expectations, their aspirations, capabilities and desires together with the way these developed within their life history. Peoples' ambitions usually get downsized in the course of psychiatric treatment [33], and no simplified outcome measures will capture such decisive outcomes.

> Wandering aimlessly down the street one day, I realized that I felt as if I'd died and gone to hell. The bright, creative, joyous, promising young person I'd been the year before – the person I used to think of as "me" – had been crushed out of existence. In her place was a debilitated mental patient, gazing through windows at women who were slinging burgers or operating cash registers for minimum wage, wishing desperately that she could pull herself together enough to do that one day. [41]

When I got out of the hospital I felt hopeless. Even though I was only twenty one years old, I felt like my life was over. [42]

Comprehensive research on coercion would need to develop criteria for judging treatment outcomes which go beyond adherence to treatment or any single quantitative data like the number of hospital re-admissions. The latter is, for instance, used commonly to assess the outcomes of community treatment orders. Interestingly enough, the possibility of suicide is never mentioned amongst the descriptions of treatment outcomes. Even just the simple numbers of suicides committed following psychiatric treatment, or in the course of it, are not publicly available. Judgements of treatment outcomes need to include suicide as well. Outcomes of treatment refer to *peoples' lives* and therefore cannot be of a technical nature. Their definition needs to be individualized, able to capture people's lives and the way they feel about them. We are aware, however, that such an approach would challenge the understanding of the purpose of psychiatric intervention, measuring its outcomes against the criteria of a fulfilled life. Investigators would need to give up their ambition to separately define what constitutes a good prospect for a person with a psychiatric diagnosis and accept that we are all entitled to the same opportunities in life. Psychiatric interventions would then be judged by their ability to assist individuals in the process of realizing those opportunities. If adopting such outcome criteria seems too ambitious or even utopian, our minimum expectation of all studies is that they become clear and transparent about the perspective they apply when judging the outcomes of coercive treatment.

## 13.9   Closing remarks

In both our review of psychiatric studies and in our attempt to come up with some principles and suggestions for comprehensive research on coercion, we have focused on empirical research as a source of knowledge. We are aware, however, that empirical research is just one form of knowledge production, and we would like to stress the importance of using other available sources of knowledge and letting them become part of what constitutes evidence. It should also be recognized that coercion in psychiatry has at no point been an evidence-based intervention. From the origins of psychiatry, coercion and actual force have been a given aspect of the incarceration and treatment system and have remained so. In the interests of genuine scientific research, as well as ethical, moral and values-based approaches, there should be an opportunity to take a step back from the assumptions and received wisdom that coercive psychiatry is 'natural' or inevitable.

If people with a psychiatric diagnosis are not to be 'objects, imprisoned with and without walls, cut-off from a meaningful dialogue' [43], then our experiential knowledge of madness, distress, treatment and force needs to find its place on equal terms with other types of knowledge.

Experiential knowledge takes more forms than those of testimonies and narratives, and nowadays includes advocacy, research and conceptual work done by mental health service users/psychiatric survivors.

We see ourselves and many of our peers in Louise Pembroke's words:

> Something was very wrong with the treatment but I didn't have the language or the analysis to articulate it beyond refusing to cooperate with it. [22]

For those of us who have experienced forced treatment, it usually takes years until we come to terms with our lives, until we comprehend what happened and find a way to integrate that experience and deal with it. It takes even longer until we complete our interrupted education and achieve formal requirements to take part in organized knowledge production, often in the form of research. We wish for service user/survivor knowledge to find a shorter and more direct way to enter and inform public debates. We are convinced of its potential to reshape mental health legislation and policy towards fostering quality improvement in services instead of merely extending coercion.

## Acknowledgments

Jasna Russo warmly thanks Toma Tasovac and Debra Shulkes for all their support, proofreading and editing.

## References

1. UN Convention on the Rights of Persons with Disabilities, Resolution A/RES/61/106 of the General Assembly of the United Nations (13 December 2006). Available at www.un.org/disabilities/default.asp?id=259 (accessed 30 April 2010)
2. Secretariat for the Convention on the Rights of Persons with Disabilities (2010) Rights and Dignity of Persons with Disabilities. www.un.org/disabilities/index.asp (accessed 7 April 2010).
3. Katsakou, C. and Priebe, S. (2006) Outcomes of involuntary hospital admission – a review. *Acta Psychiatrica Scandinavica*, **114**, 232–241.
4. Hiday, V.A., Swartz, M.S., Swanson, J. and Wagner, H.R. (1997) Patient perceptions of coercion in mental hospital admission. *International Journal of Law and Psychiatry*, **20**, 227–241.
5. McKenna, B.G., Simpson, A.I.F. and Laidlaw, T.M. (1999) Patient perception of coercion on admission to acute psychiatric services. The New Zealand Experience. *International Journal of Law and Psychiatry*, **22**, 143–153.
6. Priebe, S., Katsakou, C., Amos, T. *et al.* (2009) Patient's views and readmissions 1 year after involuntary hospitalisation. *British Journal of Psychiatry*, **194**, 49–54.
7. Rain, S.D., Williams, V.F., Robbins, P.C. *et al.* (2003) Perceived coercion at hospital admission and adherence to mental health treatment after discharge. *Psychiatric Services*, **54**, 103–105.

8. Stanhope, V., Marcus, S. and Solomon, P. (2009) The impact of coercion on services from the perspective of mental health care consumers with co-occurring disorders. *Psychiatric Services*, **60**, 83–88.
9. Steadman, H.J., Gounis, K., Dennis, D. *et al.* (2001) Assessing the New York city involuntary outpatient commitment pilot programme. *Psychiatric Services*, **52**, 330–336.
10. Gibbs, A., Dawson, J. and Mullen, R. (2006) Community treatment orders for people with serious mental illness: a New Zealand study. *British Journal of Social Work*, **36**, 1085–1100.
11. Johansson, I.M. and Lundman, B. (2002) Patients' experience of involuntary psychiatric care: good opportunities and great losses. *Journal of Psychiatric and Mental Health Nursing*, **9**, 639–647.
12. Tew, J. (2008) Researching in partnership. Reflecting on a collaborative study with mental health service users into the impact of compulsion. *Qualitative Social Work*, **7**, 71–87.
13. Katsakou, C. and Priebe, S. (2007) Patient's experiences of involuntary hospital admission and treatment: a review of qualitative studies. *Epidemiologia e Psichiatria Sociale*, **16**, 172–178.
14. Burns, T., Rugkåsa, J., Molodynski, A. *et al.* (2010) Oxford Community Treatment Order Evaluation Trial (OCTET). www.psychiatry.ox.ac.uk/research/researchunits/socpsych/research/octet (accessed 31 March 2010).
15. Faulkner, A. and Thomas, P. (2002) User-led research and evidence-based medicine. *British Journal of Psychiatry*, **180**, 1–3.
16. O'Hagan, M. (2003) Force in mental health services: international user/survivor perspectives. Keynote address, World Federation for Mental Health Biennial Congress, Melbourne, Australia, 2003. Available from www.peoplewho.org/readingroom/ohagan.force.doc (accessed 30 March 2010).
17. Campbell, P. (1996) Challenging loss of power, in *Speaking Our Minds* (eds J. Readand J. Reynolds), Macmillian Press Ltd, London.
18. Russo, J. (2008) Consultation with service users: focus groups report of the ITHACA project (Institutional Treatment, Human Rights and Care Assessment), Institute of Psychiatry, Kings College London. See www.ithaca-study.eu (accessed 3 December 2010).
19. Hoge, S., Lidz, C., Mulvey, E. *et al.* (1993) Patient, family and staff perceptions of coercion in mental health hospital admission: an exploratory study. *Behavioral Science and the Law*, **11**, 281–293.
20. Spensley, J., Edwards, D. and White, E. (1980) Patient satisfaction and involuntary treatment. *American Journal of Orthopsychiatrics*, **50**, 725–727.
21. Toews, J., El-Guebaly, N. and Leckie, A. (1981) Patients' reactions to their commitment. *Canadian Journal of Psychiatry*, **26**, 251–254.
22. Pembroke, L.R. (ed) (1994) *Self-Harm Perspectives from Personal Experience*, Survivors Speak Out, London, pp. 31–60.
23. Russo, J. and Stastny, P. (2009) Beyond involvement. Looking for a common perspective on roles in research, in *Handbook of User Involvement in Research* (eds M. Amering, B. Schrankand J. Wallcraft), John Wiley & Sons, Ltd, Chichester, UK, pp. 61–72.
24. Council of Europe (2010) CPT: European Committee for the Prevention of Torture and Inhuman or Degrading Treatment or Punishment. www.cpt.coe.int/en/about.htm (accessed 18 April 2010).
25. Office of the United Nations High Commissioner for Human Rights (OHCR) (2008) Interim Report of the Special Rapporteur on Torture and Other Cruel, Inhuman or Degrading Treatment or Punishment. Available from http://www2.ohchr.org/english/issues/disability/torture.htm (accessed 30 April 2010).

26. Davis, C. (2001) Building self-esteem, in *Something Inside so Strong. Strategies for Surviving Mental Distress* (ed J. Read), The Mental Health Foundation, London, pp. 21–25.
27. Mental Disability Advocacy Center (2008) Guardianship Reports 2006–2008. Available from www.mdac.info/en/reports (accessed 30 April 2010).
28. Gilburt, H., Rose, D. and Slade, M. (2008) The importance of relationships in mental health care: a qualitative study of service users' experiences of psychiatric hospital admission in the UK. *BMC Health Services Research*, **8**, 92.
29. Campbell, P. (2001) Crisis cards and advance directives, in *Something Inside so Strong. Strategies for Surviving Mental Distress* (ed J. Read), The Mental Health Foundation, London, pp. 77–82.
30. Penney, D. (1994) Choice, common sense, and responsibility: the system's obligations to recipients, in *Choice and Responsibility: Legal and Ethical Dilemmas in Services for Persons with Mental Disabilities* (ed C.J. Sundram), New York State Commission on Quality Care, New York, pp. 29–32. Available at http://community-consortium.org/pdfs/Choice%20Common%20Sense%20Responsibility.pdf (accessed 6 December 2010)
31. Bassman, R. (2005) Mental illness and the freedom to refuse treatment: privilege or right. *Professional Psychology: Research and Practice*, **36**, 488–497.
32. Stastny, P. and Lehmann, P. (2007) *Alternatives Beyond Psychiatry*, Peter Lehmann Publishing, Berlin.
33. Russo, J. (2009) Re-building of a life written off. Survivor perspectives on first breakdown. Working paper presented at INTAR (International Network toward Alternatives and Recovery) lead-up retreat (21–22 November 2009, Rye, New York) to Conference Rethinking Psychiatric Crisis: Alternative Responses to "First Breaks", 23 November 2009, New York.
34. Patterson, C. (2001) MindFreedom Personal Stories: Carol J Patterson. www.mindfreedom.org/personal-stories/Carol%20Patterson/ (accessed 13 April 2010).
35. Amering, M. and Schmolke, M. (2007) *Recovery. Das Ende der Unheilbarkeit*, Psychiatrie Verlag, Bonn.
36. Stastny, P. (2000) Involuntary psychiatric interventions: a breach of the Hippocratic oath? *Ethical Human Sciences and Services*, **2**, 21–41.
37. Tenney, L.J. (2000) It has to be about choice. *Journal of Clinical Psychology*, **56**, 1433–1445.
38. Bassman, R. (2007) *A Fight to Be. A Psychologist's Experience from Both Sides of the Locked Door*, Tantamount Press, Albany, NY.
39. Caplin, R. (1994) Rosalind Caplin, in *Self-Harm Perspectives from Personal Experience* (ed L.R. Pembroke), Survivors Speak Out, London, pp. 27–29.
40. Smith, C. (2002) MindFreedom Personal Stories: Clover Smith. www.mindfreedom.org/personal-stories/smithclover/ (accessed 13 April 2010).
41. Shimrat, I. (1997) *Call Me Crazy – Stories from the Mad Movement*, Press Gang Publishers, Vancouver.
42. Chamberlin, J. (2006) Judi Chamberlin, in *First Person Stories on Forced Interventions and Being Deprived of Legal Capacity* (eds T. Minkowitz and A. Dhanda), WNUSP and BAPU Trust, Pune, pp. 19–20.
43. Bassman, R. (2001) Whose reality is it anyway? Consumers/survivors/ex-patients can speak for themselves. *Journal of Humanistic Psychology*, **41**, 11–35.

# 14 Seventy years of coercion in psychiatric institutions, experienced and witnessed

## Dorothea S. Buck-Zerchin

*German Federal Association of (ex-)Users and Survivors of Psychiatry, Hamburg, Germany*

Dorothea Buck's lecture was published in revised version in the book: *Alternatives beyond Psychiatry*, edited by Peter Stastny and Peter Lehmann, Berlin/Shreswbury/Eugene: Peter Lehmann Publishing, 2007, pp. 19–28.

Listen to her speech and download the film of it from http://ki-art-multimedia.de/dresden/doro-english.htm

My name is Dorothea Buck, I am 90 years old, and a so-called historical witness. The theme of my presentation is: 'Seventy Years of Coercion in the German Psychiatric System, Experienced and Witnessed'. I will start with the forced treatment and forced sterilization that was inflicted upon me 71 years ago. In 1966, Alexander Mitscherlich wrote in his book *Krankheit als Konflikt: Studien zur psychosomatischen Medizin I (Illness as a Conflict: Studies on Psychosomatic Medicine, Volume I)*, in the chapter entitled 'On the complexity of social influences on the origin and treatment of psychoses and neuroses' about the treatment measures: 'From the days of the primitive cultures, up to present times there have always been

*Coercive Treatment in Psychiatry: Clinical, Legal and Ethical Aspects*, First Edition.
Edited by Thomas W. Kallert, Juan E. Mezzich and John Monahan.
© 2011 John Wiley & Sons, Ltd. Published 2011 by John Wiley & Sons, Ltd.

methods of torment. On closer examination, a terrible arsenal of tortures in themselves. . .'

This applies also to the present-day practices of restraints and forced medication, which continue despite the fact that much more effective and helpful treatments for schizophrenia, such as Soteria and Professor Yrjö Alanen's *need-adapted treatment* in Finland, have proven their worth for decades.

In 1936, 71 years ago, at the age of just 19, I went through the most inhumane experience of my life in a psychiatric institution. Even the experience of being buried alive during the Second World War was not as traumatic for me. I experienced the psychiatric system as being inhumane because nobody actually spoke with us. A person cannot be more devalued than to be considered unworthy or incapable of conversation. What made it even worse was the fact that this happened at the von Bodelschwinghsche Asylum Bethel in Bielefeld, which considered itself a 'Christian' institution. Bethel and its director, Pastor Fritz von Bodelschwingh, were held in high esteem and considered an embodiment of compassion in the parsonage, which was my parent's home, and by us children as well. But I got to experience a totally different Bethel, compared to the one I had heard about from the newsletter *Bote von Bethel* (*Messenger from Bethel*).

On the light green wall opposite my bed one could read in large letters the words of Jesus: 'Come unto me all you who are weary and tired and I will give you rest.' How were we to be given rest? Rest was given with buckets of cold water poured over our heads, with lengthy baths in a tub covered with canvas that bore a stiff, high collar in which my neck was fixed for 23 hours, from one doctor's rounds to the next. Rest was given with wet packs and with sedating injections of paraldehyde. A wet pack meant to be bound into cold, wet sheets so tightly that one could no longer move at all. From our body temperature, the sheets would become first warm and then hot. I would cry out in rage at this senseless restraint in these hot sheets. I just couldn't believe that the natural way of helping in the form of conversation and occupation was being replaced by these torturous 'sedative measures'. It was only natural that we got restless without occupation and diversion, without a single conversation, not even as part of the admission procedure, and from staying in bed all the time, despite being in good physical health. How were we to recognize this senseless kind of behaviour on the part of the doctors and nurses as 'helpful' for us?

These methods of Emil Kraepelin, who had lived from 1856 until 1926, influenced our German psychiatry. The medical director of our Hospital for Nervous and Mood Diseases in Bethel, as it was then called, was one of his last students. Emil Kraepelin replaced the conversations that his predecessors, such as Wilhelm Griesinger (1817–1868), and Carl Wilhelm Ideler (1795–1860), had kept going with their patients, with the silent observation of symptoms, the hallmark of clinical phenomenology or 'nosological' psychiatry. As a result he was no longer capable of recognizing his patients as fellow human beings, because that is only possible by speaking with them. The symptoms they observed took the place of the human being with his or her experiences. Kraepelin demanded 'a ruthless intervention against hereditary degeneracy, the elimination of the psychopathic degenerate, including the use of sterilization.'

Thus the director of Bethel, Pastor Fritz von Bodelschwingh, demanded the sterilization two years ahead of the National Socialist Regime at the *Protestant Specialist Conference on Eugenics* held from May 18 to 20, 1931, in Treysa. He explained his position by saying that

> ... the destruction of the Kingdom of God in any one of its members justifies the possibility or the responsibility for its eradication to take place. Therefore I would be concerned if sterilizations were only accepted as a response to an emergency. I would prefer to see these procedures as a responsibility that conforms to the will of Christ. (From the conference minutes)

A truly monstrous 'Kingdom of God' that granted us only a hopeless and idle custodial existence without the right to any communication, sanctioned by the words of the Bible.

On the other hand, Dr Carl Schneider, the medical director of Bethel from 1930 to 1933, was opposed to the sterilization law:

> He considers it an error to assume that what is biologically valuable is also mentally valuable. For example, in patients with manic-depressive disorders 'such a high level of social competence tends to be inherited,' that it is impossible 'to sterilize for purely medical reasons'. Schneider's conclusion: 'We know nothing about this issue, we are just drawing conclusions from experiments with animals and plants.' (From the conference minutes)

Two years before the Nazis came to power, Protestant physicians and clergymen were calling for sterilization:

> Those who are hereditary carriers of social[!] inferiority and need care should be prevented from procreating if possible. (From the conference minutes)

When I asked the charge nurse about the scars that my young female fellow patients had in the middle of their lower abdomens, she explained that these were 'appendectomy scars'. Did they lie to us at home when they said that the appendix is located on the right side? Concealment of the fact that the operation I had been subjected to was in fact a sterilization seemed to be common practice here, even though the genetic health law of 1933 required that those sterilized had to be informed by the physicians about the nature of the procedure.

Even after the operation, it was not a doctor or a nurse who told me what had been done to me, but a fellow female patient. I was distraught, because people who had been forcibly sterilized were not allowed to pursue a higher education nor could they marry a non-sterilized partner. I had to abandon my chosen profession as a kindergarten teacher for which I had prepared myself for such a long time. Not to mention the lifelong stigmatization of being 'inferior'.

In the January 2007 edition of the *Deutsche Ärzteblatt* (a German medical journal), one finds an article about the absence of compensation for us 'inferior individuals' up to the present day, which quoted a statement by Professor Werner Villinger, Bethel's medical director from the year 1934 on, made before a German Parliamentary Committee for Restitution on April 13, 1961:

> [Dr Villinger] claimed that by paying compensation to people sterilized under coercion they would be damaged once again: "The question arises whether this might lead to the appearance of neurotic complaints and illnesses, which would not only diminish their previous subjective wellbeing and... their capacity to be happy, but also their productive capacity?"

On the 21st of January, 1965, Pastor Fritz von Bodelschwingh's nephew and successor, Pastor Friedrich von Bodelschwingh, argued as an expert before the Committee for Restitution in a similar manner, totally ignorant of our reality: 'If one were to grant the sterilized people a right to compensation, this would cause them only unrest and considerable new suffering...'

Bethel kept on sterilizing patients long after 1945. Last year, in 2006, I received a call from someone telling me that Bethel had pressured her to be sterilized even in the 1970s. If only theologians and psychiatrists would doubt their own worth for our sake!

When some 60 asylum directors and psychiatry professors were informed for the first time about SS-Führer Viktor Brack's 'euthanasia' programme in Adolf Hitler's Berlin Chancellery in July 1939, all of them declared their willingness to cooperate in the killing of asylum patients, with the exception of Professor Gottfried Ewald from Göttingen. He explained his disapproval in detail. One single person sound in mind and soul amongst 60 professors of psychiatry and clinic directors! Where was their conscience, their courage and their compassion, the values that account for people becoming fellow human beings?

In Berlin, at Tiergartenstreet 4, regular and senior experts pronounced death sentences simply on the basis of questionnaires that had been filled out in the asylums. In six psychiatric killing centres, those who had been sentenced to death were gassed. When Hitler responded to the protest sermon of the Catholic Bishop Clemens August von Galen in Münster on 3rd August, 1941 by ordering a stop to the gassing on the 24th of August, 1941, the asylums took over and continued the killing by medication overdoses and starvation diets. According to the latest research results submitted by the historian Professor Hans-Walter Schmuhl, nearly 300 000 asylum and nursing care home patients were gassed, poisoned and starved to death. Of these, 80 000 came from Polish, French and Soviet institutions. Considering that our politicians, psychiatrists and theologians have since nearly completely repressed this most drastic kind of compulsory treatment in the form of killing people whose lives were considered 'devoid of value', it is mostly left up to us users and survivors of psychiatry to preserve the memory of those murdered in the name of psychiatry, in our hearts.

After 1943, psychiatrists, who had turned out to be adversaries of their patients and in the period from 1939 to 1945 had proven themselves to be – in the literal sense of the term – their 'mortal enemies', continued to convey to their students and to the public nothing other than an image of deficiency regarding their patients who had been classified as 'incurable'. Even on the 20th of April 1979, 40 years after the beginning of the 'euthanasia' programme in 1939, the weekly paper *Die Zeit* ran the following headline on the front page: 'A Society of Cold Hearts – In the Snake Pits of the German Psychiatric System'. The article states that 'no minority is treated as disgracefully as the mentally ill'.

The decades of backwardness of this kind of psychiatry have not been overcome despite considerable efforts in recent years. It remains devoid of conversation and uses medication even under coercion and restraint just to fight the symptoms, rather than aim for understanding.

Soteria and Professor Yrjö Alanen's need-adapted treatment in Finland have focused on the experiences and needs of patients for over 30 years, by taking them seriously and by giving immediate psychotherapy for those diagnosed with 'schizophrenia' absolute priority over antipsychotic medication. In contrast, the German Society for Psychiatry, Psychotherapy and Neurology assigns just 10 out of a total of 140 pages to the topic of psychotherapy in their draft version of *Treatment Guidelines for Schizophrenia*.

Cognitive behavioural therapy is the only form of psychotherapy they approve, but even this therapy they would only recommend when pharmacotherapy has failed. Today's German psychiatric system has fully adopted Emil Kraepelin's concept of a hereditary or genetically caused brain disease which is by definition devoid of meaning, just calling it a disorder of the brain metabolism instead.

Antipsychotic medication has existed since 1953. Since then, its immediate application has been the method of choice. A patient who is overwhelmed by his psychosis certainly wants to have his experiences taken seriously and wants to understand them. The immediate sedation with strong antipsychotic medication cannot be taken as well-intentioned help from the patient's point of view. He or she will resist. To make the patients compliant with the medication, they will often be strapped to the bed by the waist and all four extremities restrained. At the first psychiatric world congress in Germany after the Second World War, held in 1994 in Hamburg, jointly organized by Dr Thomas Bock and our Federal Organization of (ex-) Users and Survivors of Psychiatry, the Federal Association of Relatives of the Mentally Ill, and the German Society for Social Psychiatry, the artist Jutta Jentges exhibited a large expressive painting of a person with arms and legs spread-eagled and tied to the bed with the question 'Why?' She expresses the torment of being restrained even through the night. The restrained person has been furnished with a diaper, another kind of humiliating debasement. For many people who have had the agonizing experience of being restrained, it sometimes remains a life-long trauma.

During my five stays in psychiatric institutions between 1936 and 1959, this tormenting method of tying patients to bed by their hands, feet and waist did not exist yet, and body-belts were used only rarely. Up to my fourth episode in 1946, it was common practice to wait a few weeks to see if the psychosis would recede on its own accord, before Metrazol (Cardiazol – pentetrazol), insulin, or electroshock were applied. In 1936, these shock treatments were not yet available either. During my last psychotic episode in 1959, I experienced for the first time, along with all of the others on the ward, an immediate injection of high dosages of antipsychotic drugs. I considered this to be a total dictatorship which prevented us from thinking and feeling and also caused extreme physical weakness; it was deeply repulsive. I was lucky to develop a skin rash after the first two days (of injections); when pills were shoved into my mouth instead, I was able to hide them under my tongue and dump them in the toilet. Nonetheless, it took me the same amount of time as my fellow patients to be rid of the psychosis. Today, liquids are used instead of pills, to prevent behaviour like mine.

In contrast, how much more helpful, respectful and competent is the Krisenpension (Crisis Hostel) in Berlin, staffed in a 'trialogue' manner by psychiatric survivors, family members/relatives, professionals and lay people, who work without using any kind of coercion. Here a person experiencing psychosis is taken seriously instead of being dismissed and reduced to a disturbed brain metabolism. Many people are looking for a way to understand themselves and their psychotic experiences. Whoever wants to understand their psychosis or did find a way to understand it, as I did, after five episodes, at the age of 42, which enabled me to get rid of it 48 years ago, still has to find the necessary insights for this process all by themselves – even today.

For these reasons and as an attack against biological reductionist psychiatry, with its distaste for talking with patients, we started the 'Psychosis Seminars' together with Dr Thomas Bock at the Department of Psychiatry of the Hamburg University Clinic, in the winter semester of 1989/1990. We conceived them as an opportunity to exchange experiences between users of psychiatry, family members/relatives and professionals and called this a *trialogue*. In this format, people who have gone through psychoses can talk freely about their deepest experiences, without having to take higher dosages of medication as would be the case in psychiatric institutions. This is a way of exchanging experiences that gives equal rights for all and makes it possible to understand each other a lot better. In the 17 years of their existence, the 'Psychosis Seminars' were replicated in Switzerland and Austria, but far too few psychiatrists are taking part in them.

What is a psychosis? The problem of coercion and violence largely depends on this definition. The medical concept of a meaningless, genetically caused disorder of brain metabolism devalues the patient, ignores him as a person along with his experiences, and virtually provokes his resistance.

What would happen if, instead of you – the psychiatrists – we had the power to define psychosis? We would define it as an emergence of something that is normally unconscious, in an attempt to resolve a preceding crisis that we were not able to solve with our conscious capacities. We would also say that this was the reason for the obvious similarities between the well-known schizophrenic symptoms and the stuff our night dreams are made of, since they both originate from the same source – our unconscious. For example, the emergence of symbols, thinking and acting in symbolic terms are considered symptoms of schizophrenia. Our dreams are full of symbols. Or the fact that identifications with Jesus and other personalities can often be found in schizophrenic episodes. In our dreams, we also identify ourselves with the people who appear in them, which frequently signify ourselves. And the same is true with the frequent occurrence of 'ideas of reference and overvalued ideas' in schizophrenia. These can only be understood within the context of an altered experience of the world in psychosis that reveals otherwise hidden connections. The same applies to dreams. In *An Outline of Psychoanalysis*, Sigmund Freud mentioned, as regards to dreams, 'a remarkable tendency to condense, to create new entities from elements that in our waking hours we would surely have kept separate from each another.'

Consequently, the illness is based on the fact that we consider our psychotic experiences real. If we recognized them as relating to a dream level from the outset, we would not be ill. Therefore, we need to shift the contents of our psychosis to the 'dream level', which would enable us to hold on to the meaning of our psychosis without maintaining its objective reality. Our psychoses are often accompanied by emerging impulses and emotions, which also come from our subconscious. I always live by these impulses or by the inner, inaudible voice to prevent these impulses and feelings from getting bottled up. Some people do hear these voices. This definition of schizophrenia is not debasing and invites people to deal with the contents of the psychosis and the preceding crisis, in order to understand oneself better and know how to handle oneself.

We experience and regard the emergence from the unconscious as 'insertions' coming from outside ourselves. Therefore, the British psychiatrist John K. Wing refers to the 'experience of thought insertion' as a 'central schizophrenic symptom'.

It is probably this experience of thoughts inserted from the outside that provides the basis for the term 'schizophrenia'. As soon as we realize that we are dealing with an emergence from our unconscious, which we experience as coming from outside ourselves because of a completely different way of thinking and imagining, which is like 'being thought' rather than active thinking, then we can work towards an understanding of the psychosis and of the self. The fact that our psychoses are psychologically caused by preceding crises in our lives is known to nearly all who have had these experiences.

Many people are afraid of psychiatric institutions with their forced medication and absence of help in understanding either the psychosis or the self. From their very first contact with a patient, psychiatrists should prove themselves to be helpers and not opponents. My wish would be that the patients could – right from the start – present their disturbing experiences in group sessions, that they could talk about them, write about them, paint and draw them. I wish that they would be taken seriously with their experiences, without needing to fear unwanted psychiatric interventions. During this process, it would be very valuable to have the support of individuals who have experienced psychoses themselves and have overcome them, understood their meaning for their lives, and have been able to integrate these experiences into their regular lives.

Currently, there is a pilot project at the University Clinic Hamburg, Department of Psychiatry, called 'Experienced Involvement' (EX-IN), sponsored by the European Leonardo da Vinci Programme, where people who have experienced psychoses are being trained. Further details about this project can be found in the February 2007 edition of the journal *Eppendorfer*, under the title 'Vom Patienten zum Profi – Ein europäisches Projekt qualifiziert Psychiatrie-Erfahrene für die Hilfe anderer Betroffener' (From patient to professional: a European project qualifies (ex-) users and survivors of psychiatry to give peer support).

I experienced five different psychiatric hospitals from 1936 to 1959, with 23 professors of psychiatry, medical directors, senior physicians and their assistants. They all subscribed to a genetically caused, meaningless and incurable schizophrenia. As a result, I didn't experience a single conversation about the content of my psychoses or the life-crisis that led to them, and certainly not about any meaningful connections. Psychiatric inpatients today still complain about this lack of dialogue.

I was encouraged by the publicist Hans Krieger who called for more considerate treatment of psychotic patients in several outspoken reviews of psychiatric and psychological literature in *Die Zeit* during the 1960s and 1970s. He also had introduced us to foreign reform initiatives, such as Ronald Laing's Kingsley Hall and others. He is the one to be thanked for urging me to write about my experiences of psychosis and healing. In 1990, he edited my accounts in a book titled *Auf der Spur des Morgensterns – Psychose als Selbstfindung* (*On the Trail of the Morning Star: Psychosis as Self-Discovery,* currently published by Paranus (in the German language)). There you can see that I really had schizophrenia. Because, according to Kraepelin, a person who has recovered from schizophrenia never had schizophrenia.

How can we trust in a psychiatric system that rejects the concept of healing, because such healing would contradict the theory of a meaningless, incurable metabolic brain disorder? We older people, who have experienced psychoses, have paid for this genetic–somatic dogma with forced sterilization and its consequences, and the 'euthanasia' victims paid for it with their lives. Now is the time for the psychiatric system to become an empirical science, based on the experiences of patients.

# 15 Coercion – point, perception, process

## Dorothy M. Castille[1], Kristina H. Muenzenmaier[2] and Bruce G. Link[3]

[1]*National Institutes of Health, National Institute on Minority Health and Health Disparities, Bethesda, MD, USA*
[2]*Albert Einstein College of Medicine, Bronx, NY, USA*
[3]*Columbia University, New York State Psychiatric Institute, New York, NY, USA*

## 15.1 Introduction

The use of force in psychiatric treatment continues to be a hotly debated topic. Supporting the coercion-is-necessary perspective is the contention that persons with mental illness fail to behave in socially acceptable ways [1]. At the same time, they may not perceive themselves as behaving in any way outside of acceptable social norms nor find their own behaviour to be a problem to themselves, as it is to others [2,3]. Historically, physicians, legislators and others maintain that the biological condition that underlies some serious mental illnesses results in impaired insight [2,3]. Thus, for many individuals, failure to recognize the need for treatment may require their being forced to enter or remain in treatment.

*Coercive Treatment in Psychiatry: Clinical, Legal and Ethical Aspects*, First Edition.
Edited by Thomas W. Kallert, Juan E. Mezzich and John Monahan.
© 2011 John Wiley & Sons, Ltd. Published 2011 by John Wiley & Sons, Ltd.

Detracting from the coercion-is-necessary perspective are those who argue that the use of force constitutes discrimination and destroys trust in the relationships between mental health consumers and their treatment providers, and may contribute to destabilizing a person's mental health. The more negative consequences of coercive treatment as outlined by consumers are fear, anger and disempowerment, and provoking such labels as 'treatment resistant' and 'treatment noncompliant' [4]. Anger at being forced to take treatment, and fear at being treated against a person's will may trigger people to leave the treatment system or to move to another state where they have not been engaged with the mental health system.

Since deinstitutionalization in the 1970s, a number of strategies have been employed to promote treatment adherence in persons with serious mental illness, particularly those who are seen as treatment resistant. Outpatient commitment is a relatively recent strategy to ensure adherence to treatment in the least restrictive environment. How does the individual with mental illness experience court-ordered assignment to outpatient treatment? Does the order cause people to feel coerced?

Rosenberg and Pearlin [5] assert that coercion represents 'power based on compulsion, sanctions, or the threat of sanctions'. In fact, as Lovell [6] points out, mental health treatment, viewed through the lens of social control, places coercion on a 'pure coercion' to 'bilateral control or voluntarism' continuum. From the perspective of the mental health care professional, the power enlisted to ensure adherence may be persuasive, manipulative, authoritative, contractual or coercive [5]. These approaches represent the effort of one individual to control the behaviour of another; however, all such efforts are not experienced as equally coercive by the recipient [7].

While the concept of coercion is central to a consideration of policies, such as outpatient commitment, measuring it accurately and completely is difficult. Two approaches are prominent and widely used. In the first, one uses the objective fact of an event such as involuntary commitment, exposure to restraints, or assignment to outpatient commitment to gauge exposure to coercion. This approach uses objective conditions experienced by the consumer as the key evidence of coercive treatment and is exemplified in questions such as: what difference does a court order make in patient adherence to treatment? While extremely important and useful, a problem with this approach is that it misses complex processes comprising patient experience and the psychological reaction to those experiences. In the second approach, people are asked questions that reveal whether and to what extent they feel coerced. The exemplar of this latter approach is the Perceived Coercion Scale developed by the MacArthur Research Network on Mental Health and the Law [8–10]. This instrument has been translated into 42 languages [11–13] and applied to hospital admission experiences [14,15] and outpatient commitment [16–19]. Based on its widespread use, we included the MacArthur Perceived Coercion Scale in a study of Kendra's Law, New York State's outpatient commitment law, that compared a sample of people assigned to outpatient commitment and a group of people who were not.

We wondered how strongly the two methods of assessing coercion might be related and what, if anything, might drive feelings of coercion other than the objective fact of court-ordered treatment.

## 15.2   New York State's Kendra's Law

Our study of coercion in outpatient treatment was undertaken in the context of New York State's Kendra's Law. In 1999, New York became the 42nd of the 50 states to have an outpatient commitment law when the state legislature passed Kendra's Law (New York Mental Hygiene Law 9.60), allowing courts to require 'assisted outpatient treatment' (AOT) for severely ill individuals with a history of noncompliance with treatment and in need of additional support to successfully engage in treatment in an outpatient setting. Accompanying a court order to outpatient treatment may be a bundle of services which is always coordinated by an Intensive Case Manager or an Assertive Community Treatment (ACT) team, often someone with training as a Social Worker, including: clinical services and medication; blood tests or urinalysis to determine compliance with prescribed medications; individual or group therapy, day or partial day programming activities; alcohol or substance abuse treatment and counselling and periodic tests for the presence of alcohol or illegal drugs for persons with a history of alcohol or substance abuse; supervision of living arrangements; and any other service within a local or unified service plan [20]. The law has given priority access to scarce necessities of life, for example housing, clinical outpatient services and assignment to a case manager, to the proportion of the population most severely affected by mental illness and yet most difficult to engage in the treatment system.

In the present chapter we begin with a comparison between the two previously mentioned approaches to measuring coercion. We ask: does a person with a court order perceive him/herself as being more coerced than a person in outpatient treatment without a court order? As we document below, the answer we obtained surprised us, as the group court-ordered to treatment was not significantly higher than the comparison group in perceptions of coercion to outpatient treatment. This anomalous finding led us to ask about the reliability and validity of the Perceived Coercion Scale in our sample, to explore other determinants of perceptions of coercion, and to conduct in-depth qualitative interviews to deepen our understanding about the reasons for our findings.

## 15.3   Methods

### 15.3.1   Study sample

Men and women between the ages of 18 and 65 years with a history of serious mental illness, the capacity to give informed consent, and with the ability to speak either

English or Spanish were recruited from various outpatient clinics in two boroughs of New York City (Table 15.1). People court-ordered into assisted outpatient treatment (AOT Group) and people in outpatient treatment (Outpatient Group or OPT) receiving care as usual comprise the study population. Of the 184 people interviewed

**Table 15.1**    Socio-demographic characteristics of sample population by AOT and OPT status.

|  | AOT $n = 76$ (41.3%) | OPT $n = 108$ (60.3%) | Total $n = 184$ (100%) |
|---|---|---|---|
| *Age – Mean* | 35.8 | 37.8 | 37.0 |
| *Sex* | | | |
| Female | 24 (31.6%) | 49 (45.4%) | 73 (39.7%) |
| Male | 52 (68.4%) | 59 (54.6%) | 111 (60.3%) |
| *Race* | | | |
| Black | 45 (59.1%) | 53 (49.1%) | 98 (53.3%) |
| White | 6 (7.9%) | 8 (7.1%) | 14 (7.6%) |
| Hispanic | 18 (23.7%) | 35 (32.4%) | 53 (28.8%) |
| Other | 7 (9.2%) | 13 (11.1%) | 19 (10.3%) |
| *Marital* | | | |
| Married, common law | 5 (6.7%) | 12 (11.1%) | 17 (9.3%) |
| Widowed, divorced, separated | 12 (16.0%) | 25 (23.1%) | 37 (20.2%) |
| Never married | 58 (77.3%) | 71 (65.7%) | 129 (70.5%) |
| *Employment* | | | |
| Currently unemployed | 63 (86.3%) | 93 (88.6%) | 156 (87.6%) |
| No. wks unemployed in past year – Mean | 46.5 wk | 47.3 wk | 47.0 wk |
| *Income source[a]* | | | |
| Public Assistance | 10 (13.2%) | 13 (12.1%) | 23 (12.6%) |
| SSI (Gold Check) | 31 (40.8%) | 40 (37.0%) | 71 (38.6%) |
| SSD (Disability) | 24 (32.4%) | 29 (26.9%) | 53 (29.1%) |
| SSP (Pension) Medicaid | 0 (0.0%) | 1 (0.9%) | 1 (0.5%) |
| Medicaid | 62 (81.6%) | 84 (77.8%) | 146 (79.3%) |
| Medicare | 20 (26.7%) | 21 (19.6%) | 41 (22.5%) |
| Food Stamps | 21 (27.6%) | 24 (22.4%) | 45 (24.6%) |
| *Education* | | | |
| Less than High School | 33 (43.4%) | 40 (37.0%) | 73 (39.7%) |
| Completed HS or more | 43 (56.6%) | 68 (63.0%) | 111 (60.3%) |
| *Axis I diagnosis* | | | |
| Schizophrenia | 29 (40.3%) | 42 (40.0%) | 71 (40.1%) |
| Schizo-affective disorder | 30 (41.7%) | 27 (25.7%) | 57 (32.2%) |
| Major depressive disorder | 1 (1.4%) | 12 (11.4%) | 13 (7.3%) |
| Bipolar disorder | 11 (15.3%) | 22 (21.0%) | 33 (18.6%) |
| Other | 1 (1.4%) | 2 (1.9%) | 3 (1.7%) |

[+] $P < 0.1$; [*] $P < 0.05$; [**] $P < 0.01$; [***] $P < 0.001$.
[a]Percentages do not sum to 100% because respondents may have more than one source of income and service coverage.

at baseline, 39.7% are female and 60.3% are male. The ethnic distribution of the people in the sample reflects that of the clinics at which respondents were recruited; therefore, there are few respondents in our sample of white (7.6%) or other ethnicities (10.3%), the majority endorsing African descent (53.3%) and Hispanic (28.8%) ethnic identities. The AOT and OPT groups differ very little by mean age: AOT respondents, 35.8 years; and OPT respondents, 37.8 years. Fewer persons on AOT (43, or 56.6%) had completed high school or more years of education than out-patient respondents (68, or 63.0%). Most (70.5%) of the people in the sample had never married. The majority of the respondents in the sample reported being unemployed (87.6%) for an average of 47 of the previous 52 weeks. Most study participants received services reimbursed by Medicaid regardless of AOT or OPT status. While the ethnic distribution of this New York City sample differs from that published by the New York State Office of Mental Health for the entire state, it does reflect the population receiving services in the state on every other dimension and does not differ from published data for New York City recipients (http://bi.omh.state.ny.us/aot/about).

Of respondents, 59.2% reported having been arrested, AOT 50 (66.7%) vs. OPT 59 (54.6%), prior to the baseline interview and 48 (26.1%) of the total study population described a history of more than three arrests. Court-ordered consumers reported significantly more hospitalizations (an average of 9.51 hospitalizations per person) than their non-court-ordered peers (6.26 hospitalizations). These characteristics suggest a group of individuals experiencing more life difficulties than their outpatient peers (Table 15.2).

### 15.3.2 Measures

The battery of measures administered in this study used multiple-item scales measured at six time points: baseline, 1, 3, 6, 9 and 12 months; however, we report here on baseline results only. For scales containing positively and negatively worded statements, each item is scored so that a high score on the item reflects a high score

**Table 15.2** Self-reported clinical and forensic history by AOT and OPT status.

|  | AOT | OPT | Total |
| --- | --- | --- | --- |
| *Arrest history* | | | |
| Ever arrested | 50 (66.7%) | 59 (54.6%) | 109 (59.2%) |
| Arrested four or more times | 24 (31.6%) | 24 (22.2%) | 48 (26.1%) |
| *Hospitalization* | | | |
| No. of hospitalizations – Mean | 9.51*** | 6.26 | 7.88 |

$^{+}P < 0.1$; $^{*}P < 0.05$; $^{**}P < 0.01$; $^{***}P < 0.001$.

on the construct being measured. For each scale employed, we report the baseline internal consistency reliability ($\alpha$) and create scale scores by summing the scores for each item in a scale and dividing by the total number of items in that scale when values for at least two-thirds of the scale items are present. This yields scores that locate the scale mean in relation to the response categories for the items, and prevents loss of subjects due to the absence of less than one-third of the scale items. For example, a scale mean of 2 for items using a four-point 'strongly disagree' (0), 'disagree' (1), 'agree' (2) and 'strongly agree' (3) format would tell us that the average respondent is in agreement with the items in the scale.

*AOT Assignment*    Individuals experiencing a court order for mandated treatment within 90 days of the baseline interview constituted the AOT group. Of the 184 study participants, 76 experienced this form of objective coercion while 108 did not.

*Perceived Coercion Scale*    The Perceived Coercion Scale is a five-item version of a scale developed by the MacArthur Research Network on Mental Health and the Law [10,21]. In contrast to the original scale construction that used a 'true/false' response pattern, the scale items were adapted in the present study to ask whether, considering experiences of the past 12 months, the individual 'strongly disagrees = 0', 'disagrees = 1', 'agrees = 2' or 'strongly agrees = 3' with the following statements:

- '...you felt free to do what you wanted about getting outpatient mental health treatment';
- '...you chose to get outpatient mental health treatment';
- '...it was your idea to get mental health treatment';
- '...you had a lot of control over whether you got outpatient mental health treatment'; and
- '...you had more influence than anyone else on whether you got treatment'.

Items were scored such that a high score reflected high perceived coercion.

To evaluate construct validity of the Perceived Coercion Scale, we used a number of measures that, if correlated in the predicted direction, would support the validity of the scale.

Potential correlates to be used as evidence in assessing construct validity include measures of stigma, quality of life, insight, the working alliance, the severity of psychotic symptoms, and the number of involuntary hospitalizations.

Stigma, known to be associated with mental illness, may be hypothesized to correlate significantly with a court order to remain in treatment. We assessed stigma using an eight-item version of Link's [22] perceived devaluation/discrimination measure ($\alpha = 0.74$). The measure asks the extent to which respondents 'strongly agree', 'agree', 'disagree' or 'strongly disagree' with statements indicating that most people devalue or discriminate against current or former psychiatric consumers.

Quality of Life [23] ($\alpha = 0.91$) is an area in which a reduction in symptoms due to adherence to treatment may bring improvement. Therefore, better quality of life may be negatively associated with the Perceived Coercion Scale. Quality of Life is assessed using 14 items of Lehman's self report scale that asks respondents to rate as 'poor' (1), 'fair' (2), 'good' (3) or 'excellent' (4) multiple domains of life such as living conditions, employment, social life, physical health, level of independence and self-esteem. Items are summed and divided by 14 if values for two-thirds of the items are present, to yield scale scores with a maximum high point of 4 and a minimum low of 1.

The Working Alliance Inventory ($\alpha = 0.91$) [24], expected to be negatively associated with high perceived coercion because coercion is hypothesized to reduce trust between the individual and the case manager, is assessed using an eight-item measure. Respondents are asked how often ('very often', 'fairly often', 'sometimes', 'almost never' or 'never') their case manager does things for them or makes them feel a particular way. Example items are 'How often are you confident in your case manager's ability to help you?' and 'How often do you feel that your case manager appreciates you?'

Insight expected to be impaired by symptom severity may be expected to improve with treatment and thus to be associated with low perceived coercion. The Insight measure comprised a four-item scale based on three slightly modified items of the ITAQ (the Insight and Treatment Attitudes Questionnaire [25]) and one item of the ROMI (Rating of Medication Influences Scale [26]) ($\alpha = 0.73$), including these questions: 'Do you think you have mental illness now?', 'Have you ever had mental illness?', 'Have you ever needed treatment for mental illness?' and 'Do you believe that you don't have a mental illness?'

Severity of psychotic symptoms occurring in the past three months was assessed using both a fixed-format, self-report symptom scale and a scale of symptoms derived from the clinician-administered Structured Clinical Interview for Diagnosis (SCID). The fixed-format scale ($\alpha = 0.95$) is a 10-item scale designed especially for this research and targets so-called threat/control override symptoms (TCO) that have been proposed as symptoms that might lead to violence [27]. We used the clinician-administered SCID to construct a scale of psychotic symptoms ($\alpha = 0.62$) by summing ratings of the presence (1) or absence (0) of delusions of reference, persecutory delusions, delusions of control, thought broadcasting and grandiose delusions.

The number of involuntary hospitalizations is assessed by asking at baseline how many times the study participant had been hospitalized against their will. Because the resulting frequency distribution is skewed, we add one to the number of involuntary commitments and then take the natural log of the sum to create a metric that varies from 0 to 2.77.

### 15.3.3   Qualitative interviews

Open-ended interviews were conducted in conjunction with the nine-month interview with a sample of 20 respondents, 9 persons on AOT and 11 Outpatient (OPT) group members. Interviewer recommendations influenced the choice of persons to be interviewed based on the respondent's ability to speak about his or her experience and to represent as wide a range of perspectives on the experience of coercion as possible. We wanted the qualitative subsample to include both individuals who felt coerced and individuals who did not feel coerced, in both the AOT and the non-AOT groups. Interviews were audio taped, transcribed and coded thematically by two coders (the first author and a social worker with more than 30 years of experience and trained in thematic coding). Disagreements in coding were discussed until agreement was reached. The software ATLAS.ti was used to assist in the analyses of the coded transcripts and to permit some quantitative analyses of qualitative data.

### 15.3.4   Recruitment

Recruitment for the overall project proceeded when the treating psychiatrist, psychologist or social worker approached the patient about study participation. If the patient agreed to participate, a project research interviewer contacted him/her, introduced the study and extended a formal invitation to the individual to participate. No one who was incapable of giving informed consent was referred by the health care provider to project interviewers. Participants were given a small monetary compensation at the completion of the interview [28,29].

### 15.3.5   Statistical analyses

Data were analysed in the software package SPSS 14.0 [30] using basic descriptive statistics and linear regression models. Statistical significance at $P < 0.05$ or higher is indicated where appropriate.

## 15.4   Human subjects protections

The project has Institutional Review Board approval at the New York State Psychiatric Institute, Bronx Psychiatric Center, Creedmoor Psychiatric Center, Bronx-Lebanon Medical Center and the New York State Office of Mental Health. Further, all participants are covered by a Certificate of Confidentiality issued by the Federal Government Services that allowed us to treat the information obtained as privileged in any legal proceeding.

## 15.5  Results

### 15.5.1  *Perceived coercion in AOT and OPT*

We compared AOT and OPT respondent means on the Perceived Coercion Scale using two methods of calculating scores for that scale. The first method, 'non-weighted', recoded the items for a high score to represent high perceived coercion and took the mean with values for, at least, three of the five scale items. The second method, 'weighted', used a 'true–false' fixed response, recoding 'strongly disagree/disagree' responses as 0 and 'agree/strongly agree' responses as 1, and weighting the characteristics of coercion according to the salience of each item to the concept of coercion as identified by Gardner and colleagues [10]. As Figure 15.1 shows, there are no statistically significant differences in the means for AOT versus OPT for either the weighted or non-weighted calculation of the Perceived Coercion Scale. In the remaining analyses reported on here, we use the un-weighted calculation of the MacArthur measure of perceived coercion and refer to it as the Perceived Coercion Scale (PCS).

Using this scale we observe non-significantly higher perception of coercion in the AOT group (mean = 1.44) as compared with the OPT (mean = 1.33). These results differ from other comparisons of perceived coercion in groups that differ in objective coercion such as at hospital admission [15,31], in mental health courts [32], and in outpatient commitment [32,33]. In each of these instances there is a significant difference in perceived coercion between the objectively coerced group and the

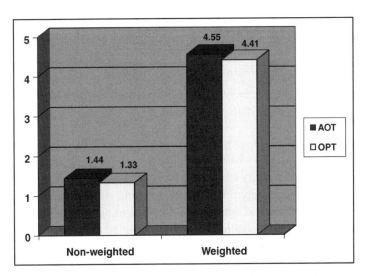

**Figure 15.1**  Comparison of AOT and OPT mean scores using two calculations of perceived coercion.

comparison group, while in the current study there is no significant difference between the groups.

### 15.5.2   Perceived coercion and AOT dose

Finding that the two groups of consumers perceived themselves as being relatively equally coerced led us to a number of further questions. Perhaps, persons with different levels of access to case management services might experience coercion differently, a discrimination obscured by the dichotomous grouping of subjects into either AOT or OPT. To examine this possibility, we compared Perceived Coercion Scale means for persons who had no case manager, persons with a case manager but no court order, and persons on court order for three months or less, with persons who had more than three months on an AOT court order. We found that those groups of individuals exposed to AOT for longer periods of time had slightly higher means on the Perceived Coercion Scale (no OPT with no case manager, mean = 1.31 ($n = 44$); OPT with case manager, mean = 1.34 ($n = 64$); AOT court order 90 days or less, mean = 1.41 ($n = 26$); AOT court order more than 90 days, mean = 1.46 ($n = 49$)). However, there were no significant differences in the means across the groups.

Further, when we compared PCS scores for persons on AOT with those not on AOT in multiple regression analyses (not shown), controlled for age at baseline, sex, race, marital status and education, the association between AOT status and perceived coercion remained non-significant.

One potential explanation for the lack of a difference between committed and not committed groups on perceived coercion could be measurement problems associated with our use of the PCS. As a result, we assess whether the PCS performs reliably and shows evidence for validity in this New York sample of people with serious mental illness. The internal consistency reliability of the PCS assessed via Cronbach's Alpha is 0.86, which reveals a high level of reliability, suggesting that the unreliability of the measure is probably not the source of the no-difference finding.

To assess construct validity, we determined whether the PCS scale correlated in this context as predicted with measures of other constructs. Again, using the concerns of consumer and human rights advocates, we expected that perception of coercion would significantly, negatively influence the working alliance between the person and the case manager. On the other hand, the competing hypothesis suggested by family members and mental health care professionals led us to expect that indicators of illness severity (lack of insight, number of prior hospitalizations and delusions of harm) should be strongly associated with higher perception of coercion. We recognize that additional factors that may have a bearing on perceived coercion, for example the stigma of mental illness and of the court order itself, may contribute to a

**Table 15.3**  Construct validity of the perceived coercion scale

|  | Perceived coercion Pearson Correlation |
|---|---|
| AOT ($N = 183$) | 0.086 |
| Working Alliance Inventory ($N = 133$) | −0.339** |
| Insight ($N = 181$) | −0.236** |
| Harm Delusions ($N = 183$) | 0.126+ |
| Prior Involuntary Hospitalizations ($N = 179$) | 0.331** |
| Stigma Devaluation-Discrimination Scale ($N = 178$) | 0.260** |
| Stigma: AOT Scale ($N = 71$) | 0.378** |
| Quality of Life ($N = 182$) | −0.223** |

$^{+}P < 0.1$; $^{*}P < 0.05$; $^{**}P < 0.01$; $^{***}P < 0.001$.

person's feeling more coerced. A positive consequence of mandated treatment may be an improvement in the individual's quality of life. Thus, we test, as well, the association of stigma and quality of life with perceived coercion.

We found:

- The event of a court order to AOT was not significantly correlated with high perceived coercion (Pearson Correlation Coefficient = 0.087; see Table 15.3)
- Coercion negatively affects the patient's relationship with the case manager.
- Perception of coercion is associated with markers of illness severity (low insight, number of prior hospitalizations and delusions of harm) and feelings of being stigmatized.
- The higher a person's perception of coercion, the lower the self-reported quality of life.
- We also examined and found no significant correlation of our measure of perceived coercion with the key demographic variables of age, sex, race/ethnicity, years of education and marital status (see Table 15.4).

In sum, the Perceived Coercion Scale, whether constructed using a weighting scheme or a simple mean with at least three of five items present, is reliable and shows evidence for construct validity in the study population.

**Table 15.4**  Comparison of AOT and OPT groups on perceived coercion by sex, age, race, marital status and education

| *Coercion* | AOT/OPT | Sex | Age | Race | Marital | Education |
|---|---|---|---|---|---|---|
| *Correlation coefficient* | 0.087 | 0.045 | −0.026 | 0.038 | 0.021 | −0.014 |
| *Significance* | 0.249 | 0.541 | 0.723 | 0.609 | 0.783 | 0.850 |
| *Ns* | 183 | 183 | 182 | 183 | 182 | 183 |

### 15.5.3    Perceived coercion and the use of leverage in outpatient commitment

Having increased our confidence that the finding of no difference between AOT and OPT groups on perceived coercion was not an artefact of poor measurement spurs us to further consideration of our finding. For example, could it be that some participants did not realize they had been court-ordered into treatment due to the direct effects of the disease process, and thus did not see themselves as coerced? Did the manner in which the judge conducted the AOT hearing or the case manager discussed treatment options effect the patient's feeling of being coerced? Is the use of force in treatment so pervasive that a court order adds nothing noticeable to the individual?

Monahan and colleagues contend that the court order is only one form of leverage used to ensure adherence to treatment [7,34–37]. Included in the battery of measures administered to study respondents were items developed by the MacArthur Violence Risk Network to measure aspects of leverage that might be used with persons with serious mental illness. 'Did you ever live somewhere where you felt you were required to stay in mental health or substance abuse treatment (or take your medication)?' assessed the use of housing as leverage. Other questions evaluated leverage of outpatient commitment and reception of benefits through a representative payee. Of the 75 individuals on AOT asked whether they felt 'required to stay in mental health treatment' to obtain housing, 56% ($n = 42$) of the respondents said they did *not* feel required to stay in mental health treatment as compared with 68.2% ($n = 73$) of the OPT respondents, significant at the $P < 0.064$ level. At the same time, some of the OPT group, 31.8% ($n = 34$), felt obligated to remain in treatment without the presence of a court order. Further, when housing, representative payee and outpatient commitment forms of leverage were summed and a comparison of means performed, there was no significant difference between persons on AOT and OPT in this sample. Nor was there a correlation between cumulative forms of mandated treatment and either court-ordered status or perception of coercion. Either an important dimension of the experience of the court order is not being tapped by the Perceived Coercion Scale, or the scale itself does not touch significant mediating aspects of coercive treatment that negatively affect treatment adherence.

### 15.5.4    Qualitative results: why is there no difference?

What does explain this lack of expected differences? To answer this question, we drew on qualitative interviews, data from participant observation and, at times, survey results, as they proved relevant to the qualitative data. Open-ended interviews were completed with a subsample of 20 men and women in AOT (9) and not in AOT (11) interviewed at the nine-month follow-up interview. All individuals approached agreed to talk about their responses with Dr Castille as part of the follow-up interview. Those discussions were transcribed and the content coded following conventions described by Miles and Huberman [38], Ryan and Bernard [39] and others, and analysed specifically to build an understanding of what does and does not make a person feel coerced. There were no significant differences between the subsample interviewed in-depth about perception of coercion and the remaining un-interviewed sample on any demographic variable. Participant observation data came from the involvement of one of us (Dorothy Castille) in conducting the quantitative study and thereby spending time in the clinical settings. Notes from these observations were recorded and reviewed for relevance to the issue of coercion. For each person quoted, we give their sex, age, group membership and their perceived coercion score as compared with the mean for their group.

We organized our results in the form of findings from our qualitative study concerning key contextual drivers of the experience and perception of coercion. Specifically, we identify three such reasons including: (i) the ubiquity of coercion; (ii) compliance over confrontation; and (iii) a valued services perspective that addresses the availability of an Intensive Case Manager, housing, employment, and the ability to achieve goals. We treat each theme in turn and support our discussion with excerpts from participant narratives.

### 15.5.5 The ubiquity of coercion

Does coercive experience form such a consistent backdrop to life that treatment feels equally coercive to those with and without a court order? A number of explanations for this are possible. All respondents in the study had considerable histories in the mental health system. As previously mentioned, we found number of prior involuntary hospitalizations to be significantly, positively correlated with high perceived coercion ($0.331^{**}$, $P < 0.01$), lending some support to this hypothesis. Additionally, having been brought to the emergency room in handcuffs by law enforcement personnel, having been subjected to restraints and/or seclusion, or having been medicated over objection, comprise significant coercion. Moreover, coercive practices take place on a daily basis throughout a hospitalization where rules narrowly constrain behaviour. The in-hospital treatment regime requires participation in scheduled activities. Certain spaces, such as a person's room, can only be used at certain times and usually under circumstances that are not private. Medication is administered at regular supervised intervals; refusal of medication may be met with court orders to medicate over the patient's objection, and so forth. For example, 'As far as taking my meds, I been taking medication for the longest time, ... they watch you take your meds so I couldn't not take them over there because that would get written up...' (*38-year-old, male, AOT, CO[1]mean = 0.80 vs. AOT CO mean = 1.44*). Coercive practices may extend to residential treatment centres and supervised housing. Thus coercion experienced daily may make the court order one more in the sequence of coercive procedures [40].

### 15.5.6   Compliance over confrontation

For some individuals, the threatening aspect of AOT carries weight in two ways: as a heavy, punitive hand – 'AOT, it's like you go or you're in trouble' or 'it were just threatening if I had missed a day or something like that, they would, um, hospitalize me again' (*30-year-old, male, AOT, CO mean = 1.00 vs. AOT CO mean = 1.44*) – and as a forced choice – 'I agreed to comply. . . They would have kept me. It would have been a big thing. So I just agreed' (*29-year-old, female, AOT, CO mean = 1.80 vs. AOT CO mean = 1.44*). Here, going along with the court order represents the path of least resistance for discharge, knowing when protest is more trouble than it is worth, and 'choosing' compliance over confrontation.

### 15.5.7   A valued services perspective – benevolent manipulation

Upon discharge, coordination of essential services including clinical services and medication management, housing, money and legal advocacy are delivered by different agencies. For example, medication and clinical services may be funded through Medicaid and Medicare; housing, provided and administered through residential services agencies; money, supplied through Supplemental Security Income; and legal advocacy, made available through organizations such as MFY Legal Services [35]. The case manager or an Assertive Community Treatment (ACT) Team, assigned via the mechanism of a court order, coordinate services that may be impossible for the patient to organize and access without that support. In addition to bridging the hospital–community gap and coordinating services located in different places, for some the treatment structure provided for the person on AOT creates a context that reduces some of the complex and confusing pressures experienced by the individual transitioning to community life: '. . .it [AOT] took a weight off of my shoulders' (*38-year-old, male, AOT, CO mean = 0.80 vs. AOT CO mean = 1.44*). Put another way,

R:   Well, AOT is something like, it put you in the right path. They have a lot to offer because if you do what you've been told and you're clean and sober, they would help you find an apartment. They will help you buy furnitures. They make sure that you get your benefits. They make sure you get your medication. . . Make sure that you are, you are responsible for yourself. You have access to have your apartment. And you know, it's pretty helpful. . . It doesn't bother me. (*39-year-old, male, AOT, CO mean = 1.40 vs. AOT CO mean = 1.44*)

The coordination of services (housing, clinical outpatient services and case management services) being offered with AOT is highly valued by consumers. Services mentioned by participants as being particularly important and influential, for example case management and housing, are discussed below along with two areas that may be facilitated by services offered through AOT: employment and attainment of goals.

## Treatment alliance and intensive case management

Intensive case management bridges inpatient and outpatient services, hospital life and life in the community. Case managers see consumers at least once weekly and are responsible for assisting the patient with clinic appointments, the coordination of vital financial support, locating appropriate housing, reviewing and applying for treatment options that provide vocational training, securing a job, and easing the transition from hospital to community. Study respondents cited case managers as one of the important reasons for feeling that the 'program did wonders' for them (*38-year-old, male, AOT, CO mean = 0.80 vs. AOT CO mean = 1.44*). For example, a case manager advocate helps a client to locate specific service and training programmes: 'Some programs, you know, don't live up to their expectations' (*36-year-old, male, AOT, CO mean = 1.20 vs. AOT mean = 1.44*). Help with negotiating the system features prominently in reduced feelings of coercion. Where a case manager can be empathic, able to hear the client's concerns and goals, and facilitate attaining those ends, the individual does perceive the interaction as empowering rather than as coercive [41].

On the other hand, the presence of a case manager who uses coercion or manipulation that is not benevolent to secure compliance with treatment may result in patient anger and frustration and the feeling that the programme is 'too strict'. These emotions may not be reflected in the person's mean score (for example, 1.40 as compared with the AOT group mean of 1.44) on the Perceived Coercion Scale because experiences may not come to mind in association with survey items, but emerge only in recounting events: 'She talk nice to everybody, but when it comes to me, she... give me a hard time... When she talk to my brother, she tell him all my personal business...' (*39-year-old, male, AOT, CO mean = 1.40 vs. AOT CO mean = 1.44*). For this respondent, when the case manager turned to family members to gain greater control over her client, the intervention injured and angered the respondent, making him less likely to comply with treatment and leaving him feeling more coerced. Breaking confidentiality, even in the service of gaining treatment adherence, may destroy rather than enhance compliance. This supports the contention that absence of perceived fairness and apparent lack of procedural justice are important components of the experience of coercion [7]. Criticism of AOT may be expressed in terms of the difficult role of the case manager, but the services represented by being assigned to a case manager are only part of the picture. While the case manager–client match on race, sex and age can contribute to strengthening the bond between case manager and client, empathy and respect between the case manager and client appear to be the key to whether a client feels empowered or coerced.

Special efforts to engage with the patient, provide education about treatment, medication and available resources, and include the patient in treatment planning can improve quality of life, and empower the patient with a sense of choice and control. These forms of more benign coercion can be experienced as helpful and supportive [6], and some of the participants were able to articulate clearly the importance of a trusting relationship with the case manager, despite the coercive practices embedded in a psychiatric hospitalization experience.

*I:* And how did. . . you come to be on AOT?

*R:* Because when I was in. . . Hospital, I think for the second or third time, the doctor there suggested that AOT would be beneficial to me, help me, because I have a violent history and they wanted me to be able to have someone to talk to on the outside, so they took me to court and I agreed to comply, because I was non-compliant with medicine and I wasn't going to my program. . . They would have kept me. It would have been a big thing. So I just agreed. . . and then when I met her [case manager]... She came to visit me in the hospital a couple of times. . . So by the time I agreed to, I agreed to it because me and her already established a good relationship. (*29-year-old, female, AOT, CO mean = 1.80 vs. AOT CO mean = 1.44*)

One outpatient respondent with a case manager but not court-ordered into treatment highlights just how significant the help of a case manager can be: 'Like, right, now I need her more than ever because I'm getting ready to move from here, so she's going to help me find housing and stuff like that' (*18-year-old, male, OPT, CO mean = 1.60 vs. OPT mean = 1.33*).

### Housing

Housing represents a valued resource to participants in this study that can be a source of coercion or an aid to community re-entry. For example, Monahan and colleagues identified outpatient commitment as one of four forms of leverage used to secure an individual's adherence with treatment requirements along with housing, money and criminal justice [35]. In New York State, an AOT order moves the individual to priority consideration for housing. As one young man who did not perceive himself as being coerced put it: '. . . in order for me to go to the B___ [a supervised residence on the hospital campus], they had to put me on AOT. . . that was the only way I could get to B___.' In this case, and that of several other men and women in this study, the court order was the pathway to secure housing, a means to force the system to provide scarce resources. What statistically amounts to multiple forms of leverage may not be perceived as coercive when the patient feels his/her needs are being met – evidence of a more nuanced reality.

## Employment

Employment is a marker of adulthood, a goal toward which men and women strive, and a vehicle for recovery and community reintegration. Work emerged as a frequently mentioned theme in both AOT and OPT interviews. Some study participants cited rigidity of the system set in place through a court order as one reason for feeling coerced by being on AOT. Where the demands of prescribed treatment, attending programmes, receiving medication interfere with the ability to find and keep a job, self-esteem is undermined and the path to recovery obstructed. A 52-year-old male on AOT (*CO mean = 1.20 vs. AOT mean = 1.44*) expressed it this way: 'Well, in a way they teach you how to have motivation, to be responsible, but in another way they don't look at your side, like for example, me, I don't have a lot of clothes so I would like to work to buy me new clothes. But they don't want me to work. That's the bad thing about AOT, you know' (*52-year-old, male, AOT, CO mean = 1.20 vs. AOT CO mean = 1.44*). A 44-year-old, male outpatient also spoke of work and treatment, 'Right now all I need is a job, a possible (*sic*) go to church, and a job, and live a normal life and they don't, they say, "Well, you're taking medication, you're doing much better, don't go too fast, go slow"' (*44-year-old, male, OPT, CO mean = 2.20 vs. OPT CO mean = 1.33*). Work and school form important connections to life in the community and 'normality':

> 'Cause I don't like being inpatient. I like having freedom. I like being free and I'm working towards having my complete freedom and returning back to society and to work. That's why I'm involved in school right now. (*29-year-old, male, AOT, CO mean = 0.80 vs. AOT CO mean = 1.44*)

Work though is a double edged sword, 'I would say that making more than $200 a week would make me lose my medical benefits' (*28-year-old, male, OPT, CO mean = 1.60 vs. OPT CO mean = 1.33*). Consumers both on and not on AOT balance recovery-orientated goals and desires with the reality of securing and maintaining stable housing, working enough to advance recovery but not too much to cause a loss in benefits, and attending treatment to retain the useful and supportive features of the mental health care system.

### Attainment of goals

The final theme emerging from participant narratives was the importance of having and attaining goals. The ability to develop and work toward achieving goals challenges the recipient of treatment for serious mental illness. Side effects of psychotropic medication include such overwhelming fatigue and lethargy that maintaining a future orientation is a difficult though important task.

> There's [sic] a lot of people in here who's not doing well...They just get their medication and come here and go to sleep or go back and go to sleep. They not aiming towards anything. I'm aiming towards getting my own apartment, you know, eventually having kids and things like that. You know, I'm aiming towards the future. . . (18-year-old, male, OPT, CO mean = 1.60 vs. OPT CO mean = 1.33)

## 15.6   Discussion

Validation of the Perceived Coercion Scale in a New York sample of persons with serious mental illness, court-ordered and non-court-ordered to remain in outpatient treatment is the primary goal of this study. We find that the Perceived Coercion Scale is a psychometrically sound instrument with high internal consistency reliability, and some evidence of construct validity. We expected to find the Perceived Coercion Scale to be significantly associated with the event of the court order, because the authoritative and official force exerted a strong impression on the patient through appearing before a judge and receiving an order from the court to remain in treatment following discharge from the hospital. We found that the scale is significantly associated with poor alliance with the case manager at baseline, poor insight into illness, poor quality of life, and endorsement of more psychotic symptoms, as predicted. It is also significantly associated with a history of a higher number of prior involuntary hospitalizations. These findings lend some support to conflicting hypotheses about the positive and negative role of the use of force in psychiatric treatment. However, in this sample, the Perceived Coercion Scale does not differentiate statistically between persons court-ordered into outpatient treatment and those not court-ordered, failing to replicate findings of other coercion researchers [14–17,42–44]. Interpretation of these complex and somewhat conflicting findings led us to use qualitative methods to deepen our understanding of the concept and process of coercion in the experiences of the men and women in the study.

Qualitative interviews with men and women court-ordered into outpatient treatment and not court-ordered suggested that perception of coercion is highly context dependent. While perceived coercion may be easily measured by a survey instrument, the experience may be more nuanced, and statistical results may not be easily interpreted. For example, the decision to accept or comply with a court order may be a 'forced choice' – agree and be discharged from the hospital or resist and remain hospitalized or, worse yet, overtly forced to comply. For the individual aware of personal needs and available options, a court order may be part of a strategy to obtain scarce and highly desirable services such as a case manager and housing, thus may not be experienced as coercive. Many people with serious and persistent mental illness have no permanent housing, in part due to their inability to manage their lives – including a job, money and relationships. The availability of supervised housing is limited, and applicants are subject to acceptance by residential providers. AOT recipients gain priority consideration for housing, a condition for hospital discharge. A court order shortens the wait for an available slot once the person has been accepted. From this perspective, the law encumbers the system to provide services to recipients. So there is potential in the system itself to assist the person needing services, changing the leverage implicit in the use of outpatient commitment and housing to secure treatment adherence into focused problem solving [35].

Case management services and the manner in which they are delivered, more than the court order, seem to influence perception of coercion. The degree of fit between the case manager and the person receiving services is very important. Specific qualities such as the ability to hear the needs of the patient and to help to meet those needs, to use personal commonalities of sex, age and race to establish or strengthen an alliance with the client, and to use persuasion, can transform a potentially demeaning and stigmatizing relationship into one of support and empowerment [41]. Broken trust between case manager and client leads the client to feelings of anger, frustration and disgust with both the case manager and the mental health system.

A culture of coercion, as has long existed in the lives of persons treated for serious mental illness, means that events, attitudes and behaviours, ways of being treated by others, comprise so much of the unspoken texture of life that it is only noticeable in contrast to a culture where coercion is not as pervasive. Men and women with numerous prior psychiatric hospitalizations, including involuntary commitment, became part of that culture long ago, starting with their early treatment, and, by the time of our study, had experienced so much coercion that it had become difficult to differentiate all coercive events in the surrounding social environment. Freedom, for them, is constructed only within the context of a culture of coercion.

Recognizing the limited good that coercive treatment practices impart, interventions can be designed to diminish the need to use coercion. In our qualitative interviews, the consumers for whom outpatient commitment appeared to work the best were those who received services from people who treated them as equal and important, deserving of respect, and as a valued member of the community; that is, where the power employed was persuasive [6] and decisions were made collaboratively.

### 15.6.1 Limitations

The findings reported on here are limited by size of the overall study sample and the sampling methods necessitated by the inability to randomly assign people to different standards of care. Outpatient and Assisted Outpatient Treatment project participants differed little on any of the demographic characteristics collected, and the demographic characteristics of the qualitative subsample do not differ from those of the larger sample. Neither do the sample characteristics reported on here differ significantly from data collected by the New York State Office of Mental Health at the state level, on a much larger group of consumers court-ordered into treatment.

## 15.7 Conclusion

The experience of coercion is more than can be measured by either a point or isolated coercive incident or through a measure using survey-type items. Coercion, rather, refers to a process that is sometimes de-emphasized in the individual's narrative about their experience, sometimes recognized for what it is, and sometimes alienates the coerced individual from other influences in their environment. The scope of the long-debated value of coercive treatment must be re-examined with a broader view of individual history and context included in the formulation. Moreover, ready access to high-quality treatment services is recognized and valued highly by consumers, suggesting that treatment emphasis be targeted toward more and better services for all consumers. This study identifies coercive treatment as a point ripe for intervention and rethinking.

## Acknowledgements

This research was funded by a contract from the New York State Office of Mental Health, Bureau of Adult Services Evaluation Research, the Center for Information Technology and Evaluation Research, Albany, New York and by support from the MacArthur Violence Research Network. We gratefully acknowledge the contribution of the men and women who responded to our interview protocols, the staff at outpatient clinics in the Bronx and Queens who facilitated all aspects of data collection, and contributions from Steve Huz, Susan Shilling, Marian Schweger, Lori Hopner, Marian Reiff, Rosalind Prince and members of the Services Research Group at New York State Psychiatric Institute. The views expressed here are ours alone.

## References

1. Good, B.J., Good, M.-J.D. and Moradi, R. (1985) The interpretation of Iranian depressive illness and dysphoric affect, in *Culture and Depression: Studies in the Anthropology and Cross-Cultural Psychiatry of Affect and Disorder* (eds A. Kleinman and B. Good), University of California Press, Berkeley, CA, pp. 369–428.

2. Torrey, E.F. and Zdanowicz, M. (2001) Outpatient commitment: what, why, and for whom. *Psychiatric Services*, **52**, 337–341.
3. Amador, X. (2000) *I Am Not Sick I Don't Need Help*, Vida Press, Peconic, NY.
4. Pollack, D.A. (2004) *Moving from Coercion to Collaboration in Mental Health Services*. DHHS Publication No. (SMA) 04-3869, Center for Mental Health Services, Rockville, MD.
5. Rosenberg, M. and Pearlin, L. (1962) Power-orientations in the mental hospital. *Human Relations*, **15**, 335–349.
6. Lovell, A.M. (1996) Coercion and social control: a framework for research on aggressive strategies in community mental health, in *Coercion and Aggressive Community Treatment: A New Frontier in Mental Health Law* (eds D.L. Dennis and J. Monahan), Plenum Press, New York, pp. 148–166.
7. Monahan, F.J., Bonnie, R.J., Appelbaum, P.S. *et al.* (2001) Mandated community treatment: beyond outpatient commitment. *Psychiatric Services*, **52**, 1198–1205.
8. Hoge, S.K., Lidz, C.W., Eisenberg, M. *et al.* (1997) Perceptions of coercion in the admission of voluntary and involuntary psychiatric patients. *International Journal of Law and Psychiatry*, **20**, 167–181.
9. Hoge, S.K., Lidz, C.W., Eisenberg, M. *et al.* (1998) Family, clinician, and patient perceptions of coercion in mental hospital admission: a comparative study. *International Journal of Law and Psychiatry*, **21**, 131–146.
10. Gardner, W., Hoge, S.K., Bennett, N. *et al.* (1993) Two scales for measuring patients' perceptions for coercion during mental hospital admission. *Behavioral Sciences and the Law*, **11**, 307–321.
11. McKenna, B.G., Simpson, A.I. and Coverdale, J.H. (2006) Outpatient commitment and coercion in New Zealand: a matched comparison study. *International Journal of Law and Psychiatry*, **29**, 145–158.
12. Lidz, C.W., Hoge, S.K., Gardner, W. *et al.* (1995) Perceived coercion in mental hospital admission: pressures and process. *Archives of General Psychiatry*, **52**, 1034–1039.
13. Lidz, C.W., Hoge, S.K. and Monahan, J. (1997) Perception of coercion: a pilot study using the Swedish version of the Admission Experience Scale: Comment. *Nordic Journal of Psychiatry*, **51**, 214.
14. Rain, S.D., Williams, V.F., Robbins, P.C. *et al.* (2003) Perceived coercion at hospital admission and adherence to mental health treatment after discharge. *Psychiatric Services*, **54**, 103–105.
15. Hiday, V.A., Swartz, M.S., Swanson, J. and Wagner, H. (1997) Patient perceptions of coercion in mental hospital admission. *International Journal of Law and Psychiatry*, **20**, 227–241.
16. Rain, S.D., Steadman, H.J. and Robbins, P.C. (2003) Perceived coercion and treatment adherence in an outpatient commitment program. *Psychiatric Services*, **54**, 399–401.
17. Monahan, J., Hoge, S.K., Lidz, C. *et al.* (1995) Coercion and commitment: understanding involuntary mental hospital admission. *International Journal of Law and Psychiatry*, **18**, 249–263.
18. Hiday, V.A. (1996) Outpatient commitment: official coercion in the community, in *Coercion and Aggressive Community Treatment: A New Frontier in Mental Health Law* (eds D.L. Dennis and J. Monahan), Plenum Press, New York, pp. 29–47.
19. Hiday, V.A. (1992) Coercion in civil commitment: process, preferences, and outcome. *International Journal of Law and Psychiatry*, **15**, 359–377.
20. New York State Office of Mental Health (2006) An Explanation of Kendra's Law. www.omh. state.ny.us/omhweb/kendra_web/ksummary.htm (accessed 12 December 2010).

21. Monahan, J., Appelbaum, P.S., Mulvey, E.P. *et al.* (1993) Ethical and legal duties in conducting research on violence: lessons from the MacArthur Risk Assessment Study. *Violence and Victims*, **8**, 387–396.
22. Link, B.G., Cullen, F.T., Frank, J. and Wozniak, J.F. (1987) The social rejection of former mental patients: understanding why labels matter. *American Journal of Sociology*, **92**, 1461–1500.
23. Lehman, A.F. (1988) A quality of life interview for the chronically mentally ill. *Evaluation and Program Planning*, **11**, 51–62.
24. Horvath, A.O. and Greenberg, L.S. (1989) Development and validation of the Working Alliance Inventory. *Journal of Counseling Psychology*, **36**, 223–233.
25. McEvoy, J.P., Aland, J., Jr, Wilson, W.H. *et al.* (1981) Measuring chronic schizophrenic patients attitudes toward their illness and treatment. *Hospital & Community Psychiatry*, **32** (12), 856–858.
26. Weiden, P., Rapkin, B., Mott, T. *et al.* (1994) Rating of Medication Influences (ROMI) in schizophrenia. *Schizophrenia Bulletin*, **21**, 419–429.
27. Link, B.G., Monahan, J., Stueve, A. and Cullen, F.T. (1999) Real in their consequences: a sociological approach to understanding the association between psychotic symptoms and violence. *American Sociological Review*, **64**, 316–332.
28. Link, B., Castille, D.M. and Stuber, J. (2008) Stigma and coercion in the context of outpatient treatment for people with mental illnesses. *Social Science & Medicine*, **67**, 409–419.
29. Phelan, J.C., Sinkewicz, M., Castille, D.M. *et al.* (2010) Effectiveness and outcomes of assisted outpatient treatment in New York state. *Psychiatric Services*, **61**, 137–143.
30. SPSS Inc. (2001) *SPSS for 14.0 for Windows*, SPSS Inc., Chicago.
31. Hoge, S.K., Bonnie, R.J., Poythress, N. *et al.* (1997) The MacArthur adjudicative competence study: development and validation of a research instrument. *Law and Human Behavior*, **21**, 141–179.
32. Poythress, N.G., Bonnie, R.J., Monahan, J., *et al.* (2002) *Adjudicative Competence: The MacArthur Studies*, Kluwer Academic/Plenum Publishers, New York, NY.
33. Swartz, M., Swanson, J., Hiday, V. *et al.* (2001) A randomized controlled trial of outpatient commitment in North Carolina. *Psychiatric Services*, **52**, 325–329.
34. Robbins, P.C., Petrila, J., LeMelle, S. and Monahan, J. (2006) The use of housing as leverage to increase adherence to psychiatric treatment in the community. *Administration and Policy in Mental Health and Mental Health Services Research*, **33**, 226–236.
35. Monahan, J., Redlich, A.D., Swanson, J. *et al.* (2005) Use of leverage to improve adherence to psychiatric treatment in the community. *Psychiatric Services*, **56**, 37–44.
36. Swartz, M.S., Swanson, J.W., Kim, M. and Petrila, J. (2006) Use of outpatient commitment or related civil court treatment orders in five U.S. communities. *Psychiatric Services*, **57**, 343–349.
37. Van Dorn, R.A., Swartz, M., Elbogen, E.B. and Swanson, J.W. (2005) Perceived fairness and effectiveness of leveraged community treatment among public mental health consumers in five U.S. cities. *International Journal of Forensic Mental Health*, **4**, 119–133.
38. Miles, M.B. and Huberman, M. (1994) *Qualitative Data Analysis: An Expanded Sourcebook*, 2nd edn, Sage Publications, Thousand Oaks, CA.
39. Ryan, G.W. and Bernard, H.R. (2000) Data management and analysis methods, in *Handbook of Qualitative Methods*, 2nd edn (eds N.K. Denzin and Y.S. Lincoln), Sage Publications, Thousand Oaks, CA, pp. 769–802.
40. Steadman, H.J. and Redlich, A.D. (2006) A scale to measure perceived coercion in everyday life: a concept to inform research on the legal issues of coerced treatment. *International Journal of Forensic Mental Health*, **5** (2), 167–171.

41. Bachelor, A. and Salame, R. (2000) Participants' perceptions of dimensions of the therapeutic alliance over the course of therapy. *Journal of Psychotherapy Practice & Research*, **9**, 39–53.

42. Lidz, C., Mulvey, E., Hoge, S.K. *et al.* (1998) Factual sources of psychiatric patients' perceptions of coercion in the hospital admission process. *American Journal of Psychiatry*, **155**, 1254–1260.

43. Elbogen, E.B., Swanson, J.W. and Swartz, M. (2003) Effects of legal mechanisms on perceived coercion and treatment adherence among persons with severe mental illness. *The Journal of Nervous and Mental Disease*, **191**, 629–637.

44. Monahan, J., Hoge, S.K., Lidz, C. *et al.* (1995) Coercion and commitment: understanding involuntary mental hospital admission. *International Journal of Law and Psychiatry*, **18**, 249–263.

# Endnote

[1] CO is the coercion measure, designating the mean of the respondent as compared with the mean for the group.

# Section 5

## Coercion and undue influence in decisions to participate in psychiatric research

# 16 Ethical issues of participating in psychiatric research on coercion

## Lars Kjellin

*Örebro University, School of Health and Medical Sciences, Psychiatric Research Centre, Örebro, Sweden*

Even though psychiatric empirical research has evolved in recent years, further research efforts are needed to achieve increased knowledge regarding mental illnesses, the suffering of individuals affected by mental illnesses, and the effects of individual and system-level interventions to reduce suffering. At the same time there has been an evolution in the field of psychiatric research ethics, influenced by efforts from professional associations, medical ethicists, legislators, service users and others.

The use of coercion in mental health care services is a field of controversy in the professional as well as the public debate. Mental health care law reforms regarding involuntary hospitalization and treatment, compulsory outpatient care, and advance directives have been implemented in many countries recently. Psychiatric research on coercion has expanded during the last decades, but the knowledge of the use and effects of coercive interventions is still insufficient, and further research is greatly needed. This need is emphasized by the fact that coercive interventions have a potential for doing harm. In Scandinavian studies, a majority of involuntarily admitted patients reported being subjected to integrity violations [1] and

*Coercive Treatment in Psychiatry: Clinical, Legal and Ethical Aspects*, First Edition.
Edited by Thomas W. Kallert, Juan E. Mezzich and John Monahan.
© 2011 John Wiley & Sons, Ltd. Published 2011 by John Wiley & Sons, Ltd.

feeling humiliated [2]. An expansion of psychiatric research on coercion, however, highlights the need to properly address the ethical issues of psychiatric research in general and research on coercion in particular.

Much has been written about general medical research ethics and about ethics in psychiatric research, but less about the specific ethical issues of research on the use of coercion in mental health services. The question of whether people suffering from mental illnesses have the capacity to make an informed decision, for example, is a different issue from whether involuntarily hospitalized psychiatric patients are able to make a free choice to participate in research [3].

To put the ethical issues of psychiatric research on coercion into context, this chapter will start by briefly going through some important international declarations on ethics of medical research in general and some aspects of general psychiatric research ethics. After that, issues of research on the use of coercion in psychiatry and ethical aspects of such research will be dealt with. Experiences from a large European multi-centre study and a Nordic study of coercion in psychiatry will be described, and specific issues of randomized controlled trials and some particularly vulnerable research populations will be discussed. Some related cultural aspects and further research efforts will be commented on, and finally some short concluding remarks will be presented.

## 16.1    International codes of medical research ethics in general

### 16.1.1    The Nuremberg Code

The first international code of ethics for research with human beings is the Nuremberg Code [4]. It was drawn up after 'the Doctors' Trial' in 1946, one of the Nuremberg Trials where former Nazi leaders were convicted as war criminals. Mentally ill persons were principal victims of the criminal Nazi research programmes, where psychiatrists played a central role [5]. Before the Second World War there was little systematic international attention to the ethical dimensions of psychiatric research. The Nuremberg Trials showed the need for explicit safeguards for research subjects, and the aim of the Nuremberg Code was to prevent any repeat of the medical crimes committed in Nazi Germany.

The Nuremberg Code emphasizes in its first standard that voluntary consent of the human research subject is essential and that the person should have legal capacity to give consent, be able to exercise free power of choice without any kind of constraint or coercion, and have sufficient knowledge and comprehension to be able to make a rational decision. To what degree persons receiving psychiatric treatment for different mental illnesses have decisional capacity for such decisions is a crucial question for psychiatric research ethics.

### 16.1.2    The Declaration of Helsinki

The basic requirement of the Nuremberg Code – informed consent – has been accepted worldwide, but still the Nuremberg Code showed to be insufficient to protect research subjects. Unethical research was reported from the area of physical medicine [6], and institutional abuse of psychiatry has taken place not only in countries with totalitarian regimes, but also in democratic countries [5]. The need for further protection of human research subjects was reflected in the World Medical Association (WMA) Declaration of Helsinki [7], a general statement of ethical principles for medical research involving human subjects adopted in 1964. The declaration has been amended several times, the latest by the WMA General Assembly in Seoul in 2008.

According to the Declaration of Helsinki, 'no competent individual may be enrolled in a research study unless he or she freely agrees' (Principle 22). Unlike the Nuremberg Code, however, the Declaration of Helsinki includes statements about research on persons who are regarded as incompetent to give an informed consent. A legally authorized representative may be asked for consent, if '. . . the research cannot instead be performed with competent persons, and the research entails only minimal risk and minimal burden' (Principle 27). If the person later on regains decisional capacity, he or she then should be asked for assent, and a refusal to participate should be respected (Principle 28).

### 16.1.3    CIOMS

The Council for International Organizations of Medical Sciences (CIOMS) is an international nongovernmental organization connected to the World Health Organization (WHO). CIOMS has worked on biomedical research ethics since the 1970s, and updated in 2002 its International Ethical Guidelines for Biomedical Research Involving Human Subjects [8]. Guideline 9 deals with research involving individuals who are not capable of giving informed consent. The risk of research interventions should not be more likely or greater than the risk of routine medical and psychological examination of such persons, but 'slight or minor increases above such risk may be permitted when there is an overriding scientific or medical rationale for such increases and when an ethical review committee has approved them.' If the persons involved in such research later on become capable of making independent decisions, they should be asked for informed consent to continued participation.

## 16.2    Some aspects of psychiatric research ethics

### 16.2.1    WPA work on ethics

Initiated by the disclosure of political abuse of psychiatry in the former Soviet Union, the World Psychiatric Association (WPA) in 1977 adopted the declaration of Hawaii, updated in Vienna in 1983 [9]. The declaration prohibits the use of psychiatry for political purposes in diagnosing, classification and treatment. Unless psychiatric illness has been established, professional psychiatric methods must under no circumstances be used. Patients' participation in psychiatric research must be voluntary and based on informed consent, and the balance between calculated risks and benefits of the research must be reasonable.

Further concerns for professional ethics in relation to changing attitudes and medical development resulted in the WPA Declaration of Madrid [9], adopted in 1996 and last amended in 2005. The declaration addresses the specific ethical demands of psychiatry and states that, in spite of cultural and social differences over the world, there is a need for universal ethical standards. The seventh guideline of the Declaration of Madrid is about research ethics. Research should be approved by recognized research ethics committees, national and international research rules should be followed, and researchers should be properly trained. Since psychiatric patients are particularly vulnerable, the declaration stresses the need to assess their competence to participate and to protect their autonomy and integrity. In an additional guideline, genetic research on mental disorders is addressed.

### 16.2.2   Informed consent and decisional capacity

All international codes of research ethics include informed consent as a basic requirement for research involving human subjects. Persons asked to participate in research must be informed about the nature of the study, its aims, risks, advantages, alternatives, confidentiality and any other condition of relevance for an informed decision, and they should know that participation is voluntary. To be able to make a rational decision based on this information, the person needs to have a decisional capacity, that is capacity to make and express a choice, understand the information, evaluate the situation and possible consequences, and handle information rationally [10,11]. Laura Weiss Roberts [3] describes a third element of informed consent, voluntarism, encompassing 'ability to act in accordance with one's authentic sense of what is good, right, and best in light of one's situation, values, and prior history. Voluntarism involves the capacity to make this choice freely and in the absence of coercion.'

Information about research procedures has to be formulated carefully, and decisional capacity is a complicated issue, especially in clinical research. In a study of a general population sample, 25% did not know the meaning of the word 'placebo', 83% could not define 'double blind', and 78% did not understand the meaning of 'randomly' [12]. Furthermore, even if the basic concepts are understood, subjects asked for informed consent may not realize that research sometimes conflicts with best possible treatment for the individual. Treatment is performed in the interest of the individual patient, the aim of treatment is individual improvement, and treatment measures are individual. On the other hand, research is conducted in the interest of future patients, the aim is to gain knowledge that can be generalized, and the research methods are standardized. The so-called therapeutic misconception occurs when a research participant fails to appreciate this distinction between clinical research and ordinary treatment [13]. In an interview study of 155 participants in 40 clinical trials, 24% reported no risks or disadvantages of trial participation, and only 14% reported any risks or disadvantages of the research design itself. The authors conclude: 'It appears that subjects often sign consents to participate in clinical trials with only the modest appreciation of the risks and disadvantages of participation' [14].

### 16.2.3   Mental illness and decisional capacity

Regardless of the therapeutic misconception, much has been written about mental illness and decisional capacity for informed consent and will just briefly be discussed here. The MacArthur Competence Assessment Tool – Clinical Research, MacCAT-CR, has been developed for assessing competence to consent to research [15,16], and has been used by several researchers. For example, William Carpenter *et al.* [17] found that patients with schizophrenia performed poorer on the MacCAT-CR than a healthy comparison group. However, most subjects increased their capacity through an educational informed-consent process, suggesting that a single brief research study presentation may not be sufficient. In an interview study of patients diagnosed with schizophrenia, at least a subgroup showed abilities to decide whether to participate in research or not [18]. In another study it was found that patients with diabetes mellitus performed better on the capacity instruments than patients with schizophrenia, who in turn performed better than patients with Alzheimer disease [19]. Persons with psychiatric diagnoses other than schizophrenia have been studied too. In a study of women with major depression, almost all scored adequately on the MacCAT-CR and maintained this level of performance over time [20].

   Most studies are based on small samples, but the main conclusion relevant for this chapter is that many individuals with mental illnesses have full or partial capacity to consent or not to consent to research. The important point when assessing decisional capacity to provide informed consent is not whether there is a psychiatric diagnosis or not, but whether the patient has the mental abilities to make an informed decision. However, people who, because of mental disorders, are judged to be incapable of giving adequately informed consent should not be deprived of the possible benefits of research. In these cases, researchers may resort to proxy decision-making.

### 16.2.4   Research on individuals not capable of giving informed consent

As mentioned above, the Declaration of Helsinki [7] states that a legally authorized representative of the research subject may be asked for consent, on condition that the research cannot be conducted with competent persons and there are only minimal risks and burdens of participation. If the person later is regarded to have gained decisional capacity, he or she should be asked for informed consent. Furthermore, the research must be intended to promote the health of the population that the potential research subject represents, and the condition preventing capacity for informed consent should be a necessary characteristic of the research population.

Also, CIOMS [8], Guideline 15, deals with research involving individuals who by reason of mental disorders are incapable of giving informed consent. Such research should not be carried out if it equally well could be done on persons with decisional capacity. The consent of such persons should be sought to the extent that their mental state permits. A refusal to participate should be respected, unless in exceptional cases there is no reasonable medical alternative and the refusal can be set aside according to local law. When potential research subjects lack capacity to consent, permission from a responsible family member or a legally authorized representative should be sought. It should be recognized, however, that family proxies might have interests of their own, not primarily concerned with the rights and welfare of the patients.

Thus, international codes of research ethics do not, under certain conditions, prohibit research on individuals who due to mental disorders are regarded as incapable of giving an adequate informed consent. Amongst individuals who are subject to the use of coercion in mental health services, there may be both persons who are, and persons who are not, regarded to have decisional capacity for giving an informed consent to research.

## 16.3    Research on the use of coercion in mental health services

Coercion is used in mental health care worldwide. Given the serious nature of deprivation of a person's liberty for the purpose of giving psychiatric treatment, and the controversies coercive measures in psychiatry have generated in professional and public debates, an extensive research on involuntary psychiatric care could be expected. The international research literature on coercion in psychiatry is relatively sparse, however, even though there has been a remarkably growing research interest in this field during the last decades.

One of the basic assumptions underlying the use of coercion in psychiatry is that coercion in specific situations will lead to a better outcome than if the patients were not coerced into treatment. In a paper published in 1998, Charles W. Lidz phrased the following crucial question: 'Is it advisable for society to have a policy in which an individual can be forced to receive mental health treatment? (and then, of course, under what circumstances, what types of treatment, for how long, etc.).' He concluded that there was no clear evidence that the personal or social burdens of mental illness are reduced by the use of coercive treatment, neither was there any evidence that voluntary treatment is more effective than coercive [21]. Ten years later, Georg Høyer stated that we still have insufficient knowledge about the use of involuntary hospitalization, and that we lack evidence on how coercive interventions in psychiatry influence outcome [22]. In a review of 18 outcome studies it was found that most involuntarily admitted patients show substantial clinical improvement, and that retrospectively between 33 and 81% found the admission as justified and/or the treatment as beneficial. The authors concluded that it is not possible to determine whether the differences in results reflect true differences or different methodologies, and that data on predictors of outcomes is limited [23]. Thomas Kallert *et al.* reviewed the literature on the outcome of acute involuntary and voluntary psychiatric hospitalization of adults in general psychiatry, and found differentiated results on a range of outcome domains. They considered the methodological level to be generally low, and a huge variety of methodological aspects was found in the studies. They concluded that there still is a need to perform methodologically sound studies in clinical settings [24].

One explanation of this lack of knowledge could be the problem of designing studies of high scientific quality in this field of research. Random admission or discharge of patients fulfilling the legal criteria for compulsory psychiatric care raises serious ethical questions and could probably not be approved by a research ethics committee, and might also imply that researchers waive the legal statutes for compulsory psychiatric care [25]. Still, occasional randomized controlled trials of involuntary outpatient commitment have been performed [26,27], which will be discussed below.

## 16.4 Some general aspects of ethics and psychiatric research on coercion

The literature on ethics in psychiatric research is extensive, but not so much has been written about the specific issues of research on the use of coercion in mental health services. Ethical problems of psychiatric research in general may be even more challenging in research on coercion, and additional ethical questions may be raised when the research subject is undergoing psychiatric treatment against his or her own will. The general ethical issue of competence to consent to research amongst persons with mental illnesses is of course highly valid in research including patients in compulsory psychiatric care. In national mental health laws, psychotic conditions or other serious mental disorders are common basic legal criteria for involuntary admissions in psychiatric care. As noted above, this does not imply that involuntarily admitted patients in psychiatry by definition lack decision-making capacity. However, at least at the time of admission, all involuntary patients are presupposed to suffer from serious states of mental illnesses, and the more serious nature of the mental disorder, the higher the probability that the person is in part or fully incapable of giving an informed consent to participate in research.

An additional important aspect in this context is the concept of voluntarism [3], which requires that the individual can make a free choice without coercion. Issues of coercion and undue influence in decisions to participate in psychiatric research are elaborated in chapter 17 of this volume.

The risk of harm caused by lack of decisional capacity and undue influence to participate in research must be balanced against the need for further research in specific fields and the importance of giving all patient groups possibilities to participate in research and to gain from the development of evidence-based clinical practices. As mentioned above, we have insufficient knowledge about many aspects of the use of compulsory psychiatric care and, above all, we lack evidence on the outcome of coercive interventions in mental health services. Given the serious nature of such interventions, including deprivation of liberty and violation of individual autonomy, and the worldwide practice of coercion in psychiatry, it could be considered unethical not to perform scientifically sound studies on the use of coercion and its outcomes.

Support to include involuntarily admitted psychiatric patients in research is found in the Declaration of Helsinki [7]. It states that populations, underrepresented in medical research, should be given appropriate access to research participation. However, those who cannot give an informed consent and those who are subjected to coercion or undue influence are, according to the Declaration, particularly vulnerable and need special protection. Research on disadvantaged and vulnerable populations can be justified only if it is in the interest of these populations and it is likely that they will benefit from the results.

The concept 'vulnerable populations' is applicable to many psychiatric patients in general and to involuntarily admitted psychiatric patients in particular. Principle 26 of the Declaration of Helsinki states:

> When seeking informed consent for participation in a research study the physician should be particularly cautious if the potential subject is in a dependent relationship with the physician or may consent under duress. In such situations the informed consent should be sought by an appropriately qualified individual who is completely independent of this relationship.

As noted above, for a potential incompetent research subject, consent should be sought from a legally authorized representative.

To my view, however, proxy decision-making regarding participation in research should generally be avoided for research subjects who are involuntarily admitted to psychiatric care. If incompetent persons, already coerced to treatment, are to be included in research, it would be particularly important to clarify the ethical considerations. There is a risk for harm when these persons, when regaining competence, understand that someone else has consented to participation on their behalf.

After these general remarks I will now present two international studies on coercion in psychiatry and some ethical considerations in these studies.

## 16.5 The EUNOMIA study

A major international research initiative in order to gain increased knowledge regarding the use and outcome of coercive measures is EUNOMIA (European Evaluation of Coercion in Psychiatry and Harmonisation of Best Clinical Practise), a multi-centre prospective study conducted in 12 countries (Bulgaria, Czech Republic, Germany, Greece, Israel, Italy, Lithuania, Poland, Slovakia, Spain, Sweden and the United Kingdom) [28]. Between one and five hospitals were included in each country. Coercive psychiatric treatment measures studied were: forced admission to a psychiatric hospital, involuntary detention after voluntary admission, seclusion, restraint and forced medication.

Two groups of patients were included: legally involuntarily admitted patients, and legally voluntarily admitted patients who felt coerced to admission as measured by the MacArthur Perceived Coercion Scale [29]. The aims of the study were to investigate the two patient groups regarding socio-demographic and clinical characteristics, the frequency and intensity of perceived coercion, coercive treatment measures applied, the medium-term outcome (three months after admission), baseline predictors of more or less favourable medium-term outcome, and the international variation in all these respects. Data were collected between 2003 and 2006 and were obtained from case records and from assessments and interviews of the patients within the first week of admission and at follow-up at one and three months.

Patients were asked for participation if they were between 18 and 65 years of age, lived in the catchment areas of the participating hospitals, had not been admitted to a special unit only for forensic psychiatric or intoxicated patients, were able to speak the national language, and were not already included in the study. Patients with all diagnoses of mental disorders, except patients with substance abuse disorders and dementia, were eligible if the rest of the inclusion criteria were fulfilled, but could be excluded because the clinical situation did not allow the obtaining of reliable information. The patients should be considered to be able to give informed consent.

### 16.5.1 Some ethical aspects of the EUNOMIA study

No standardized method, like the MacCAT-CR [15,16], was used to assess the competency of the patients to provide informed consent. Thus, an ethical problem of the study might be that researchers at the different centres have assessed competence differently and that incompetent patients have been included. In the study as a whole, the total number of eligible involuntarily admitted patients was 4651, and 728 absconded or were discharged before they could be asked for participation. Of the remaining 3923 patients, 771 (20%) were assessed as clinically too unwell to be asked for consent, with a variation from 13 to 32% between centres [30]. It is not known whether this variation was due to real differences in patients' clinical conditions or in differences in assessments of competence to provide informed consent.

For educational purposes at the University of Örebro, Sweden, a survey regarding some ethical issues connected to the EUNOMIA study was performed amongst the national principal investigators at the end of the data collection period. They were asked to describe national laws and regulations on research ethics, the procedure for ethical approval applications, and the status of the decisions of the ethical committees – advisory or mandatory. Regarding the EUNOMIA study, they were asked to describe how the patients were approached and informed about the study and asked to participate, the content of the information given to the patient, how informed consent was obtained, and if they had noticed any kind of ethical problems related to the study. A majority of the principal investigators responded, and some experiences from the survey will be presented in the following.

In most centres the researchers performed the assessments of the patients' decisional capacity to provide informed consent, but in some of the participating centres the assessments were done by clinical staff. There are no indications, however, that the latter centres in general had higher or lower proportions of patients assessed as clinically too unwell.

The EUNOMIA study was approved by national or regional research ethics committees according to the regulations in force in each country. Even though the international ethical declarations are valid in all countries, national legislation differs. Some countries have specific laws regulating medical research ethics, while other countries have incorporated such rules in the general health acts. Furthermore, the professional background of ethical committee members and the procedures of the committees differ between countries. In most cases the decision of the ethical committee is binding, while in others the committee has a consultative function.

In all centres, eligible patients assessed as competent were given oral and written information about the study by researchers or clinicians specially assigned and trained for the EUNOMIA research interviews. Written informed consent was obtained from all participating patients. A common standard for the content of the written information was developed within the project, but was adapted to national preconditions in each country. The length and content of the information sheets differed, even though the most important information was included in all cases.

Economic reimbursement was given to participating patients in some centres. The amount varied from €9 to €30 when taking part in all three interviews (within one week, one month and three months of admission). In other centres no reimbursement was given. Economic compensation to patients for participating in research was prohibited by law in at least one of the participating countries, and not approved by the ethical committees in another.

Of involuntarily admitted patients asked for informed consent in the EUNOMIA study, 26% refused to take part. The proportion of refusing patients varied from 5 to 54% between the participating centres. There were no obvious associations between the ways in which the patients were approached, how the written information was drawn up, and if the patients were reimbursed or not, and the percentage of patients not consenting. There are no data to explain the differences between centres, but cultural and clinical differences, and the way the oral information was given, might be contributing factors. In the Swedish centre, which had the highest proportion of refusals, the patients were approached by clinical psychologists, psychiatric nurses, and social workers in clinical psychiatry. They were not involved in the treatment of the patients they informed and asked for consent, and they were specially trained for doing research interviews in the EUNOMIA study. No reimbursement for participation was given to the patients. The Swedish written information was quite long and detailed in order to follow Swedish regulations and practices of the ethical review boards. On the written informed consent form, the patient declared that he or she had been given oral and written information, that participation was by his or her own free choice, and that he or she understood that without specifying the reason he or she could break off at any time and that this would not have an effect on his or her treatment and care. The interviewer declared on the same form that, as far as he or she could judge, the patient had understood the information and had freely made his or her decision.

This careful process of information and consent might be of importance for the high number of refusing patients in the Swedish centre. An experience reported by the interviewers was that quite a few patients declared that they were willing to participate, but that they did not want to sign any paper. However, these patients could not be included according to the research protocol and the ethical approval of the study.

Thus, in spite of a common research design and common procedures agreed upon in this international study, there were substantial differences in the informed consent processes and the inclusion of patients in the different countries. An important ethical problem is that we could have included patients not competent to provide informed consent. However, EUNOMIA is a non-intervention study, based on data collected from case records, staff assessments and personal interviews. The possible risk of harm to patients caused by study participation is considered to be low, and there are possible important benefits from the results of the study regarding improvement of involuntary psychiatric treatment and its outcomes across Europe [30]. Despite the general ethical issue of research being done on coercively treated patients, no matter the 'naturalistic' and non-interventional design, and the possibility that incompetent patients might have been included, actually no ethical problems were reported by the principal investigators.

There is a substantial variation in involuntary hospitalization rates between countries, probably at least partly due to differences in legal framework and procedures [31]. However, there are substantial variations also within countries [32]. Differences within the same jurisdictions might be associated with differences in structure and resources of mental health services and/or with local traditions and attitudes towards the use of coercion in psychiatry [22]. Similarly, the differences in competency assessments, research information and informed consent procedures between countries, as found in the EUNOMIA study, might occur between centres and local or regional ethical committees within countries, with a uniform legal and procedural framework. In a national Swedish study of the use of coercion in child and adolescent psychiatry, the regional ethical review boards in some essential aspects judged the application for ethical approval differently, and an extensive communication was needed to reach consensus on information procedures [33]. Since then, however, a new Swedish law on research ethical approval and a new organization of the regional ethical review boards have come into force.

## 16.6   The Nordic study on the use of coercion in the mental health care system

In a study on coercion in psychiatry performed in 12 psychiatric services in Denmark, Finland, Iceland, Norway and Sweden, more than 400 involuntarily admitted and close to 500 voluntarily admitted patients were assessed and interviewed, amongst other things about their experiences of coercion during the admission process [34]. Like in the EUNOMIA study, eligible patients were approached, informed about the study and asked for consent to participate, and no major ethical problems connected to the study were reported from any of the participating centres.

Knut-Ivar Iversen [35] has described the informed consent process in the Norwegian part of the Nordic study. The research programme was presented at the participating wards, and the practical procedures and how the patients should be approached were discussed with the staff. A two-step approach was used to ensure that given consent would be reliable and valid. Eligible patients were approached by a research assistant and informed verbally and in writing. To give the patient time for consideration, the research assistant returned the next day and asked for written informed consent. The experience was that most patients found the second step unnecessary and were already willing to express a clear opinion on whether to

**Table 16.1** Patients' views on the Swedish coercion study and on the voluntariness of participation (percentages).

|  | Voluntarily admitted patients $n = 116$ | Involuntarily admitted patients $n = 117$ | Total $n = 233$ |
|---|---|---|---|
| *What's your opinion about the fact that we're doing a study like this?* |  |  |  |
| It's good | 90.5 | 88.9 | 89.7 |
| It's bad | 0.0 | 0.9 | 0.4 |
| Don't know | 7.8 | 6.8 | 7.3 |
| No answer | 1.7 | 3.4 | 2.6 |
| *Do you feel that your participation in the study is entirely voluntary?* |  |  |  |
| Yes | 94.8 | 85.2 | 90.0 |
| Hesitant/don't know | 3.4 | 4.3 | 3.9 |
| No | 1.7 | 7.8 | 4.8 |
| No answer | 0.0 | 2.6 | 1.3 |

participate or not after the first approach. In the Swedish part of the study, a clear expression of opinion by the patient at the first contact was accepted, and the two-step approach was applied only when the researcher assessed that it was needed due to the response of the patient.

In the Swedish part of the Nordic study, a follow-up patient interview was performed at discharge (alternatively, after three weeks from admission if the care was still ongoing by then). At the end of this interview, which was quite long and could take up to an hour to go through, the patients were asked about their opinion about the study and if they experienced their participation as entirely voluntary. About 90% of the patients stated that it was good that the study was done and that they felt they participated voluntarily, with similar responses from both voluntarily and involuntarily admitted patients (Table 16.1). Still, 15% of the involuntary patients said they did not participate voluntarily, or gave hesitant answers, or didn't answer at all. This gives a reminder that researchers should be careful not to take the expressed opinion of the patient for granted too easily, and that patient attitudes may change over time.

## 16.7 Randomized controlled trials

To my knowledge, no randomized controlled trials (RCTs) have been performed to study outcomes of involuntary psychiatric hospitalization. In most jurisdictions it would probably be illegal, and not be approved by ethical committees, to randomly assign patients to compulsory psychiatric care or to voluntary psychiatric care, with a risk that no care at all would be brought about if a patient who is randomized to voluntary care refrains from receiving any kind of treatment. RCTs have been performed, however, to evaluate compulsory outpatient care or outpatient commitment [26,27], with conflicting results.

Marwin Swartz *et al.*, who performed one of these studies, have discussed the ethical challenges involved [36]. As a starting point, they argue that random assignment in clinical trials is ethically acceptable if clinicians have no reason to prefer either of the treatments in the study. As previous research had shown mixed results regarding the effectiveness of outpatient commitment, they considered this precondition to be fulfilled. Eligible patients in the study they designed were involuntarily hospitalized patients who were ordered into outpatient commitment upon discharge by a court. They were randomly assigned either to a group who received outpatient commitment and case management, or a group receiving case management only. The authors raise a number of important and complex ethical issues connected to this design. For example: who would legally and ethically be responsible for adverse outcomes of the study, such as suicide and violence to others? How should situations be handled where clinicians in the individual cases found random assignment unethical? Is it ethical to ask patients for consent to be coerced? The authors argue that the ethical dilemmas can be successfully addressed.

Even if this is the case, there are severe legal, ethical and practical problems of performing randomized controlled trials to study the effectiveness of legally coercive interventions. Forthcoming studies will in most cases have to rely on alternative research designs.

## 16.8   Particularly vulnerable populations

Populations that could benefit from research should not be excluded because of gender, age, specific diagnoses, or ethnicity, for example, as long as their inclusion is motivated by the aims of the study and for scientific reasons, and the possible risk/ benefit ratio of participation does not weigh against inclusion. Ethical issues of research on coercion may be even more complex, however, when it comes to specific populations like children and adolescents, elderly, mentally ill offenders, and substance abusers.

### 16.8.1   Children and adolescents

Involuntary hospitalization of minors is probably, in most jurisdictions, not so frequent, even if very few data have been presented. In Finland, however, a leading country regarding psychiatric research on coercion of children and adolescents, an increase in the number of coercively treated individuals under 18 years of age has been reported [37]. To force someone to psychiatric treatment by deprivation of liberty is one of the most serious interventions of a society towards its citizens. Such interventions are even more serious when directed towards young people, possibly affecting their trust in grownups and in society. Most often parents or guardians are involved in the decisions, assessments of need for care are complex, and there are potential risks of psychological stigmatization of the young person. Still, few studies have focused on coercion in child and adolescent psychiatry.

Jinger Hoop *et al.* [38] have argued that the scientific evidence base in child psychiatry is modest, and that this scientific neglect of childhood mental and emotional illnesses is an ethical failure; a lack of beneficence towards the population representing the future of humanity. Research on psychiatric conditions amongst minors and on psychiatric treatment of young people, however, involves special ethical issues, and even more so when studying involuntary psychiatric care of children and adolescents. Scientific issues, risks and benefits, confidentiality, recruitment issues, informed consent, incentives, ethical review, and data protection issues have to be carefully scrutinized in designing such studies. For example, to what extent do children and adolescents with mental illnesses have the capability to understand research information, decisional capacity, and the ability to make a free, uncoerced decision? Are there circumstances and situations when it would be acceptable to leave the consent decision to the parents or to a guardian?

According to CIOMS [8], Guideline 14, a deliberate objection by a child against taking part in research should normally be respected even if the parents have consented. In specific cases, however, particularly for a very young or immature child, a parent or a guardian may override the child's refusal. If children during research become capable of independent informed consent, they should be asked for informed consent to continued participation, and their decision should be respected.

Despite these ethical challenges, it should be feasible to conduct ethically sound research on the use of coercion against minors in psychiatric care. For example, qualitative interviews with involuntarily admitted teenagers in child and adolescent psychiatric inpatient care about their care experiences have been performed without any reports of unfavourable effects on the participants or their families. In order not to interfere with treatment, an inclusion criterion in the study was that clinicians at the ward should assess the young person not to be too clinically unwell to participate in the interviews. A staff member gave the first information about the study to the patient, and asked for consent to participate. If the young person accepted participation, the parents were contacted and informed about the study. There was no legal obligation to ask the parents, at least not for subjects over 15 years of age, but the intention was to inform them about what happened to their child during care and that he or she would be contacted by a researcher. Then, when permission was obtained from the young patient and the parents, the researcher contacted the patient by telephone, gave further information and again asked for consent. It was stressed that whether the young person agreed to participate or not did not in any way influence his or her treatment. If he or she consented, time and place for the interview were agreed upon [39].

### 16.8.2  Other vulnerable populations

Forensic patients possess dual vulnerabilities regarding voluntary participation in research, being both 'prisoners' and psychiatric patients. 'Prisoners' are in this context defined as individuals sentenced to institutions under criminal or civil law, including patients in forensic mental health facilities [40]. Research on court-supervised persons with addictive disorders faces similar ethical challenges, with a variety of potentially coercive factors possibly influencing the research subjects' ability to provide informed consent [41]. Applying the CIOMS guidelines [8] to these fields of research, studies have to be intended to obtain knowledge that will lead to improved diagnosis, prevention or treatment of diseases or other health problems of either the actual subjects or other forensic patients.

Like prisoners and forensic psychiatric patients, psychiatric patients who are involuntarily hospitalized according to mental health law are deprived of their liberty, too. Thus, basically the same ethical demands should be applicable on research involving involuntary psychiatric patients in general psychiatry, mentally ill offenders, and court-supervised subjects who suffer from drug dependence.

## 16.9   Mainstream bioethics and cultural aspects

Informed consent is a central concept in current international codes of ethics and recommendations regarding medical research ethics. It is closely related to the concept of autonomy, which is emphasized in liberal bioethics. The most influential authors in the field, Tom Beauchamp and James Childress, have had an enormous impact on current bioethics with the four basic ethical principles they have presented: autonomy, beneficence, non-maleficence and justice [42]. Beauchamp and Childress express no particular ranking of these principles, but usually the principle of autonomy is emphasized in the literature. The right to individual self-determination comes to the front, and the main ethical task of clinicians and researchers is to respect the wishes of the individual.

Beauchamp and Childress focus on the autonomous choice rather than the autonomous person. Autonomous individuals may temporarily lack the capacity to make their own choices, for example due to illness, and individuals with impaired autonomy may sometimes be able to make autonomous choices. An autonomous choice is made intentionally, with comprehension and without controlling influences affecting it.

The implementation of international codes of ethics in which the individual is in focus, however, requires cultural sensitivity and understanding of the social context. The family, not the individual, is the unit of society in many cultures, where social integration is emphasized rather than individual autonomy. The community collective may be valued more highly than the individuality of its members in some cultures. How can the international ethical guidelines be applied without disregarding local values and norms? How can respect for local culture be shown without disregarding the codes of ethics and the patients' rights? Ahmed Okasha suggests that patients could be asked if they want to be informed about their illnesses and take part in decisions regarding their care, or if they prefer that information is given to and decisions handled by their families. By respecting the patient's wishes of a family-orientated decision process, respect for individual autonomy and informed consent will not be abandoned [43].

In the CIOMS commentaries to Guideline 4 [8], dealing with informed consent, cultural issues are addressed. It is stated that in some cultures, permission should be obtained from community leaders or some other kind of authorities before potential research subjects are approached. This should be respected, but such permission may in no case be a substitute for individual informed consent. To my view, the suggestion by Okasha does not rule out informed consent but shows a way to apply individual autonomy in a culturally sensitive way. This approach should be possible to apply also to psychiatric research on the use of coercion, even though in these cases careful attention should be paid to the fact that the patient's family might have been highly involved also in the treatment decisions.

## 16.10   Other research initiatives

There are further important research efforts in the field of coercion in psychiatry that have not been discussed in this chapter. Advance directives [44] and so-called Ulysses arrangements [45] are legally possible in several jurisdictions. Evaluations of arrangements based on the expressed will of the patient, at a time when competent, on the use of involuntary admission and treatment during a future episode when not competent, call for further ethical considerations. This is true also for studies of coercion in psychiatry using participant observations [46].

Even if no RCTs of involuntary psychiatric hospitalization have been reported, an interesting study with an experimental design was published in 1978. To study if involuntary hospitalization was overused, the requirements for involuntary hospitalization were made more stringent than usual during a 'no-commitment week'. Only patients in absolute need of hospitalization, according to a detailed protocol, and with every commitment decision co-signed by a specially assigned senior psychiatrist, were committed during this week. The number of involuntarily hospitalized patients during the no-commitment week was compared with the week before and the week after at the same hospital. No significant differences were found, but the authors recommended replication on a larger scale [47]. To my knowledge, no such replication has been performed so far.

Values-based medicine (VBM) has been introduced as a complement, but not an alternative, to evidence-based medicine (EBM). Whereas the EBM concept gives priority to objective facts, the emphasis in VBM is on subjective information. Legitimately, people have different values that have to be taken into account. Values should in this context be understood in a wider sense than ethical values, and include any kind of positive or negative value judgements. Possible value conflicts between therapists and patients cannot be solved by referring to the 'right' answer but should be handled in a process of mutual discussion. Values-based practice is an approach to balanced decision-making in situations involving complex and conflicting values. While ethics is mainly focused on outcome, values-based practice is process orientated [48].

Researchers and service users tend to prioritize different research topics and outcomes of services [49], and there is a growing interest and great potential benefits in service-user or consumer involvement in mental health research. The use of coercion in mental health services has inherent value conflicts. A challenging and important issue in order to enhance the evidence base for compulsory psychiatric treatment would be to apply service-user involvement and values-based practice on psychiatric research on coercion.

## 16.11 Some final remarks

Medical ethics have to balance the conflicting aims of protecting research subjects and not excluding vulnerable populations from the benefits of research. Transparency of research procedures is essential. Publications should include descriptions of informed consent procedures, how competency to provide informed consent was assessed, and considerations regarding risks and burdens for participants [50].

To obtain an evidence base for compulsory psychiatric care, further research on the use and outcome of coercion in mental health services is greatly needed. Such research requires participation from individuals who are legally coercively admitted and treated in psychiatry, as well as from formally voluntary patients who feel coerced to admission and/or treatment [28,34]. An experience from the EUNOMIA and the Nordic studies on coercion in psychiatry, referred to above, is that many patients appreciated being asked for participation and found it positive and helpful to get the opportunity to speak about their experiences and perceptions. A majority of patients were found to be competent to provide informed consent.

Even so, researchers have to be careful and sensitive when approaching involuntarily admitted patients, in particular, to ask for informed consent to participate in research. In the admission process, they have been considered not capable of making treatment decisions of their own, and they are in a dependent position likely to impact on the possibility of making free choices without undue influences. There is a risk that some patients not competent to provide informed consent have been included in psychiatric research on coercion.

On the other hand, the therapeutic misconception might occur with competent subjects in all fields of research, and no serious ethical problems or harm to participating patients have, to my knowledge, been reported from 'naturalistic' studies of coercion in psychiatry with non-interventional designs. The possible benefits for future psychiatric patients, subjected to coercive measures in psychiatric care, from high quality and scientifically and ethically sound studies of this kind, will most likely be greater than the possible risks for harm to patients participating in such studies. It is more questionable if controlled trials with random assignment to involuntary or voluntary admission, or studies on involuntarily admitted patients including interventions with risks of negative side effects, could be performed with adherence to international ethical research standards.

# References

1. Kjellin, L., Andersson, K., Candefjord, I.L. *et al.* (1997) Ethical benefits and costs of coercion in short-term inpatient psychiatric care. *Psychiatric Services*, **48**, 1567–1570.
2. Svindseth, M.F., Dahl, A.A. and Hatling, T. (2007) Patients' experiences of humiliation in the admission process to acute psychiatric wards. *Nordic Journal of Psychiatry*, **61**, 47–53.
3. Weiss Roberts, L. (2002) Informed consent and the capacity for voluntarism. *American Journal of Psychiatry*, **159**, 705–712.
4. Green, S.A. and Bloch, S. (eds) (2006) *An Anthology of Psychiatric Ethics*, Oxford University Press, Oxford, p. 448.
5. López-Muñoz, F., Alamo, C., Dudley, M. *et al.* (2007) Psychiatry and political-institutional abuse from the historical perspective: The ethical lessons of the Nuremberg Trial on their 60th anniversary. *Progress in Neuro-Psychopharmacology & Biological Psychiatry*, **31**, 791–806.
6. Beecher, H. (1966) Ethics and clinical research. *New England Journal of Medicine*, **274**, 1354–1360.
7. World Medical Association (2010) WMA *Declaration of Helsinki – Ethical Principles for Medical Research Involving Human Subjects*. www.wma.net/en/30publications/10policies/b3/index.html (accessed 15 February 2010).
8. Council for International Organizations of Medical Sciences (CIOMS) (2010) *International Ethical Guidelines for Biomedical Research Involving Human Subjects*, CIOMS, Geneva. http://www.cioms.ch/publications/guidelines/guidelines_nov_2002_blurb.htm (accessed 7 December 2010).
9. World Psychiatric Association (WPA). (2010) *The Declaration of Hawaii and the Declaration of Madrid*. www.wpanet.org/detail.php?section_id=5&content_id=31 (accessed 13 December 2010).

10. Appelbaum, P.S. and Grisso, T. (1988) Assessing patients' capacities to consent to treatment. *New England Journal of Medicine*, **319**, 1635–1638.
11. Berghmans, R.L.P. and Widdershoven, G.A.M. (2003) Ethical perspectives on decision-making capacity and consent for treatment and research. *Medicine and Law*, **22**, 391–400.
12. Waggoner, W.C. and Mayo, D.M. (1995) Who understands? A survey of 25 words or phrases commonly used in proposed clinical research consent forms. *IRB*, **17**, 6–9.
13. Lidz, C.W. and Appelbaum, P.S. (2002) The therapeutic misconception. Problems and solutions. *Medical Care*, **40** (Supplement), V55–V63.
14. Lidz, C.W., Appelbaum, P.S., Grisso, T. and Renaud, M. (2004) Therapeutic misconception and the appreciation of risks in clinical trials. *Social Science & Medicine*, **58**, 1689–1697.
15. Grisso, T., Appelbaum, P.S. and Hill-Fotouhi, C. (1997) The MacCAT-T: a clinical tool to assess patients' capacities to make treatment decisions. *Psychiatric Services*, **48**, 1415–1419.
16. Appelbaum, P.S. and Grisso, T. (2001) *MacCAT-CR: MacArthur Competence Assessment Tool for Clinical Research*, Professional Resource Press, Sarasota, FL.
17. Carpenter, W.T., Gold, J.M., Lahti, A.C. *et al.* (2000) Decisional capacity for informed consent in schizophrenia research. *Archives of General Psychiatry*, **57**, 533–538.
18. Roberts, L.W., Warner, T.D., Brody, J.L. *et al.* (2002) Patient and psychiatrist ratings of hypothetical schizophrenia research protocols: assessment of harm potential and factors influencing participant decisions. *American Journal of Psychiatry*, **159**, 573–584.
19. Palmer, B.W., Dunn, L.B., Appelbaum, P.S. *et al.* (2005) Assessment of capacity to consent to research among older persons with schizophrenia, Alzheimer disease, or diabetes mellitus. *Archives of General Psychiatry*, **62**, 726–733.
20. Appelbaum, P.S., Grisso, T., Frank, E. *et al.* (1999) Competence of depressed patients for consent to research. *American Journal of Psychiatry*, **156**, 1380–1384.
21. Lidz, C.W. (1998) Coercion in psychiatric care: what have we learned from research? *Journal of American Academy of Psychiatry and Law*, **26**, 631–637.
22. Høyer, G. (2008) Involuntary hospitalization in contemporary mental health care. Some (still) unanswered questions. *Journal of Mental Health*, **17**, 281–292.
23. Katsakou, C. and Priebe, S. (2006) Outcomes of involuntary hospital admission – a review. *Acta Psychiatrica Scandinavica*, **114**, 232–241.
24. Kallert, T.W., Glöckner, M. and Schützwohl, M. (2008) Involuntary vs. voluntary hospital admission. A systematic literature review on outcome diversity. *European Archives of Psychiatry and Clinical Neuroscience*, **258**, 195–209.
25. Dawson, J., King, M., Papageorgiou, A. and Davidson, O. (2001) Legal pitfalls of psychiatric research. *British Journal of Psychiatry*, **178**, 67–70.
26. Swanson, J.W., Swartz, M.S., Borum, R. *et al.* (2000) Involuntary out-patient commitment and reduction of violent behaviour in persons with severe mental illness. *British Journal of Psychiatry*, **176**, 324–331.
27. Steadman, H.J., Gounis, K., Dennis, D. *et al.* (2001) Assessing the New York City involuntary outpatient commitment pilot program. *Psychiatric Services*, **52**, 330–336.
28. Kallert, T.W., Glöckner, M., Onchev, G. *et al.* (2005) The EUNOMIA project on coercion in psychiatry: study design and preliminary data. *World Psychiatry*, **4**, 168–172.
29. Gardner, W., Hoge, S.K., Bennet, N. *et al.* (1993) Two scales for measuring patients' perception for coercion during mental hospital admission. *Behavioral Sciences and the Law*, **11**, 307–321.
30. Priebe, S., Katsakou, C., Glöckner, M. *et al.* (2010) Patients' views of involuntary hospital admission after 1 and 3 months: a prospective study in 11 European countries. *British Journal of Psychiatry*, **196**, 179–185.

31. Salize, H.J. and Dressing, H. (2004) Epidemiology of involuntary placement of mentally ill people across the European Union. *British Journal of Psychiatry*, **184**, 163–168.
32. Priebe, S., Badesconyi, A., Fioritti, A. *et al.* (2005) Reinstitutionalisation in mental health care: comparison of data on service provision from six European countries. *British Medical Journal*, **330**, 123–126.
33. Engström, I. (ed) (2006) *Tvingad till hjälp. Om tvång, etik och tillit i barn- och ungdomspsykiatrisk vård* (in Swedish) [*Forced to Help. On Coercion, Ethics And Trust In Child- And Adolescent Psychiatric Care*], Studentlitteratur, Lund.
34. Kjellin, L., Høyer, G., Engberg, M. *et al.* (2006) Differences in perceived coercion at admission to psychiatric hospitals in the Nordic countries. *Social Psychiatry and Psychiatric Epidemiology*, **41**, 241–247.
35. Iversen, K.-I. (2008) Coercion in the delivery of mental health services in Norway. Dissertation. Institute of Community Medicine, Faculty of Medicine, University of Tromsø, Norway.
36. Swartz, M.S., Burns, B.J., George, L.K. *et al.* (1997) The ethical challenges of a randomized controlled trial of involuntary outpatient commitment. *The Journal of Mental Health Administration*, **24**, 35–43.
37. Kaltiala-Heino, R. (2004) Increase in involuntary psychiatric admissions of minors. A register study. *Social Psychiatry and Psychiatric Epidemiology*, **39**, 53–59.
38. Hoop, J.G., Smyth, A.C. and Roberts, L.W. (2008) Ethical issues in psychiatric research on children and adolescents. *Child and Adolescent Psychiatric Clinics of North America*, **17**, 127–148.
39. Engström, K. (2008) *Delaktighet under tvång. Om ungdomars erfarenheter i barn- och ungdomspsykiatrisk slutenvård* (in Swedish) [*Participation under coercion. On young people's experiences in child and adolescent psychiatric inpatient care*]. Dissertation. Örebro Studies in Education, Örebro, Sweden.
40. Regehr, C., Edwardh, M. and Bradford, J. (2000) Research ethics and forensic patients. *Canadian Journal of Psychiatry*, **45**, 892–898.
41. DuVal, G. and Salmon, C. (2004) Research note: ethics of drug treatment research with court-supervised subjects. *Journal of Drug Issues*, **34**, 991–1005.
42. Beauchamp, T. and Childress, J. (2001) *Principles of Biomedical Ethics*, 5th edn, Oxford University Press, New York.
43. Okasha, A. (2005) The impact of Arab culture on psychiatric ethics, in *Ethics, Culture, and Psychiatry. International Perspectives* (eds A. Okasha, J. Arboleda-Flórez and N. Sartorius), American Psychiatric Press, Washington, DC, pp. 15–28.
44. Campbell, L.A. and Kisely, S.R. (2009) Advance treatment directives for people with severe mental illness. *Cochrane Database of Systematic Reviews*, 1 (Art. No.: CD005963). doi: 10.1002/14651858.CD005963.pub2
45. Gremmen, I., Widdershoven, G., Beekman, A. *et al.* (2008) Ulysses arrangements in psychiatry: a matter of good care? *Journal of Medical Ethics*, **34**, 77–80.
46. Sjöström, S. (1997) *Party or Patient? Discursive Practices Relating to Coercion in Psychiatric and Legal Settings*, Boréa, Umeå.
47. Zwerling, I.M., Conte, H.R., Plutchik, R. and Karasu, T.B. (1978) "No-commitment week": a feasibility study. *American Journal of Psychiatry*, **135**, 1198–1201.
48. Fulford, K.W.M. and Wallcraft, J. (2009) Values-based practice and service user involvement in mental health research, in *Handbook of Service User Involvement in Mental Health Research* (eds J. Wallcraft, B. Schrank and M. Amering), John Wiley & Sons, Ltd, Chichester, pp. 37–60.

49. Del Vecchio, P. and Blyler, C.R. (2009) Identifying critical outcomes and setting priorities for mental health services research, in *Handbook of Service User Involvement in Mental Health Research* (eds J. Wallcraft, B. Schrank and M. Amering), John Wiley & Sons, Ltd, Chichester, pp. 99–112.

50. I-Ping Tsao, C., Layde, J.B. and Weiss Roberts, L. (2008) A review of ethics in psychiatric research. *Current Opinion in Psychiatry*, **21**, 572–577.

# 17 Coercion and undue influence in decisions to participate in psychiatric research

Paul S. Appelbaum,[1,2] Charles W. Lidz[3] and Robert Klitzman[4,5]

[1]*Columbia University, Department of Psychiatry, New York, NY, USA*
[2]*New York State Psychiatric Institute, Division of Law, Ethics, and Psychiatry, New York, NY, USA*
[3]*Center for Mental Health Services Research, Department of Psychiatry, University of Massachusetts Medical School, Worcester, MA, USA*
[4]*Columbia University, Department of Psychiatry and Mailman School of Public Health, New York, NY, USA*
[5]*New York State Psychiatric Institute, HIV Center, Ethics, Policy and Human Rights Core, New York, NY, USA*

Voluntariness of consent has been considered an essential aspect of participation in research at least since the decision of the Nuremberg Tribunal in the Doctor's Trial. After declaring that 'the voluntary consent of the human subject is absolutely essential,' the judges elaborated on the concept by suggesting that the subject 'should

*Coercive Treatment in Psychiatry: Clinical, Legal and Ethical Aspects*, First Edition.
Edited by Thomas W. Kallert, Juan E. Mezzich and John Monahan.
© 2011 John Wiley & Sons, Ltd. Published 2011 by John Wiley & Sons, Ltd.

be so situated as to be able to exercise free power of choice, without the intervention of any force, fraud, deceit, duress, over-reaching, or other ulterior form of constraint or coercion' [1]. Although the tribunal's opinion overstated its case in some ways (e.g. if taken at face value, it would absolutely preclude participation in research by incompetent persons), it illustrates the importance accorded in the Western legal tradition to voluntariness of choice with regard to research.

Government regulation of research with human subjects, which accelerated in the last third of the twentieth century, followed the lead of the Nuremberg decision in highlighting the importance of voluntary consent. The federal regulations in the United States, for example, charge institutional review boards (commonly known as IRBs, but referred to as 'research ethics committees' in much of the world) with determining that for a research protocol in which 'some or all of the subjects are likely to be vulnerable to coercion or undue influence, such as children, prisoners, pregnant women, mentally disabled persons, or economically or educationally disadvantaged persons... additional safeguards have been included in the study to protect the rights and welfare of these subjects' [2]. However, embedded in many regulatory approaches, including this one, are assumptions about which subjects are particularly likely to face coercive influences and about the efficacy of prophylactic measures, the empirical bases for which are thin at best.

Added to these regulatory approaches – which notably single out 'mentally disabled persons'– are the rules of thumb formulated by many research ethics committees as to those situations likely to evoke coercion and as to possible remedies, often reflected in the literature on research ethics. These include studies in which:

- substantial compensation is offered to research subjects [3];
- subjects are recruited by their own physicians or in facilities on whose care they have become dependent [3–5];
- subjects have been involuntarily committed for mental or behavioural disorders, including substance abuse [6];
- persons targeted for recruitment would otherwise lack access to medical care in general or to the kind of care being studied in particular [7];
- the research is taking place in a society in which members are generally subordinate to traditional leaders, including where women generally do not make decisions independently of their husbands [8–10]; or
- access to substances of abuse is afforded to persons dependent on those substances [11–13].

The prevalence of circumstances involving persons with psychiatric disorders, including substance abuse, is striking.

In response, investigators have been required to: reduce the amount of compensation being offered [14–17]; avoid recruiting their own patients; exclude involuntarily committed patients from their studies; include additional safeguards (e.g., consent monitors); and offer forms of compensation that are less likely to lead to abuse of substances (e.g., food and clothing vouchers). United States federal regulations also restrict the kinds of research that can be performed with prisoners [18] – although some relaxation of these rules has been suggested [19] – and, less rigidly, with children and pregnant women [20,21]. Many of these approaches, however, especially restrictions on compensation, have been criticized as misguided [3,22,23]. Often lacking in these well-meaning efforts is a clear conceptualization of what constitutes coercion or undue influence and how it can be prevented.

The goal of this chapter is to outline a theory of voluntary consent to research and of those factors that may constrain it; to review approaches to the assessment of coercion and undue influence in research settings; and to present an overview of the existing research on the nature and prevalence of constraints on voluntariness, including our own, along with an indication of gaps in current knowledge. Where relevant, we highlight in particular the applicability of these theories and data to research subjects with psychiatric and substance use disorders.

## 17.1 Understanding voluntariness from the perspective of the legal doctrine of informed consent

Given its importance as one of the three pillars of informed consent – along with disclosure of relevant information to patients or research subjects and decisional competence or capacity [24] – voluntariness of consent has been under-conceptualized. This is true despite a large philosophical literature on the related concept of free choice [25], and a growing number of investigations of conscious control of behaviour in the psychological and neuroscience literatures [26]. Because informed consent originated as a legal construct, however, only later becoming a cornerstone of bioethics, for our purposes the law's approach may be particularly instructive. Western legal traditions generally presume that people are able to act freely and that their actions reflect their free choices – unless constraints exist that would render those choices involuntary [27]. Thus, the law's test is essentially a negative one: in the absence of relevant constraining conditions, voluntariness will be presumed. This approach is reflected in the Anglo-American legal tradition's approach to torts [28], contracts [29] and criminal law [30], amongst other areas.

Not all constraints, though, qualify to negate the legal voluntariness of an act. The law of consent recognizes, to begin with, that no decisions or subsequent actions are completely uninfluenced [31]. Persons' decisions are typically shaped, often without their conscious awareness, by aspects of character, situational considerations and the influence of other people. The mere presence of influences *per se* does not trump the presumption that the person is the ultimate decision maker and that the final decision will reflect that person's desires, taking into account all of the relevant aspects of the person's situation. Thus, in the context of a decision about participation in research, common influences may include attitudes towards science and medicine in general; desires to advance knowledge of particular disorders; risk-averse or risk-seeking personality traits; desires for personal benefits that may be obtained through research participation; opinions of other influential people in a person's life; and realistic aspects of the person's situation (e.g., a need for medical treatment that may only be available by means of enrollment in a research study) [32]. None of these considerations ordinarily will make it impossible for a potential research subject to make a voluntary choice.

Rather, as implied by the Nuremberg Tribunal's language, and as reflected in other areas of law, those influences that vitiate voluntariness are of a very particular type. As will be explicated at greater length below, legally problematic influences have four key characteristics; they:

- derive from sources external to the person;
- are applied with the intention of determining the person's choice;
- are not the sorts of influences that ordinarily would be recognized as legitimate; and
- have a causal impact on the decision of the research subject [33].

Influences that fail to meet all four of these criteria usually will not be deemed to have coerced or unduly influenced a subject's decision.

The first of the key considerations is that a voluntariness-impairing influence must originate from a source external to the person. This rules out internal drives, mood states, affects and even addictions as legally relevant considerations, though they all unquestionably influence the choices that people make. Decisions about engaging in sexual intercourse are not involuntary because a person has a strong desire for sex, nor are decisions about financial affairs presumed to be beyond the control of someone who is extremely anxious about a serious financial situation. Were it to be otherwise, for example for the purpose of determining the voluntariness and therefore the validity of a contract, courts would be forced to inquire into difficult-to-ascertain and often imponderable aspects of a person's motivation. Similarly, for the sake of deciding on a person's criminal responsibility for an act committed under the influence of financial pressure, finders of fact would need to ascertain when such pressures were not resistible as opposed simply to not having been adequately resisted. In the service of avoiding this quagmire, the law has declined to consider internal influences as relevant to issues of impaired voluntariness, focusing instead on external constraints. This is most graphically illustrated by the decision of the US Supreme Court in a case involving a confession of murder by a defendant who claimed that he had heard the voice of God instructing him to confess and thus could not make a voluntary decision. Despite the defendant's psychotic state at the time of the confession, the court declined to declare his admission involuntary, since evidence was not presented of any coercive behaviour by the police [30].

In addition to an influence being external to the person, the second criterion for a voluntariness-negating effect is that it must be intended to influence the person's decision. Most obviously, this requirement eliminates situational constraints as vitiating voluntariness, except perhaps in the most extreme cases. The fact that someone is poor or has no other means of obtaining treatment does not render the person's choices – even if they are strongly affected by these considerations – involuntary. The alternative approach would deprive all indigent persons of the right to make decisions and perhaps bar from research those people who, because of a lack of other options, most desire to participate in it. For similar reasons, influences of organizational culture, for example in a total institution or a work place, though potentially potent, do not by themselves vitiate the power to choose. They may, however, create the conditions in which deliberate efforts may be made to influence a person's choice [34]. This concern may provide a legitimate basis, for example, for restrictions of certain kinds on prison-based research (as opposed to more simplistic notions that prisoners are *ipso facto* incapable of making voluntary decisions).

Influences can be external and intentional without impairing voluntariness, as reflection on common situations that arise in the research setting will suggest. Physicians encourage patients to enter studies; families exert pressures to forego experimental options; disease advocacy groups urge participation. Such influences are generally considered legitimate because they are the sorts of behaviours that are expected of other people with whom one interacts. When people exert influences that are outside of their accepted roles, they may cross the border into illegitimate – and hence voluntariness-denying – behaviour. An example is a doctor who suggests to a patient that she will not continue to treat him if he decides not to enter a research study. Since physicians owe ongoing duties to care for their patients, that is an influence that is not just external and intentional, but also illegitimate.

However, to consider an influence as negating the voluntariness of a decision, one more criterion must be met: the influence must have a causal relationship with the person's choice. Even illegitimate influences deliberately exerted by third parties will not invalidate a subsequent decision unless they were closely linked to the outcome. Thus, when pressure from a treating physician is irrelevant – either because the patient successfully resists it or because the patient was inclined to follow the physician's direction anyway – the patient's choice is valid, though the physician's behaviour may still warrant reprimand.

Given these characteristics of influences that negate voluntariness – external, intentional, illegitimate and causal – what special considerations may exist for research on persons with psychiatric disorders, including substance abuse? Although psychotic disorders may lead to internally generated stimuli, that is, delusions and hallucinations, that can affect decisions, and although some decisions in such circumstances may not be competent ones, the decisions will still be voluntary in the usual sense in which that word is used in legal contexts. Similarly, the craving of a cocaine addict or the withdrawal symptoms of an alcoholic may also affect capacity, but will not usually be deemed to have negated free choice. From these perspectives, psychiatric disorders are unlikely to impact voluntariness one way or the other. The US federal research regulations quoted above do appear to suggest that persons with 'mental disabilities,' a term otherwise unspecified, may be particularly prone to coercion and undue inducement, though the reasons for such a belief are unclear and there is no empirical support in the literature as far as persons with psychiatric disorders are concerned. Perhaps the drafters had in mind the well-known suggestibility of persons with mild to moderate mental retardation (now often referred to as intellectual disability); if so, research ethics committees appear to have extended its implications well beyond the original intent.

## 17.2 Manifestations of constraints on voluntariness in research – undue influence and coercion

In practice, as we have elaborated elsewhere, influences on a subject's decisions by third parties are likely to manifest themselves in one of four ways: as appeals for participation based on shared values (e.g., the desire to find an effective treatment for an illness), offers, pressures and threats [33]. The first of these is likely always to be legitimate, unless there is deception involved, and hence is likely not to meet criteria for impairing voluntary choice. Thus, the discussion here will focus on the latter three types of influence.

Offers are common in research, since they are thought to be important in motivating participants, particularly when the prospect of beneficial and desired treatment is absent (e.g., in non-therapeutic studies of disease physiology or when non-ill volunteers are required). Offers typically come in the form of financial compensation or its equivalent (e.g., vouchers), but may also include free diagnostic procedures or treatment, including medications, or unusually close monitoring and follow-up. Given that offers generally expand options rather than constrict them – that is, people always have the option of rejecting a genuine offer – we follow Wertheimer's influential analysis in construing them as legitimate and unlikely to vitiate voluntariness [27].

There may be situations, however, in which offers are problematic. Should an offer be of such magnitude relative to the effort required (e.g., $5000 for participation in a one-day study) or of such importance to the person (e.g., parole for a prisoner) that it is likely to overwhelm all other considerations, then such an offer is often considered to constitute an undue inducement. In particular, many commentators are concerned that a person offered such an incentive for participation would neglect the usual countervailing considerations, such as the nature and probability of harms stemming from the research. When an offer is substantial enough that it should evoke such concerns is a question on which agreement is lacking. Research ethics committees often have guidelines for the amount of money that can be offered subjects, with the assumption that greater amounts would play an undue role in subjects' decisions (though the situation is often mistakenly referred to as 'coercive') [14–17]. However, as discussed below, data on the benefits of such arbitrary compensation limits are absent; what data do exist have failed to suggest undue influences at reasonable levels of compensation; and some commentators have argued that no offer, regardless of magnitude, should be considered to be unduly influential [35].

A second form of influence that may be of concern is pressure. The line between legitimate persuasion and illegitimate pressure is a fine one, and may relate in part to whether an intellectual appeal is being made ('You can help us find a cure for this disease more quickly') or interpersonal or organizational pressure is being applied. An example of interpersonal pressure might be a physician who uses his relationship with a patient to raise repeatedly the issue of enrolling in research, suggesting that he very much desires that the patient participate. Faden and Beauchamp call this phenomenon 'psychological manipulation' [36]. Pressures can also be exerted organizationally, for example in the transmittal of an expectation that all psychology students will serve as their instructors' research subjects. Not all pressures will negate voluntariness, but as a group they are more likely to do so than are offers. Pressures too can rise to the level of undue influence if they lack legitimacy and causally affect the decision.

Finally, research subjects can be the target of threats, that is, declarations of intent to take actions that are detrimental to them, if they fail to perform a desired act – here, to enroll in a research study. Wertheimer's moralized approach to coercion holds that threats are coercive when they are illegitimate, as they almost always will be when they are made by treatment or research staff [27]. (In contrast, other people in a person's life may be entitled to make certain threats, for example a spouse threatening to leave if the other spouse doesn't stop drinking.) Illegitimate threats are generally considered coercive and invalidate a subject's decision when they are causally implicated.

Note should also be taken of the distinction between objective and subjective coercion. Objective coercion relates to actual offers, pressures and threats that generally would be considered lacking in legitimacy. Subjective coercion, sometimes called perceived coercion, describes the perspective of the target of the behaviour in question, who may or may not identify it as unduly influential or coercive [37]. Both are important in an analysis based on legal approaches to voluntariness, since an action will not be considered to impair voluntariness unless it is objectively external, influential and illegitimate and subjectively affects the outcome of the decision. In the following section, we consider approaches to assessing voluntariness and its impairment from both an objective and subjective perspective.

## 17.3 Measuring voluntariness

To measure any concept involves fixing its exact status at a place and time. Whether one is using a binary category, a seven-point ordinal scale, or a continuous visual analogue scale, one is establishing and fixing a value for a concept for some person or group at a point in time. This is essential for many purposes but it is not without inherent difficulties, especially when measuring legal or ethical concepts, which are inherently ambiguous [38]. If they were clear, many legal decisions such as when a person is responsible for her criminal acts or whether a dying man was competent to rewrite his will would be much more readily susceptible to determination [39]. Consider a concept like 'undue influence.' What sorts of influences are appropriate and when do they become undue? Does it matter whether the goals of the influencer are benign? Whether the influencer and the person being influenced have a relationship and what type of relationship they have? As will be seen below, we would suggest that all of these considerations may be critical in determining both the objective and subjective components of coercion.

The problems with measuring voluntariness derive directly from two of the four features of acts that undermine voluntariness that we have described above, specifically that an act:

- has a causal impact on the decision of the research subject; and
- is not the sort of influence that ordinarily would be recognized as legitimate.

Whether an act is external to the individual is not difficult to determine, but whether that act has a causal impact is difficult to assess because determining causation in non-experimental contexts is inherently problematic. One can depend either on the account of an observer who must determine what motivates the actions of the subject or on the report of the subject, both of which have their own biases.

Even more difficult is determining whether the act is a legitimate one. Although we may often feel that we know what is a legitimate act, brief consideration will make clear that the perception of the legitimacy of an action depends in part from which side of the act one is observing the behaviour. For the psychiatrist who tells the patient that it is critical that he join the study of a new intervention – for the patient's own benefit – because no other treatment exists that is likely to be helpful, this may seem an appropriate and legitimate part of her role as a clinician. The patient, however, may see this as an implicit threat that the psychiatrist will give up on him if he does not enroll in the study. Other clinicians might feel that they would be overstepping their boundaries to be so forceful about a patient's joining a clinical trial, whereas other patients might see the same act as a helpful suggestion. With such a diversity of perspectives, legal and ethical concepts are not easily locked down into scorable categories, complicating the development of measures that exhibit stability across contexts.

## 17.4   Context-free measures?

One might object, with some justification, that the analysis above is overly simplistic. If an individual is hung by his toes and beaten with a hose until he consents to participate in a trial, is not his voluntariness compromised? More realistically, do not involuntary legal status, pending legal cases, threats by a psychiatrist to abandon the patient, and so on, inherently compromise voluntariness? Are these not adequate measures of coercive pressures and thus context-free measures of voluntariness? Can an individual who is hospitalized against her will possibly give a voluntary consent to research? Are not large participant payments to subjects who are economically deprived inherently coercive? What about studies involving access to substances of choice for addicted clients? Or treatment access for those who have no insurance, a common problem in the United States? Conversely, is not the decision of a person who has a choice of treaters and of whether to participate in research, inherently voluntary? Could these not be components of a context-free measure of voluntariness?

There are several problems with such a categorical approach. First, it is too inclusive. Per the typology described above, for example, although involuntary hospitalization is an external influence, it is not invoked with the intent to influence decisions about research but for entirely different purposes. Indeed, the absence of coercive effect in practice is demonstrated by the many people who are involuntarily hospitalized yet turn down research project participation. Moreover, some people who are involuntarily hospitalized are grateful that they were hospitalized and do not feel coerced [40]. In the addiction context, as Timmermans and McKay report, people with severe addiction problems may find participation in research to be a great opportunity to manage their addiction, rather than a chance to obtain funds to purchase more drugs or alcohol, an observation that corresponds with our impressions from the study described below [41].

Second, the context-independent approach to assessing impaired voluntariness is not inclusive enough. Many people who have no objective restrictions on their freedom, access to medical care, or other influences that are often evoked as a *sine qua non* of coercion might feel that they have no choice about entering a research protocol. This might reflect the way in which their physician discussed the project or the tone of voice that the research nurse used in describing possible options. Thus, they may perceive and act as persons who are under coercive influences, even though objectively they are not. We may choose – as the law generally does – not to consider such persons as having been subject to coercion, but there may still be concerns about the acceptability of decisions made under such circumstances, and a desire to alter the situation to permit a subjectively freer choice.

Finally, such an approach conflates measures with findings. There are, indeed, objective events that, in our culture at the present time, will generally be seen by almost everyone as undermining free choices about participating in research protocols. Confinement in a penal institution may be one such example. But how widely these events undermine perceptions of voluntariness, and for whom, is an empirical matter. The measurement must be independent of that.

## 17.5 The importance of context

It is a critical feature of voluntariness in consent to psychiatric research, that assessing the pressures that interfere with voluntariness, with regard both to legitimacy and causal impact, involves context-dependent judgments. In a very important paper, Bennett *et al.* [42] described the different contextual features that affected patients' judgments about whether they had been coerced into admission to a psychiatric hospital. In open-ended interviews with patients about their admission, Bennett and her colleagues identified three themes that substantially affected the perception of whether they had been coerced into the hospital.

- **Inclusion**  Even if the decision about hospitalization was not to their liking, patients wanted to be included in the decision-making. They wanted a chance to have their views heard and to have those views taken seriously. To the extent that these desires were satisfied, perceptions of coercion were diminished.
- **The motivation of others**  Attributing the cause of another's actions to beneficent motivation had a strong positive effect on patients' views of the decision and its consequences. In essence, they felt that if someone were trying to work in their interests, pressures and even involuntary commitment were at least partially acceptable and were experienced as non-coercive.
- **Acting in good faith**  This aspect involved the actor who exerted influence being entitled, either by personal relationship or formal position, to do what he or she did;

being open about intentions and not deceitful; and treating the person with respect. Again, all of these aspects led to reduced beliefs that one had been coerced.

These features of a situation are not easily objectified and, even if they were, it is not clear that they would be important factors in other decisions, including whether to participate in research.

How can one measure a phenomenon that varies with the context in which it occurs? We noted above that one has only two choices. One can depend on the account of an observer who knows (or learns) all of the contextual features, or one can take the account of the participant. These appear to be the basic approaches that have been used to study the related issue of coercion in mental health treatment decisions. Three different methods have been employed. Ethnographic observation is almost a pure method of producing external, ostensibly objective information about the contextual meaning of an activity. Structured scales of perceived coercion are at the opposite end of the spectrum, offering a wholly subjective account. They rely almost entirely on the subject providing his description of the phenomenon, at least within the cognitive framework of the structured instrument. In between the two is the semi-structured interview, in which the interviewer explores the perspectives of the subject while attempting to follow-up and clarify the subject's descriptions.

Ethnographic observation has considerable power in studying voluntariness of consent. It is possible to observe the interaction between the consenter and the subject. What is stated and implied in the interaction becomes visible in a way that no report from any participant can provide. It allows the trained ethnographer to notice things that the research subject might not think to report (e.g., the person obtaining consent was wearing a white coat; on the wall of the psychiatric ward was posted a document signed by the local governor, urging participation in research). Moreover, because ethnographic observation often includes unstructured and semi-structured interviews, it provides an opportunity for the subject and the consenter both to describe their understanding of the decision-making process and for the research team to integrate their understandings with contextual features that the ethnographer observes. Finally, ethnography provides an optimal method for discovering the unexpected. Because the ethnographer is focused on the particular issue in a way that no one else is, he or she has the opportunity to see and appreciate what others may see as irrelevant to the practical concerns of the participants [43–46].

Ethnography, however, has some severe limitations as well. To begin with, it requires highly skilled personnel and is time consuming if it is to be done well. It is thus prohibitively expensive for any study in which voluntariness is other than the central focus. Moreover, it does not produce a score that can be included in a systematic quantitative analysis, something that is important for many studies and allows easier comparisons across studies. Another difficulty with ethnography is that it is typically limited to one or two sites. It is thus possible to say that research consents are voluntary or not voluntary for a small number of locations and projects, but a comprehensive picture of the voluntariness of research consents is not possible to obtain. Finally, of course, ethnography depends on a single observer and, given the resource commitment, is unlikely to be done frequently, so that the knowledge gained will not easily be subject to confirmation or disproof.

Semi-structured interviews have many of the strengths and weaknesses of ethnography, although perhaps a little less intensely. Like ethnography, semi-structured interviews generally give the subjects opportunities to express their opinion and the interviewer a chance to explore their dimensions in some detail. Moreover, they provide the interviewer some access to explore the particular individual and cultural contexts in which the decision to participate or not in the research was made [47,48]. On the other hand, data from semi-structured interviews also are relatively time-consuming and expensive to collect. They are, in addition, much more expensive to analyse since they need to be transcribed, read, and often coded, before analysis is completed. These resource needs mean that the sample size of any study using semi-structured methods is likely to be limited. Finally, it takes considerable work to produce a score from the transcripts that can be analysed quantitatively. Rules either must be generated anew for the particular context, or prior rules for coding voluntariness must be adapted to the specific context of the decisions. Then, at least two coders must be trained and their level of agreement measured. Continuous training must go on until the coders reach acceptable inter-rater reliability, and this reliability must be periodically reassessed [49].

Perhaps obviously, few researchers will be willing or able to commit such resources to assessing voluntariness of research consents unless that is the primary focus of the research. Without a less resource-intensive procedure, it will not be possible, for example, for researchers conducting a large multi-site clinical trial of a new psychotropic medication to monitor the extent to which their participants' decisions are acceptably voluntary. Likewise it would be prohibitively expensive for an institutional review board or research ethics committee to assess the voluntariness of subjects in research at its institution. For this reason there is much to recommend in the use of more structured measures or scales for assessing voluntariness. Such measures can involve the subject answering four or five simple questions (e.g., [49]) or even assigning a score in response to a single question [50]. Another advantage of such a scale is that it produces a simple score that can be included in more complex analyses. Are Latinos in the United States more or less voluntary participants in research than European-Americans? Are differences in perceived voluntariness accounted for by differences in research design? These and thousands of other questions are much more easily answered with a valid scale.

However, if simple scales have advantages, their disadvantages are also significant. First, they are inherently independent of context. Since the questions are fixed, they cannot be adjusted to specific issues in particular research projects. More broadly, one learns nothing about why subjects think that their consents were voluntary or not. Likewise, scales offer only the subject's perspective on voluntariness. Although an individual's experience is a critical component of voluntariness, there are sometimes pressures of which they may not be aware, but that may be influential nonetheless. There may also be pressures that the subject considers legitimate but an external observer may not, for example few subjects in research projects are likely to complain about excessive payments to participate, but some ethicists and IRBs consider 'excessive' payments to constitute an undue influence on participants' decisions.

## 17.6   Prior empirical studies

Only a few empirical studies have examined voluntariness and its constraints in research, with most of those taking place in the developing world, perhaps because research subjects in those countries are thought to be at great risk for coercion and undue influence. Generally, these investigations have used one or a few simple questions to explore subjects' perceptions of influences on their decisions [51], rather than ethnographic or interview-based approaches. Several of these studies have shown that participants in protocols in the developing world often do not know that they are free to decide about participation (i.e., that the decision is up to them) or that they can withdraw from the study if they wish [52]. However, when asked directly about coercive pressures, subjects tend to demur. Thus, in a Ugandan malaria study, for example, only 6% of subjects reported that they had felt pressure from researchers, 5% from other doctors or nurses, and 4% from the health center's staff, but none felt that this pressure impeded their ability to refuse participation if they so chose [53]. Similarly, in a Thai study, 2% of participants felt pressure from their doctor or clinic, but none did from research staff [54].

In one of the few studies of voluntariness in the developed world, more than 75% of adolescents in an emergency room research study in the United States felt that they had consented freely [55]. Similarly, in a study of prisoners, only 1 of 30 reported feeling threatened or forced to participate in a survey study, and all felt that they themselves had made the final decision [56]. Interpretation and integration of these findings is difficult since the studies used different methods and employed measures without well-established reliability and validity. In addition, major differences exist in language and culture across the locations at which studies were performed, related to concepts of autonomy, freedom, decision-making, authority and rights, and further complicating comparisons of the research data.

Several studies have explored the influences of financial incentives on participation decisions regarding hypothetical research protocols. Pharmacy students reported that levels of financial incentives and risk would influence their decisions about participating in a study, with higher incentives also associated with less willingness to disclose activities that might result in exclusion from the study [57]. Amongst subjects in a hypertension clinic, levels of incentives and risk also affected probable decisions to participate in a study [58]. But these studies did not find that incentives affected perceptions of risk, and both concluded that incentives did not distort the informed consent decision process. Relatedly, of members of a jury pool, most reported that a $500 incentive to enroll in an antihypertensive treatment protocol would affect *other people's* decisions, but not their own [59]. The only studies that were not based on hypothetical scenarios found that higher payments (in a range from $10 to $160) improved attendance at follow-up appointments, but did not – according to subjects' self-report – unduly influence decisions [60,61].

Given the paucity of research on voluntariness of consent in the research context, it is of interest to note that patients' perceptions of coercion in clinical settings also have been examined. The MacArthur Perceived Coercion Scale (PCS) was developed for that purpose, consisting of five true/false questions, indicating increased perceptions of coercion, and yielding a score from 0 to 5. The PCS was originally developed and tested regarding consent to psychiatric hospitalization [50], but modified versions may be relevant in the present context. This scale does not, however, examine several critical aspects of coercion, such as the nature and perceived legitimacy of these influences on participants' choices.

Kjellin and colleagues [51] also developed a Coercion Ladder concerning perceptions of coercion in psychiatric care. This measure employs a 10-point 'ladder' to assess subjects' perceptions of the degree to which they feel their decisions were free or constrained. Subjects indicate on this scale the point that best represents the freedom with which they experienced their choices as having been made. This instrument, too, could potentially be modified for use in research settings.

In short, despite some prior empirical research, many questions remain about the kinds and degrees of constraints on voluntariness in participants' decisions. In the absence of more data, bodies providing oversight to research studies have tended to arrive at their own 'rules of thumb' concerning the threats to voluntary consent and how they can best be avoided. Yet these subjective, *ad hoc* guidelines vary widely between institutions [16] in ways that empirical research may not wholly justify.

## 17.7  Our empirical approach

Given the needs to understand these complex issues empirically, we decided to study these phenomena further, using several approaches.

First, we conducted semi-structured interviews with 15 research staff whose responsibilities included obtaining informed consent, and with 20 recently enrolled research subjects. With both groups, we aimed to identify the kinds of motivations that lead subjects to agree to participate in studies or alternatively to decline to consent. Additionally, we explored directly the roles of offers, pressures and threats. We also sought to explore whether variations occurred across populations, and if so, how and why. The interviews were audio-recorded, transcribed and content-analysed. In brief, these interviews suggested several important themes. Subjects have diverse reasons for entering research studies, and the effect of external influences may be difficult to predict. For instance, monetary incentives can have varying roles in participants' lives. They may serve as income, if individuals are unemployed, or as a replacement for income foregone as a result of study participation. Although concerns exist about offering money to substance users, lest it be used to procure drugs, for some such subjects a cash incentive was seen as income to 'get my life together,' 'helping me to be a better parent,' or assist them in supporting their families.

Based on our prior literature reviews and these open-ended interviews, we then drafted a preliminary instrument to assess quantitatively the range of determinants of decisions, to explore subjects' views of limitations on voluntariness that they experienced, and to elicit their evaluations of the impact and legitimacy of these constraints. Though only offers, pressures and threats that are perceived as illegitimate or morally problematic may constitute coercion or undue influence, we decided to explore all such constraints to understand the phenomena and their implications as fully as possible. We circulated this draft of the instrument to five experts to solicit additional items, other aspects of constraint that we had overlooked, other independent variables, and general comments. We then pilot-tested this instrument with 10 subjects already enrolled in various research projects, to identify any problems in wording, organization or content.

As we have reported in further detail elsewhere [62], we recruited 88 subjects, of whom approximately one-third each were recently enrolled in studies in oncology (breast and prostate cancer), substance abuse, or other areas (psychiatry, cardiology and HIV). Participants in these 'parent' studies were approached by a staff member from those projects to see if they would be interested in participating in this additional protocol, examining voluntariness. To those individuals who agreed to enroll in this additional study, we administered the questionnaire that we had developed.

Subjects were asked whether their decision to participate in the parent study was at all influenced by one of 14 possible motivators, ranking each of these on a scale from 1 (not at all important) to 10 (extremely important). We also asked participants whether they had received offers, pressures or threats, and if so, to tell us what had happened, the extent (on scales of 1 to 10) to which these influenced their decisions, and the degree to which they appeared to them to be unfair. They were queried, in addition, about the risks they perceived with the parent study, and the roles of offers, pressures or threats in counterbalancing these risks. Subjects then completed modified versions of the MacArthur Perceived Coercion Scale [50] and the Coercion Ladder [51] (which we termed the 'Voluntariness Ladder').

On the questionnaire examining 14 possible motivations, all three diagnostic groups of respondents ranked highly the possibility of better care, trust in the researchers, and the reputation of the host institution. However, amongst the three groups, several differences arose. The availability of free treatment was rated highest in importance amongst those in substance abuse studies and lowest amongst those in oncology protocols. Seriously needing help with their condition was rated highest in importance by those in oncology, and lowest amongst those in substance abuse research. Desire to help patients with the same condition similarly was strongest in oncology, and weakest in substance abuse. We also conducted a factor analysis of possible motivations, and identified two factors over all – 'help and trust' (which reflected the possibility of getting better care, access to otherwise unavailable treatment, and trust in researchers) and 'free treatment' (which reflected the availability of free treatment and the absence of altruistic motives). The first factor was uniformly influential across all groups, while the second was strongest amongst those in substance abuse and weakest amongst those in oncology research projects.

Offers were reported by 35% of respondents, pressures by 3%, and threats by none. Most of those who mentioned offers said that these had little importance in their decisions to participate. The Perceived Coercion Scale showed little evidence of coercion (e.g., 75% of respondents had a score of 0). Similarly, on the Voluntariness Ladder, over 90% of respondents reported that their decision was completely voluntary. These scales were significantly inter-correlated.

In all, these data suggest little evidence of constraints on voluntariness amongst these research participants. Offers, when present, were almost never seen as having been significant influences on decisions. Moreover, even if subjects had considered these offers to be significant, it is not clear whether these would have led to undervaluation of research risks. Rather, subjects appear to have had diverse reasons for participating in research. We found that subjects, regardless of category of disease, were often motivated by need for help with their disease, wishes for better care, and trust in the researchers and their institutions. This finding is consistent with research by Wendler *et al.* that more than one factor usually drives subjects in their decisions [63]. Of note, those subjects in substance abuse studies were motivated most by free treatment – which might otherwise have been unavailable to them – though availability of care is usually not considered an incentive in discussions of regulation of research.

Thus, our findings are consistent with a small but increasing literature that suggests that the potential for incentives to constrain voluntariness appears overrated. Our findings also indicate that higher scores on the Perceived Coercion Scale were correlated with more altruism. Those who feel 'compelled' to help others (for altruistic reasons) may experience themselves as less free to say 'no' to opportunities to participate in research. Yet, as a motivation to participate in research, altruism is not usually seen as a problem. When advice from health care workers played a more important role in decisions, individuals had higher scores on the Perceived Coercion Scale. Thus, this source of input may also lead individuals to feel less completely free to say 'no'. However, one of the questions on the scale may have been interpreted differently than intended by respondents, perhaps falsely elevating the rate of subjects who reported some loss of voluntariness. (Participants were asked to respond whether the statement 'it was my idea to sign up for the research project' was true or false. Respondents may have interpreted this statement as reflecting the source of the idea to participate, rather than the presence of actual pressure.)

This study has several limitations. For instance, we only examined these issues amongst a relatively small number of research subjects in a single, large academic medical center. But these data, if confirmed, suggest that the extent of concerns about coercion or undue influence in research amongst regulatory authorities and research ethics committees may be unwarranted. Importantly, these results should not be seen as vouchsafing the absence of undue influence from all monetary incentives, since very large amounts (which were not offered in the parent studies we examined) may indeed unduly affect subjects' decisions. Moreover, it remains important to explore these issues amongst other groups of subjects who may be vulnerable, or may be perceived as vulnerable, for various reasons – for example, persons with mental disorders, prisoners and children. Future research should focus on these populations, using our measures as well as other approaches, and can also explore perceptions of coercion not only amongst subjects themselves, but other participants in the consent process, including family members and investigators, who may be situated to provide complementary, alternative perspectives.

Particular needs also remain to explore these issues more fully amongst study subjects in the developing world, where an increasing amount of clinical research is being conducted. In these countries, these instruments may need to be modified, given linguistic and cultural differences that may exist. Defining and measuring these concepts in developing-world settings can pose several added challenges. For example, in societies where women are traditionally less empowered than men, they may not feel free to make decisions in a wide variety of spheres in everyday life, not merely regarding research participation. Questions thus emerge of whether women in these circumstances should be permitted to engage in research, and what the consequences would be of their systematic exclusion. Additional empirical research and normative analysis may help to clarify these issues and situations; for example whether the fact that women may feel that constraints on their choices imposed by men are legitimate may alleviate concerns in certain types of research, and if so, when and to what degree. Clearly, these questions merit far fuller discussion. We introduce them here merely to suggest the need to assess these issues in other, diverse cultures, and the challenges of doing so. Such further investigation also presents important opportunities to explore these vital concepts of limitations of voluntary choice in other critical contexts.

## 17.8  Conclusion

Explorations of voluntariness in the research setting are in their infancy. Frameworks for understanding voluntariness must be faithful to the legal concepts that underlie informed consent, yet sensitive to ethical considerations that may go beyond the legal rules (e.g., perceptions of coercion by subjects in the absence of objective indicators). Moreover, such theoretical frameworks must be susceptible to being put into operation in actual research settings if they are to enhance our knowledge of limitations on voluntariness in practice. The development of scales to assess impairments of voluntariness, despite their limitations, holds considerable promise for permitting studies to be replicated and results compared across sites and amongst different research groups. But the value of qualitative approaches based on ethnographic and interview methods should also be recognized, since they offer perspectives that may allow quantitative data to be placed in a more meaningful perspective. We are likely perched at the very beginning of an era of systematic study of the concepts of voluntariness, coercion and undue influence in research, which promises to provide answers to many of the important questions in research ethics.

## References

1. Nuremberg Military Tribunals (1949) *USA* v. *Karl Brandt et al.*, in *Trials of War Criminals before the Nuremberg Military Tribunals under Control Council Law No. 10*, Volume 2, US Government Printing Office, Washington, DC.
2. Protection of Human Subjects, 45 C.F.R. 46.111 (2009).
3. Kuczewski, M.G. and Marshall, P. (2002) The decision dynamics of clinical research: the context and process of informed consent. *Medical Care*, **40**, V45–V54.
4. Office of the Inspector General, US Department of Health and Human Services (2000) *Recruiting Human Subjects: Pressures in Industry-Sponsored Clinical Research*, Report No. OEI-01-97-00195, US Department of Health and Human Services, Boston, MA.
5. Shimm, D.S. and Spece, R.G. (1982) Rate of refusal to participate in clinical trials. *IRB: A Review of Human Subjects Research*, **14** (2), 7–9.
6. Appelbaum, P.S. (1995) Consent and coercion: research with involuntarily treated persons with mental illness or substance abuse. *Accountability in Research*, **4**, 69–79.
7. De Zoysa, I., Elias, C.J. and Bentley, M.E. (1998) Ethical challenges in efficacy trials of vaginal microbicides for HIV prevention. *American Journal of Public Health*, **88**, 571–575.
8. Marshall, P.A. (2006) Informed consent in international health research. *Journal of Empirical Research on Human Research Ethics*, **1**, 25–41.

9. Upvali, M. and Haswani, S. (2001) Negotiating the informed-consent process in developing countries: a comparison of Swaziland and Pakistan. *International Nursing Review*, **48**, 188–192.
10. Tindana, P.O., Kass, N. and Akweongo, P. (2006) The informed consent process in a rural African setting: a case study of the Kassena-Nankana district of northern Ghana. *IRB: Ethics and Human Research*, **28** (2), 1–6.
11. Charland, L.C. (2002) Cynthia's dilemma: consenting to heroin prescription. *American Journal of Bioethics*, **2** (2), 37–47.
12. McCrady, B.S. and Bux, D.A. (1999) Ethical issues in informed consent with substance abusers. *Journal of Consulting and Clinical Psychology*, **67**, 186–193.
13. Cohen, P.J. (2002) Untreated addiction imposes an ethical bar to recruiting addicts for non-therapeutic studies of addictive drugs. *Journal of Law, Medicine, and Ethics*, **30**, 73–81.
14. Grady, C., Dikert, N., Jawetz, T. *et al.* (2005) An analysis of U.S. practices of paying research participants. *Contemporary Clinical Trials*, **26**, 365–375.
15. Letterman, J. and Merz, J.F. (2001) How much are subjects paid to participate in research? *American Journal of Bioethics*, **1** (2), 45–46.
16. Dickert, N., Emanuel, E. and Grady, C. (2002) Paying research subjects: an analysis of current policies. *Annals of Internal Medicine*, **136**, 368–373.
17. Weise, K.L., Smith, M.L., Maschke, K.J. *et al.* (2002) National practices regarding payment to research subjects for participating in pediatric research. *Pediatrics*, **110**, 577–582.
18. Protection of Human Subjects, 45 C.F.R. 45 Subpart C (2009).
19. Institute of Medicine (2007) *Ethical Considerations for Research Involving Prisoners*, National Academies Press, Washington, DC.
20. Protection of Human Subjects, 46 C.F.R. 45 Subpart B (2009).
21. Protection of Human Subjects, 46 C.F.R. 45 Subpart D (2009).
22. Orentlicher, D. (2005) Making research a requirement of treatment: why we should sometimes let doctors pressure patients to participate in research. *Hastings Center Report*, **35** (5), 20–28.
23. Foddy, B. and Savulescu, J. (2006) Addiction and autonomy: can addicted people consent to the prescription of their drug of addiction? *Bioethics*, **20**, 1–15.
24. Berg, J.W., Appelbaum, P.S., Lidz, C.W. *et al.* (2001) *Informed Consent: Legal Theory and Clinical Practice*, 2nd edn, Oxford University Press, New York.
25. Searle, J.R. (2002) *The Rediscovery of the Mind*, MIT Press, Cambridge, MA.
26. Wegner, D.M. (2003) *The Illusion of Conscious Will*, MIT Press, Cambridge, MA.
27. Wertheimer, A. (1987) *Coercion*, Princeton University Press, Princeton, NJ.
28. American Law Institute (1979) *Restatement of the Law (Second), Torts*, American Law Institute, St Paul, MN.
29. American Law Institute (1981) *Restatement of the Law (Second), Contracts*, American Law Institute, St Paul, MN.
30. *Colorado* v. *Connelly*, 497 U.S. 157 (1986).
31. Morse, S.J. (2004) New neuroscience, old problems, in *Neuroscience and the Law: Brain, Mind, and the Scales of Justice* (ed B. Garland), Dana Press, New York, pp. 157–198.
32. Verheggen, F., Nieman, F. and Jonkers, R. (1998) Determinants of patient participation in clinical studies requiring informed consent: why patients enter a clinical trial. *Patient Education & Counseling*, **35**, 111–125.
33. Appelbaum, P.S., Lidz, C.W. and Klitzman, R. (2009) Voluntariness of consent to research: a conceptual model. *Hastings Center Report*, **39** (1), 30–39.
34. Council for International Organizations of Medical Sciences (CIOMS) (2002) *International Ethical Guidelines for Biomedical Research Involving Human Subjects*, CIOMS, Geneva.

Available at www.cioms.ch/publications/guidelines/guidelines_nov_2002_blurb.htm (accessed 8 December 2010).

35. Emanuel, E.J. (2005) Undue inducement: nonsense on stilts? *American Journal of Bioethics*, **5** (5), 9–13.

36. Faden, R.R. and Beauchamp, T.L. (1986) *A History and Theory of Informed Consent*, Oxford University Press, New York.

37. Monahan, J., Lidz, C.W., Hoge, S.K. *et al.* (1999) Coercion in the provision of mental health services: the MacArthur studies, in *Research in Community and Mental Health*, Volume 10 (eds J.P. Morrissey and J. Monahan), JAI Press, Westport, CT.

38. American Educational Research Association (1999) *Standards for Educational and Psychological Testing*, American Educational Research Association, Washington, DC.

39. Levi, E. (1948) *An Introduction to Legal Reasoning*, University of Chicago Press, Chicago.

40. Gardner, W. and Lidz, C. (2001) Gratitude and coercion between physicians and patients. *Psychiatric Annals*, **31**, 125–129.

41. Timmermans, S. and McKay, T. (2009) Clinical trials as treatment option: bioethics and health care disparities in substance dependency. *Social Science and Medicine*, **69**, 1784–1790.

42. Bennett, N., Lidz, C., Monahan, J. *et al.* (1993) Inclusion, motivation and good faith: the morality of coercion in mental hospital admission. *Behavioral Sciences and the Law*, **13**, 295–306.

43. Bodgan, R. and Taylor, S. (1975) *Introduction to Qualitative Research Methods*, John Wiley & Sons, Inc., New York.

44. Adler, P. and Adler, P. (1998) Observational techniques, in *Collecting and Interpreting Qualitative Materials* (eds N. Denzin and Y. Lincoln), Sage, New York, pp. 79–109.

45. Adler, P. and Adler, P. (1987) *Membership Roles in Field Research*, Sage, Newbury Park, CA.

46. Agar, M. (1986) *Speaking of Ethnography*, Sage, Newbury Park, CA.

47. Sudman, S. and Bradburn, N. (1982) *Asking Questions: A Practical Guide to Questionnaire Design*, Jossey-Bass, San Francisco, CA.

48. Fontana, A. and Frey, J.H. (1998) Interviewing: the art of science, in *Collecting and Interpreting Qualitative Materials* (eds N. Denzin and Y. Lincoln), Sage, Thousand Oaks, CA, pp. 47–78.

49. Tesch, R. (1990) *Qualitative Research: Analysis Types and Software Tools*, Falmer Press, New York.

50. Gardner, W., Hoge, S.K., Bennett, N. *et al.* (1993) Two scales for measuring patients' perceptions of coercion during hospital admission. *Behavioral Sciences and the Law*, **11**, 307–322.

51. Kjellin, L., Høyer, G., Engberg, M. *et al.* (2006) Differences in perceived coercion at admission to psychiatric hospitals in the Nordic countries. *Social Psychiatry and Psychiatric Epidemiology.*, **41**, 241–247.

52. Krosin, M.T., Klitzman, R., Levin, B. *et al.* (2006) Problems in comprehension of informed consent in rural and peri-urban Mali, West Africa. *Clinical Trials*, **3**, 306–313.

53. Pace, C., Talisuna, A., Wendler, D. *et al.* (2005) Quality of parental consent in a Ugandan malaria study. *American Journal of Public Health*, **95**, 1184–1189.

54. Pace, C., Emanuel, E.J., Chuenyam, T. *et al.* (2005) The quality of informed consent in a clinical research study in Thailand. *IRB: Ethics and Human Research*, **27** (1), 9–17.

55. Cohn, J.M., Ginsburg, K.R., Kasam-Adams, N. *et al.* (2005) Adolescent decisional autonomy regarding participation in an emergency department youth violence interview. *American Journal of Bioethics*, **5** (5), 70–74.

56. Moser, D.J., Arndt, S., Kanz, J.E. *et al.* (2004) Coercion and informed consent in research involving prisoners. *Comprehensive Psychiatry*, **45**, 1–9.
57. Bentley, J.P. and Thacker, P.G. (2004) The influence of risk and monetary payment on the research participation decision making process. *Journal of Medical Ethics*, **30**, 293–298.
58. Halpern, S.D., Karlawish, J.H.T., Casarett, D. *et al.* (2004) Empirical assessment of whether moderate payments are undue or unjust inducements for participation in clinical trials. *Archives of Internal Medicine*, **164**, 801–803.
59. Casarett, D., Karlawish, J. and Asch, D.A. (2002) Paying hypertension research subjects: fair compensation or undue inducement? *Journal of General Internal Medicine*, **17**, 651–653.
60. Festinger, D.S., Marlowe, D.B., Croft, J.R. *et al.* (2005) Do research payments precipitate drug use or coerce participation? *Drug and Alcohol Dependence*, **78**, 275–281.
61. Festinger, D.S., Marlowe, D.B., Dugosh, K.L. *et al.* (2008) Higher magnitude cash payments improve research follow-up rates without increasing drug use or perceived coercion. *Drug and Alcohol Dependence*, **96**, 128–135.
62. Appelbaum, P.S., Lidz, C.W. and Klitzman, R. (2009) Voluntariness of consent to research: a preliminary empirical investigation. *IRB: Ethics & Human Research*, **31** (6), 10–14.
63. Wendler, D., Krohmal, B., Emanuel, E.J. *et al.* (2008) Why patients continue to participate in clinical research. *Archives of Internal Medicine*, **168**, 1294–1299.

# Index

Note: Page numbers in *italics* refer to Figures; those in **bold** to Tables.

*Coercive Treatment in Psychiatry: Clinical, Legal and Ethical Aspects*, First Edition.
Edited by Thomas W. Kallert, Juan E. Mezzich and John Monahan.
© 2011 John Wiley & Sons, Ltd. Published 2011 by John Wiley & Sons, Ltd.

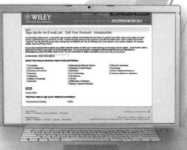